THE SCIENCE OF RUGBY

The Science of Rugby is the only book to examine the scientific principles underpinning the preparation of rugby players for high performance. Drawing on the very latest scientific evidence and covering both codes (union and league), the book explores every aspect of preparation and performance and introduces best practice by leading sports science professionals and practitioners from around the rugby world.

The book covers key topics such as:

- physical preparation and conditioning;
- strength and power training;
- monitoring match and training demands;
- match-day strategies for enhancing physical and technical performance;
- management of fatigue and recovery;
- training and playing in the heat;
- travel and jet lag;
- injury epidemiology;
- psychological preparation;
- performance analysis;
- biomechanics;
- nutrition;
- talent identification and youth development.

The book also incorporates several case-studies to demonstrate how scientific principles have been applied in practice. No other book bridges the gap between theory and applied practice in rugby, from grass-roots to elite international standard, and therefore this is essential reading for any student, researcher, sport scientist, coach, physiotherapist, or clinician with an interest in the game.

Craig Twist is Reader in Applied Exercise Physiology at the University of Chester, UK. His primary research interests revolve around the applied physiology of rugby league and recovery after fatiguing exercise. Craig is an accredited Sport and Exercise Scientist with the British Association of Sport and Exercise Sciences, and also serves as a consultant to the Rugby Football League and several elite sports teams.

Paul Worsfold is Head of Biomechanics at the English Institute of Sport and a senior lecturer in Sports Biomechanics and Performance Analysis at the University of Chester, UK. Paul is a consultant for the Rugby Football Union where he is leading research projects assessing the playing demands of the English Premiership and investigating talent development within the English national squad system.

THE SCIENCE OF RUGBY

Craig Twist and Paul Worsfold

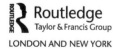
Routledge
Taylor & Francis Group

LONDON AND NEW YORK

First published 2015
by Routledge
2 Park Square, Milton Park, Abingdon, Oxon OX14 4RN

and by Routledge
711 Third Avenue, New York, NY 10017

Routledge is an imprint of the Taylor & Francis Group, an informa business

British Library Cataloguing-in-Publication Data
A catalogue record for this book is available from the British Library

Library of Congress Cataloging in Publication Data
The science of rugby / edited by Craig Twist, Paul Worsfold.
pages cm
Includes bibliographical references and index.
1. Rugby football. 2. Rugby football–Physiological aspects. 3. Sports
sciences. I. Twist, Craig. II. Worsfold, Paul.
GV945.S345 2014
796.333–dc23
2014022481

ISBN: 978-0-415-65627-6 (hbk)
ISBN: 978-0-415-65628-3 (pbk)
ISBN: 978-0-203-07801-3 (ebk)

Typeset in Bembo
by Cenveo Publisher Services

Printed and bound by CPI Group (UK) Ltd, Croydon, CR0 4YY

Craig Twist
To my family, for their love, inspiration, and support.

Paul Worsfold
For dad – Trevor Worsfold (1947–2013)

CONTENTS

CONTRIBUTORS

Graeme L. Close, *Liverpool John Moores University, UK*

Steve Cobley, *University of Sydney, Australia*

Christian J. Cook, *Bangor University, Bangor, UK*

Simon Eaves, *Manchester Metropolitan University, UK*

Ben J. Edwards, *Liverpool John Moores University, UK*

Niki Gabb, *University of Bath, UK*

Tim J. Gabbett, *Australian Catholic University, Australia; The University of Queensland, Australia*

Nicholas D. Gill, *New Zealand Rugby Union, New Zealand*

Jamie Highton, *University of Chester, UK*

Liam P. Kilduff, *Swansea University, Swansea, UK*

Doug McClymont, *New Zealand Rugby Union, New Zealand*

Michael R. McGuigan, *AUT University, Auckland, New Zealand*

Daniel Travis McMaster, *AUT University, Auckland, New Zealand*

Rudi Meir, *Southern Cross University, Australia*

James P. Morton, *Liverpool, John Moores University, UK*

Adam R. Nicholls, *University of Hull, UK*

Colin M. Robertson, *University of Bolton, UK*

Mark Russell, *Northumbria University, UK*

Keith Stokes, *University of Bath, UK*

Dave Sykes, *Heriot-Watt University, UK*

Kevin Till, *Leeds Beckett University, UK*

Grant Trewartha, *University of Bath, UK*

Craig Twist, *University of Chester, UK*

Jim M. Waterhouse, *Liverpool John Moores University, UK*

Mark Waldron, *University of New England, Australia*

Paul Worsfold, *University of Chester, UK; English Institute of Sport, UK*

CASE STUDY CONTRIBUTORS

James Bell, *Cleveland Browns, AFC, USA*

James Bickley, *Changing Minds Limited, UK*

Warren Bradley, *School of Sport and Exercise Sciences, Liverpool John Moores University, UK*

James Brown, *UCT/MRC Research Unit for Exercise Science and Sports Medicine, University of Cape Town, South Africa*

Dario Cazzola, *Department for Health, University of Bath, UK*

Michael E. England, *Rugby Football Union*

Mike I. Lambert, *UCT/MRC Research Unit for Exercise Science and Sports Medicine, University of Cape Town, South Africa*

Ezio Preatoni, *Department for Health, University of Bath, UK*

Clint Readhead, *South African Rugby Union*

Andrew Rogers, *Changing Minds Limited, UK*

Matt Thombs, *Rugby Football Union*

Wayne Viljoen, *South African Rugby Union*

INTRODUCTION

The application of science by coaches, practitioners, and medical staff is now commonplace in most rugby programmes worldwide. Indeed, rugby science is an emerging field of research that is used to inform the practice, performance, health, well-being, and development of rugby players and coaches at all standards.

This book critically examines the scientific principles underpinning the preparation and management of rugby players in both codes. Applied examples are also provided throughout to understand the practical application of the material in a real-world context. The intention of this book is to offer a significant contribution to the field of rugby science that will act as a useful resource to scientists, coaches, practitioners, and students interested in rugby.

Key topics include:

- physical and psychological preparation for rugby;
- planning and monitoring of training;
- managing fatigue, recovery, and nutrition;
- effects of environmental conditions and travel on performance;
- the mechanics of rugby techniques and injury;
- young players and talent identification.

ABOUT THE EDITORS

Craig Twist is Reader in Applied Exercise Physiology at the University of Chester, UK. His primary research interests revolve around the applied physiology of rugby and recovery after fatiguing exercise. Craig is an accredited Sport and Exercise Scientist with the British Association of Sport and Exercise Sciences, and also serves as a consultant to the Rugby Football League and several elite rugby teams.

Paul Worsfold is Head of Biomechanics at the English Institue of Sport and a senior lecturer in Sports Biomechanics and Performance Analysis at the University of Chester, UK. Paul is a consultant for the Rugby Football Union where he is leading research projects assessing the playing demands of the English Premiership and investigating talent development within the English national squad system.

1

PHYSICAL PREPARATION FOR RUGBY

Tim J. Gabbett

1.1 Introduction

Rugby union and rugby league are two collision sports played worldwide. Although the 'purists' would argue that the sports are vastly different in rules, history, and 'culture', the two codes share commonalities (e.g. running, carrying and passing a football, high-intensity tackling and collisions, and wrestling). The rugby codes (i.e. rugby league and rugby union) are characterised by frequent bouts of high-intensity exercise (e.g. striding, sprinting, tackling, wrestling, and grappling), interspersed with periods of lower-intensity activity (e.g. standing, walking, and jogging). During the course of match-play, players will cover ~68 (rugby union) (Cahill *et al.* 2013) to ~100 m·min^{-1} (rugby league) (Austin and Kelly 2014; Gabbett *et al.* 2012b; Sykes *et al.* 2011; Waldron *et al.* 2011). Although these movement demands are considerably lower than that reported for Australian football (129 m·min^{-1}) and soccer (104 m·min^{-1}) (Varley *et al.* 2013), the demands of rugby are significantly increased through the large frequency of collisions players are required to perform throughout a match. Indeed, recent evidence has shown that rugby league players engage in a significantly greater number of accelerations and collisions, and have a greater frequency of repeated high-intensity effort bouts (involving sprinting and collisions) than Australian football players (Varley *et al.* 2013). Consequently, conditioning players to perform high-intensity movements and collisions and to recover from these activities represents an important pursuit for rugby strength and conditioning coaches.

1.2 Movement demands of rugby

Early video-based time-motion analyses reported that rugby players covered approximately 6,500 m to 7,900 m during match-play, depending on playing position (Meir *et al.* 1993). The majority of time (88-95%) is spent in low-intensity activities (e.g. standing, walking, and jogging), and approximately 2.2–3.6% of time is spent in high-intensity activities (e.g. striding, sprinting, tackling, rucking/mauling, and static efforts) (Duthie *et al.* 2005). High-intensity activities have been reported to account for 11.9% of front row, 13.7% of back row, 5.9% of inside backs, and 4.1% of outside backs total match-play (Duthie *et al.* 2005). Recently, researchers have employed global positioning system (GPS) technology to investigate the locomotor demands of match-play (Cahill *et al.* 2013; Waldron *et al.* 2011). Differences in movement demands have been reported between forwards and backs in international rugby union players, with front row (5,158 m; 62.3 m·min⁻¹), second row (5,755 m; 64.7 m·min⁻¹), and back row (6,038 m; 65.3 m·min⁻¹) positions covering considerably less distance than the scrum half (7,098 m; 78.5 m·min⁻¹), inside backs (6,545 m; 71.4 m·min⁻¹), and outside backs (6,276 m; 66.9 m·min⁻¹) positions (Cahill *et al.* 2013). No differences were found among hit-up forwards (3,569 m; 94 m·min⁻¹), wide-running forwards (5,561 m; 96 m·min-1), adjustables (6,411 m; 101 m·min⁻¹), and outside backs (6,819 m; 93 m·min⁻¹) for the relative amount of distance covered in elite rugby league players (Gabbett *et al.* 2012b). However, the amount of high-speed running has been shown to differ between hit-up forwards (235 m; 6.2 m·min⁻¹), wide-running forwards (418 m; 7.2 m·min⁻¹), adjustables (436 m; 6.9 m·min⁻¹), and outside backs (583 m; 8.0 m·min⁻¹) (Gabbett *et al.* 2012b). A novel aspect of the study by Gabbett *et al.* (2012b) was the comparison of group means with the most extreme demands for each positional group. The greatest total distances covered by the hit-up forwards, wide-running forwards, adjustables, and outside backs were, respectively, 87%, 47%, 98%, and 40% greater than the mean value for each positional group. Furthermore, the physical demands of defence are consistently greater than attack (Gabbett *et al.* 2014). Moderate to large differences are reported between defence and attack for distance covered (109 ± 16 m·min⁻¹ *vs.* 82 ± 12 m·min⁻¹), low speed distance (104 ± 15 m·min⁻¹ *vs.* 78 ± 11 m·min⁻¹), frequency of collisions (1.9 ± 0.7 per min *vs.* 0.8 ± 0.3 per min), and frequency of repeated high-intensity effort bouts (1 every 4.9 ± 5.1 min *vs.* 1 every 9.4 ± 6.1 min) in professional rugby league. The amount of high-speed running performed whilst defending in the opposition's 30 m zone has been shown to be 6–8 times greater than when defending the middle third or the team's own try-line. The smallet amount of high-speed running in attack occurs when players are attacking from their own try-line, with moderately greater amounts of high-speed running occurring in the middle third of the field and when attacking the opposition's try-line. Collectively, these findings suggest that reporting mean values alone might underestimate the most intense physical demands of match-play. In addition, coaches and conditioning staff can use this information to develop game-specific drills to replicate the attacking and defensive demands of different field positional zones in rugby.

Whilst most studies investigate the physical demands of 15-a-side rugby union and 13-a-side rugby league, researchers have also studied the activity profiles of competitors in rugby sevens match-play (Higham *et al.* 2012; Suarez-Arrones *et al.* 2012). Higham *et al.* (2012) reported that male rugby sevens players ran greater distances at high-speed and performed a greater number of accelerations and decelerations during international matches than they did during domestic matches.

Moreover, the relative distance covered was reduced from the first to the second half, with substitute players exhibiting higher activity profiles for all movement variables than whole-game players. Suarez-Arrones *et al.* (2012) documented the physical demands of female rugby sevens players during international match-play, where players covered an average distance of 111 m·min⁻¹; this average distance was comprised 16.4% (256 m) striding, 3.7% (57 m) high-intensity running, and 5.4% (84 m) sprinting. For ~75% of a game, players' heart rates were greater than 80% of their maximal value. The authors concluded that the demands of rugby sevens were different than those experienced in other rugby codes (i.e. 15-a-side, 13-a-side) and that coaching, conditioning, and testing for rugby sevens should reflect the specific demands of match-play.

Repeated sprints, with short recovery between efforts, occur infrequently during competition (Gabbett 2012b). On average, players performed one repeated-sprint bout (defined as three or more sprints with less than twenty-one seconds between sprints [Spencer *et al.* 2004]) during match-play. Whilst these findings suggest that the importance of repeated-sprint ability to rugby league physical performance may have been overstated (Clark 2002), repeated-sprint training should still form part of the physical training programmes for rugby players. Indeed, it is likely that some repeated-sprint training might assist players in performing the high-speed running demands of match-play.

1.2.1 Collision and repeated high-intensity effort demands

The hit-up forwards and wide-running forwards perform a greater absolute amount of moderate and heavy collisions than the adjustables and outside backs, and are consequently engaged in significantly more collisions per minute of match-play (Gabbett *et al.* 2011b; Gabbett *et al.* 2012b; Gissane *et al.* 2001a, 2001b). Hit-up forwards and wide-running forwards are involved in a collision approximately each minute, whilst the adjustables and outside backs are involved in a collision approximately every two minutes (Gabbett *et al.* 2012b). Hit-up forwards, wide-running forwards, adjustables, and outside backs perform a heavy collision every 2.5, 3.3, 5, and 5 minutes, respectively (Gabbett *et al.* 2012b). The repeated high-intensity effort demands of rugby match-play have been investigated (Austin *et al.* 2011; Gabbett *et al.* 2012b) and are defined as three or more high-speed, high-acceleration, or contact efforts with less than twenty-one seconds between efforts (Gabbett *et al.* 2012 b).

Whilst there are no differences among playing positions for the absolute number of repeated high-intensity effort bouts performed in a match, the hit-up forwards and wide-running forwards perform more repeated high-intensity effort bouts per minute of match-play. Hit-up forwards complete, on average, one repeated high-intensity effort bout every 4.8 minutes, whilst the wide-running forwards perform, on average, one repeated high-intensity effort bout every 6.3 minutes. Conversely, repeated high-intensity effort bouts occur on average every 7.7 and 9.1 minutes for the adjustables and outside backs, respectively (Gabbett *et al.* 2012b). These repeated high-intensity effort bouts occur more frequently when defending the team's own try-line and the opposition's 30 m zone, as well as attacking the opposition's try-line (Gabbett *et al.* 2014).

Collisions and tackles are widely acknowledged as the most demanding aspect of rugby league match-play (Brewer and Davis 1995). In addition, research from our laboratory has recently shown that repeated high-intensity effort exercise (sprinting and tackling) is associated with greater heart rate and perceived exertion and poorer sprint performance than repeated-sprint exercise alone (Johnston and Gabbett 2011), demonstrating that the addition of tackling significantly increases the physiological response to repeated-sprint exercise and has the potential to reduce physical performance. These findings, coupled with the repeated high-intensity effort demands, suggest that repeated sprinting and physical collisions are necessary to adequately prepare hit-up forwards for the demands of competition (Gabbett *et al.* 2010a), whilst repeated high-speed sprinting is critical for outside backs (Gabbett 2012b). In rugby union, forwards are involved in 11–22 tackles per game compared to 10–16 for backs (Quarrie *et al.* 2013) and spend approximately three and half times longer in contact situations compared to inside (fly half and scrum half) and outside backs (wing, centre, and fullback) (Austin *et al.* 2011; Quarrie *et al.* 2013). Austin *et al.* (2011) have also reported that work-to-rest ratios are lower for forwards (~1:4) compared to inside (1:5) and outside backs (1:6). In a study of Super 14 rugby union competitions, Austin *et al.* (2011) defined a repeated high-intensity effort bout as ≥3 sprints, and/or tackles, and/or scrum/ruck/maul activities within 21 seconds during the same passage of play. Front row forwards had fifteen repeated high-intensity effort bouts, whilst back row forwards had seventeen, inside backs had sixteen, and outside backs had seven. The average duration of these repeated high-intensity effort bouts was 45 to 52 s for forwards and 26 to 28 s for backs. The individual, longest-repeated, high-intensity effort bout for front row forwards (118 s), back row forwards (165 s), inside backs (64 s), and outside backs (53 s) was considerably greater. The shortest recovery duration between repeated high-intensity effort bouts was 64 s for front row forwards, 25 s for back row forwards, 26 s for inside backs, and 44 s for outside backs. Collectively, the findings of Austin *et al.* (2011) and Gabbett *et al.* (2012b) demonstrate the extreme physical demands placed on rugby players, suggesting that training for the average demands of match-play will result in players being underprepared for the most demanding passages of play.

1.2.2 Activity and recovery cycles of match-play

Examination of ball-in-play periods (i.e. match activity cycles) provides insight into the physical demands of rugby competition. The ball-in-play demands have been used by coaches to train the ability of players to compete for long passages of play. Colloquially, long ball-in-play periods might be perceived as an 'arm wrestle', as teams battle for field position in an attempt to force an error from their opponent.

Gabbett (2012a) investigated the ball-in-play periods of senior elite and junior elite matches, coding time when the ball was continuously in play, and any recovery periods that occurred (e.g. for scrums, penalties, line drop-outs, tries, and video referee decisions). The total time the ball was in play was ~55 minutes and ~50 minutes for senior elite and junior elite matches, respectively. In comparison to junior elite matches, senior elite matches had longer average activity cycles (81.2 ± 16.1 s *vs.* 72.0 ± 14.7 s). The average longest activity cycle was also higher in senior elite (318.3 ± 65.4 s) than junior elite (288.9 ± 57.5 s) matches. The longest activity cycle was 667 s for senior elite matches and 701 s for junior elite matches. Senior elite matches had a smaller proportion of short duration (<45 s) activity cycles and a greater proportion of longer duration (91–600 s) activity cycles.

A novel aspect of this study was the inclusion of activity–recovery ratios. Rolling calculations of two sequential activity cycles and the intervening recovery periods were performed, in order to gain an understanding of the longest activity periods, shortest recovery periods, and the potential influence these passages might have on the onset of fatigue and performance. Using this definition, the activity–recovery ratio was 13:1. A wide range of activity–recovery cycles were found, with values as low as 1:1 and as demanding as 704:1 demonstrating the stochastic nature of professional rugby league.

Collectively, these findings suggest that the ability to perform prolonged high-intensity exercise, coupled with the capacity to recover during brief stoppages in play, is a critical requirement of professional rugby league match-play. Furthermore, from a practical perspective, these findings could be used to develop game-specific testing protocols and training programmes to replicate the most demanding passages expected during professional rugby league competition. The ball-in-play time of professional rugby league competition (~55 minutes) is considerably greater than that reported for international rugby union, with reports that the ball is in play between 29 and 31 minutes (McLean 1992; Eaves *et al.* 2005) during an 80 minute rugby union match. Moreover, the average duration of work periods (81.2 s) and longest ball-in-play period (667 s) in professional rugby league is considerably greater than previously reported for international rugby union (19 s and 70 s, respectively) (McLean 1992). The finding of longer ball-in-play periods in rugby league reflects the greater emphasis on stoppages (e.g. penalties, lineouts, and scrums) in rugby union. Whilst similarities clearly exist between the codes, based on the findings from ball-in-play studies, it can be concluded that rugby league and rugby union are fundamentally different games, with markedly different physical demands placed on players.

The influence of league position on ball-in-play and recovery periods in senior elite competitive matches has also been investigated (Gabbett 2013). In comparison to matches involving lower standard teams, there was a greater proportion of long duration (>91 s) and a smaller proportion of short duration (<45 s) ball-in-play periods when top four teams were competing against other top four teams. No meaningful differences were found between teams of different league positions for the proportion of short and long recovery periods. In comparison to fixture matches involving the top four teams, finals matches had a smaller proportion of long duration activity periods, and a greater proportion of short duration activity periods. Only small differences were found between finals matches and matches involving the top four teams for the proportion of short and long recovery periods. These findings suggest that the competitive advantage of the best senior elite teams is closely linked to their ability to maintain a higher playing intensity than less success-ful teams. Furthermore, long ball-in-play periods in high-standard fixture matches (i.e. involving top four teams) ensure that players are adequately prepared for the ball-in-play demands of finals matches.

1.3 Physical qualities required for competition success in rugby

Researchers have assessed the relative importance of physical qualities to playing success by comparing rugby league players who were selected to participate in a team (i.e., starters) with players from the same squad that were not selected (i.e., non-starters) (Gabbett et al. 2009, 2011d). Starters tended to be taller, have faster change of direction speed, and greater playing experience than non-starters. Moderate to large differences were also detected between starters and non-starters for acceleration, maximum velocity, and estimated maximal aerobic power (Gabbett et al. 2009). More recently, the relative importance of physical, anthropometric, and skill qualities to team selection in professional rugby league has been investi-gated. Players selected to play in the first National Rugby League game of the season were older, more experienced, leaner, and had faster 10 m and 40 m sprint times, superior vertical jump performances, and greater aerobic power than non-selected players (Gabbett et al. 2011d). Collectively, these results suggest a relation between physical fitness and the playing level attained, and that selected physical and anthropometric qualities may influence team selection in professional rugby league.

1.3.1 Relationship between physical qualities and the activity profiles of rugby

Studies exploring the relationship between tests of physical qualities and physical match performance have shown that team sport players with better developed repeated-sprint ability and better Yo-Yo intermittent recovery test performances completed more very high-speed running and sprinting during match-play than their peers (Castagna et al. 2009; Krustrup et al. 2005; Rampinini et al. 2007a). Despite the high collision demand, and the importance of repeated high-intensity effort ability to rugby performance, generic tests of physical qualities (e.g. repeated-sprint ability, prolonged high-intensity intermittent running ability, and maximal aerobic power) are commonly used to assess training adaptations and readiness to play (Gabbett et al. 2011c). Gabbett and Seibold (2013) investigated the physical qualities that discriminated state-based rugby league players competing for selection in a semi-professional rugby league team, and also determined the relationship between tests of physical qualities and physical match performance in these players. Players selected to compete in the semi-professional team had greater lower-body strength and power, upper body strength and endurance, and prolonged high-intensity intermittent running ability than non-selected players. In addition, after controlling for playing position, measures of lower body strength were significantly and positively associated with the distance covered at low and high speeds and the number of repeated high-intensity effort bouts performed in competition. These results highlight the importance of lower-body strength, upper body strength and endurance, and prolonged high-intensity intermittent running ability to team selection in semi-professional rugby league. Furthermore, these findings suggest that well-developed lower-body strength contributes to effective physical match performance in semi-professional rugby league players.

Previous studies have reported a significant, but modest association ($r = 0.38$) between measures of lower-body muscular power and tackling proficiency in rugby league players (Gabbett et al. 2011a). Given the large amount of collision activity performed in repeated high-intensity effort bouts (Gabbett et al. 2012b), the findings of Gabbett and Seibold (2013) particularly highlight the importance of lower-body strength to repeated-effort performance in rugby players. These results suggest that improvements in lower-body strength might facilitate greater repeated high-intensity effort work rates in rugby players. Moreover, whilst important to team selection, these findings suggest that upper body strength, strength endurance, and prolonged high-intensity intermittent running ability contribute minimally to repeated effort performance in rugby league players.

Gabbett et al. (2013) examined the relationship between physical qualities and physical match performance in elite rugby league players. Players with better, prolonged high-intensity intermittent running ability covered greater total distance and greater distance in high-speed running during match-play. However, inconsistent relationships were found between tests of running abilities and other match performance variables, with prolonged high-intensity running ability (negative), maximal aerobic power (positive), and repeated-sprint ability (no relationship) differentially associated with the total number of collisions and repeated high-intensity effort bouts performed in matches. These findings demonstrate the importance of prolonged high-intensity running ability to the match running performance of elite rugby league players, but also highlight the need for game-specific conditioning to prepare players for the high-intensity collision and repeated-effort demands of the game.

Game-simulated, contact conditioning of players is clearly required to adequately prepare them for the repeated high-intensity effort nature of rugby match-play. Based on previous findings (Gabbett et al. 2012b), these rugby league-specific, repeated high-intensity effort bouts should include a minimum of six efforts, each of at least 6 s duration, using a work–rest ratio of 1:1. A rugby union-specific repeated high-intensity effort drill for front row forwards would involve sustained repeated high-intensity exercise for ~120 s. Players would cover a total distance of 140 m and complete two sprints of up to 20 m in distance. At least one tackle and four scrummaging, rucking, or mauling contact efforts should also be included (Austin et al. 2011). Finally, the lack of association between repeated-sprint ability and repeated high-intensity effort performance in matches suggests that repeated-sprint and repeated high-intensity effort ability are two distinct and different qualities. The need for a test of repeated high-intensity effort ability for rugby players in order to assess their preparedness for competition is therefore warranted.

1.4 What happens in the 'real world'?

Researchers have compared the efficacy of 'traditional conditioning' (involving interval running without the ball) and 'game-based training' (involving small-sided games) programmes for rugby (Gabbett 2006; Gamble 2004) and other team sports (Buchheit et al. 2009; Hill-Haas et al. 2009; Impellizzeri et al. 2006). Results of these studies are equivocal, with some (e.g. Buchheit et al. 2009; Gabbett 2006) reporting greater relative improvements in selected physical qualities (e.g. repeated-sprint ability, speed, and vertical jump height), and others (Hill-Haas et al. 2009; Impellizzeri et al. 2006) reporting that traditional conditioning and game-based training were equally effective at improving physical fitness.

An understanding of the physical demands of competition and the physical qualities required to perform these activities is necessary before strength and conditioning programmes can be implemented to meet the individual needs of players. Without an understanding of the demands of match-play, it is impossible for strength and conditioning coaches to prepare players to meet these specific demands. Table 1.1 shows selected activity profiles of professional rugby league match-play and a comparison of two approaches (traditional conditioning and game-based training) used to replicate these demands.

The running demands are easily met using either traditional conditioning (e.g. interval running) or game-based training (in this instance, 'off-side touch with intermittent wrestling'). However, the remaining two panels of data clearly demonstrate how the demands are poorly replicated by traditional conditioning activities, or when strength and conditioning coaches have a poor understanding of the demands of the game. Including wrestling bouts within the game-based training activities had the effect of replicating the collision demands of match-play and exceeding the repeated high-intensity effort demands. Conversely, traditional conditioning activities were unable to replicate the collision or repeated high-intensity

TABLE 1.1 Physical demands of traditional conditioning, game-based training, and match-play

	Elite competition	Traditional conditioning	Game-based training
Distance (m/min)	96 ± 1	164 ± 2	137 ± 2
Collisions (no./min)	0.7 ± 0.1	n/a	0.8 ± 0.1
Repeated Effort Bouts (no./min)	1 every 6.9 min	1 every 192.0 min	1 every 4.5 min

Data are mean ± SE.

effort demands of match-play. These findings have important implications. Given the high-intensity of traditional conditioning (i.e. 164 m·min⁻¹), it is likely that this activity is adequate to prepare players for the running demands of competition. However, given that these running training activities are achieved in isolation (i.e. without collisions), and that running in rugby is normally closely preceded or followed by some contact-related activity (e.g. tackling, wrestling, grappling, rucking, or mauling), it is unlikely that these activities adequately prepare players for the collision and repeated high-intensity effort demands of competition.

It is important to keep in mind that not all traditional conditioning activities need to replicate the most demanding passages of match-play. Some activities are correctly used to develop the underpinning physiological capacities required before further progressing training volume and intensity. Equally, whilst some small-sided games can be used to effectively replicate the demands of competition, some game-based activities are more 'game-specific' than others. Table 1.2 shows the physical demands of a small-sided game commonly used by rugby league and rugby union coaches. The game ('off-side touch') allows each team to have three 'plays' whilst in possession of the ball. A 'play' is ended when the player in possession of the ball is touched by a defender with two hands. The ball is turned over when the attacking side has completed three 'plays', makes an error, or scores a try. Unlike a regular small-sided rugby game, during the 'off-side' game, the ball can be passed in any direction (i.e. to 'off-side' players). The game is typically played on a pitch of 30 to 40 m width and 70 m length, although depending on player numbers, this field size can be reduced.

Rule changes can be implemented to training games, resulting in modifications of the physical (Gabbett et al. 2012a; Kennett et al. 2012) and physiological (Foster et al. 2010; Kennett et al. 2012) demands. One such rule change is the implementation of intermittent wrestling bouts within the 'off-side' game. At random or predetermined intervals, coaches blow a whistle at which point the game stops and players must wrestle an opponent for 5–10 seconds and force the opponent onto his or her back. Whilst the running demands of 'off-side touch' that includes intermittent wrestling will obviously be reduced due to the additional time that the ball is out-of-play, this type of rule change also has the effect of increasing the repeated high-intensity effort demands (Gabbett et al. 2012a). Indeed, it could be argued that game-based training activities that employ contact and wrestling periods are better able to replicate the repeated high-intensity effort demands of match-play than

TABLE 1.2 Physical demands of game-based training activities, with and without intermittent wrestling

	Without wrestling	With wrestling
Distance (m/min)	153 ± 2	117 ± 2
High-Speed (m/min)	23 ± 2	16 ± 2
Repeated Effort Bouts (no./min)	1 every 80 min	1 every 8 min

Data are mean ± SE.

game-based training activities relying solely on running activities (Table 1.2). Other modifications to small-sided game design, including increasing or decreasing player numbers, field size, and coach encouragement will also influence the physical and physiological demands of these activities (Foster *et al.* 2010; Kennett *et al.* 2012; Rampinini *et al.* 2007b). Indeed, reducing player numbers and increasing field size results in greater relative distance covered, more high-speed running, a greater number of sprint efforts, higher heart rates, greater blood lactate concentrations, and higher rating of perceived exertion than games played on smaller fields or with greater numbers (Foster *et al.* 2010; Kennett *et al.* 2012).

Although studies have compared the efficacy of traditional conditioning and game-based training activities, these comparisons are often dictated by the strict experimental guidelines imposed by the majority of peer-reviewed journals. In reality, successful coaches will use a combination of traditional conditioning and game-based training to develop physical qualities and promote the transfer of these physical qualities to the high pressure and fatiguing environments of competition.

Figure 1.1 shows the successful integration of coaches, physiologists, and skill acquisition specialists in the high performance rugby environment. Whilst the head coach is responsible for the overall performance of the team, different staff within the team work closely with the coach and players in order to develop physical qualities and the transfer of skill. The physiologist and strength and conditioning coach are responsible for understanding the physical demands of the sport. Their role includes identifying and developing the individual musculoskeletal and physiological limitations of players in order to adequately prepare players for the most demanding passages of play. Ultimately, their goal is to observe these physical qualities expressed in game-specific passages of play. Equally, assistant coaches (and skill acquisition specialists) are responsible for identifying the factors (e.g. fatigue, pressure) that might influence the execution of skill, and developing training scenarios that regularly expose players to these demands. The goal is to maximise transfer of learning from the training environment into the high pressure environment of competition.

Gabbett *et al.* (2010b) compared the physical and skill demands of 'on-side' (i.e. where the ball must be passed backwards) and 'off-side' (i.e. where the ball can be passed in any direction) small-sided games with junior elite rugby players. The research highlights the importance of effectively integrating conditioning and skill activities within the high performance rugby environment. In comparison to 'on-side' games, 'off-side' games had a greater number of involvements ('touches'), passes, and effective passes. 'Off-side' games resulted in a greater total distance covered, greater distance covered in mild and moderate accelerations, and greater distance covered in low, moderate, and high-velocity efforts. There were also a greater number of short duration recovery periods between efforts in 'off-side' games. The results of this study demonstrate that 'off-side' games provide greater physical and skill demands than 'on-side' games, providing a practical alternative for the development of skill and fitness in elite rugby league players. However, an

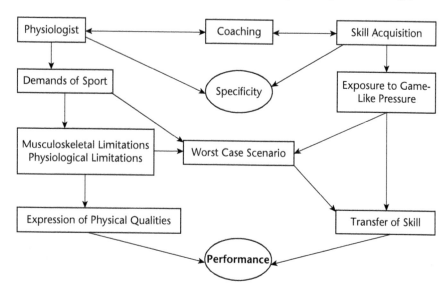

FIGURE 1.1   Integration of coaches, assistant coaches (or skill acquisition specialists), and physiologists (or strength and conditioning coaches) in the preparation of rugby players

equally important consideration in the development of conditioning programmes is the implementation of adequate recovery between intense bouts of training. Coaches often use low-intensity small-sided games as a means of reducing the physical and mental 'load' on players. Whilst 'on-side' games reduce the skill demands of training (by reducing the volume of skill executions), they also reduce the total distance covered, the number of high-acceleration and high-velocity sprint efforts, and the number of short duration recovery periods between high-intensity efforts. These results suggest that if low-intensity activity and recovery is a goal of the training session, then 'on-side' games are preferential to 'off-side' games.

1.5 Conclusion

In summary, this chapter highlights the complex activity profiles of rugby, and the challenges facing applied sport scientists and strength and conditioning staff employed to prepare players for the game- and position-specific demands of match-play. Although the locomotor demands are lower than for other team sports, rugby players are often required to perform these running activities either immediately before or after intense collisions and wrestling bouts. In addition, whilst the average ratio of high–low intensity activity is low, matches also include frequent repeated high-intensity effort bouts, with minimal recovery between efforts. Furthermore, ball-in-play analysis has shown that on occasion, players will be required to compete for extended passages of play with minimal recovery periods. Unless players are exposed to the most demanding passages of play in training, then it is highly likely that they will be under-prepared for the 'worst case scenario' expected during match-play.

Finally, researchers have attempted to determine the efficacy of traditional (e.g., interval running without the ball) and game-based (e.g. small-sided games) training for improving physical qualities and performance. Whilst a comparison between the two training modes is an interesting research pursuit, rugby coaches typically employ both traditional and game-based conditioning to improve the physical qualities of players and maximise the transfer of these qualities to the competitive environment.

Case study : recognising the value of physically hard training

Introduction

Adaptations to exercise training may be both positive and negative. Generally, higher training loads are associated with greater improvements in fitness. However, the negative consequences of training are also dose-related, with the highest incidence of illness and injury typically occurring with higher training loads (Morton 1997).

Recent studies have shown a positive relationship between training load and injury rates in rugby players (Gabbett 2004; Gabbett and Jenkins 2011). These findings suggest that the harder rugby players train, the more injuries they will sustain. Because it is critical to have the maximum number of players free from injury and available for selection in as many games as possible throughout the season, some strength and conditioning staff have begun to 'manage players away' from training in order to reduce the risk of injury. Clearly, this type of approach constrains the amount of physical training that players perform. Given that selected physical qualities (e.g., prolonged high-intensity running ability and upper body strength) protect against injury (Gabbett *et al.* 2012c), it could be argued that players should be prescribed high training loads in order to develop the physical qualities that protect against injury.

This case study reports on the value of exposing players to physically hard training, and the potential negative consequences of focusing solely on injury prevention in a high-performance environment.

Case presentation

Participants consisted of a professional rugby league team, competing in the elite National Rugby League competition. At the time, the author was employed as the Head of Sport Science for the club, working alongside skill coaching staff, physiotherapists, and strength and conditioning coaches.

Training programmes were devised and delivered by the strength and conditioning coaches. Players underwent a running-based training programme, focussed heavily on speed and agility. Repeated high-intensity effort ability was largely untrained, with skills and game-based training providing the greatest opportunity for players to perform repeated efforts (Gabbett *et al.* 2012b). Injury prevention was a major focus of the strength and conditioning coaches.

The form of the team during pre-season trial matches was poor and in the team's final trial, they marginally defeated a local reserve grade team. Thereafter, the team won their first fixture match 30–24, after leading 24–0, and after eight competition rounds, the team had won two matches (25% wins–losses). In addition, over 85 per cent of the matches missed through injury for the season occurred in this period (Figure 1.2).

A change in conditioning philosophy occurred. Training loads were increased, with players performing additional maximal aerobic speed and repeated high-intensity effort training sessions. These sessions were integrated with 'up-tempo', small-sided games so that players were competing in every session, and executing skill under pressure and whilst fatigued. These sessions were conducted early in the morning in winter. Players found the early morning sessions particularly uncomfortable, but they were working hard; they were becoming a football team again!

In the next 14 competition rounds, the team won 9 matches (75% wins–losses, and also received an additional 4 points from 2 bye rounds). During the middle and end stages of the season (where players were training the hardest), the total proportion of matches missed through injury was 5.5% and 7.5%, respectively.

Discussion

Whilst having players available for competition each week is important, it is of little use if the available players are not physically and mentally prepared for the demands of match-play. Conditioning staff need to be mindful that training programmes must be physiologically and psychologically appropriate to allow players to perform at the level of the demands of competition (Scrimgeour et al. 1986). Exposing the brain to hard physical work and fatigue on a regular basis appears to improve the body's ability to cope with fatigue; physically intense training improves appropriate physical qualities but, equally important, it also increases the mental durability of players (Noakes et al. 2005). Physically (and mentally) unfit players are more likely to pace themselves as a self-preservation and protection strategy (Noakes et al. 2005). If players have not been exposed to hard physical work on a regular basis, the brain instructs the body to stop exercise earlier to prevent exhaustion (Noakes et al. 2005). With this in mind, it may be argued that high (yet not excessive) training loads should be prescribed to players in order to determine answers to the following:

1. Which players are most susceptible to injury under physically stressful situations? (These players most likely will not tolerate the intensity and fatigue of competition.)
2. Which players are not susceptible to injury under physically stressful situations? (These players are more likely to tolerate the intensity and fatigue of competition.)

In summary, when prescribed low training loads, the rugby players of this case study experienced high injury rates and poor playing performance. Increases in training loads resulted in marked reductions in injury rates, presumably mediated through

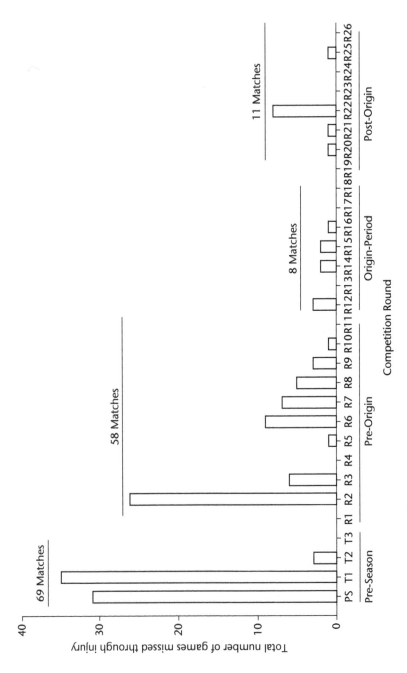

FIGURE 1.2 Matches missed through injury

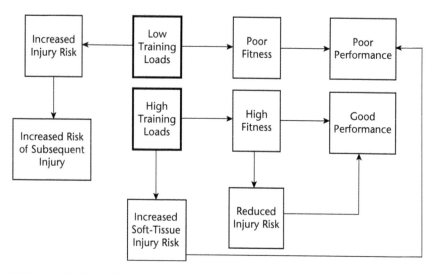

FIGURE 1.3   Relationship between physical qualities, training load, injury risk, and performance in rugby players

the development of greater physical qualities. The increased training loads also coincided with greater playing performance suggesting that physically hard training developed the physical qualities necessary for competition and the mental toughness to deal with the 'worst case scenarios' associated with match-play. Importantly, physically hard training also appeared to increase, rather than decrease, injury risk (Figure 1.3).

References

Austin, D., Gabbett, T., and Jenkins, D. (2011). Repeated high-intensity exercise in professional rugby union. *Journal of Sports Sciences*, 29, 1105–12.

Austin, D.J. and Kelly, S.J. (2014). Professional rugby league positional match-play analysis through the use of global positioning system. *Journal of Strength and Conditioning Research*, 28, 187–93.

Brewer, J. and Davis, J. (1995). Applied physiology of rugby league. *Sports Medicine*, 20, 129–35.

Buchheit, M., Laursen, P.B., Kuhnle, J., *et al.* (2009). Game-based training in young elite handball players. *International Journal of Sports Medicine*, 30, 251–8.

Cahill, N., Lamb, K., Worsfold, P., *et al.* (2013). The movement characteristics of English Premiership rugby union players. *Journal of Sports Sciences*, 31, 229–37.

Castagna, C., Impellizzeri, F., Cecchini, E., *et al.* (2009). Effects of intermittent-endurance fitness on match performance in young male soccer players. *Journal of Strength and Conditioning Research*, 23, 1954–9.

Clark, L. (2002). A comparison of the speed characteristics of elite rugby league players by grade and position. *Strength and Conditioning Coach*, 10, 2–12.

Duthie, G., Pyne, D., and Hooper, S. (2005). Time motion analysis of 2001 and 2002 Super 12 rugby. *Journal of Sports Sciences*, 23, 523–30.

Eaves, S.J., Hughes, M.D., and Lamb, K.L. (2005). The consequences of the introduction of professional playing status on game action variables in international northern hemisphere rugby union football. *International Journal of Performance Analysis in Sport*, 5, 58–86.

Foster, C.D., Twist, C., Lamb, K.L., *et al.* (2010). Heart rate responses to small-sided games among elite junior rugby league players. *Journal of Strength and Conditioning Research*, 24, 906–11.

Gabbett, T.J. (2004). Influence of training and match intensity on injuries in rugby league. *Journal of Sports Sciences*, 22, 409–17.

Gabbett, T.J. (2006). Skill-based conditioning games as an alternative to traditional conditioning for rugby league players. *Journal of Strength and Conditioning Research*, 20, 309–15.

Gabbett, T.J. (2012a). Activity cycles of National Rugby League and National Youth Competition matches. *Journal of Strength and Conditioning Research*, 26, 1517–23.

Gabbett, T.J. (2012b). Sprinting patterns of National Rugby League competition. *Journal of Strength and Conditioning Research*, 26, 121–30.

Gabbett, T.J. (2013). Activity and recovery cycles of National Rugby League matches involving higher- and lower-ranked teams. *Journal of Strength and Conditioning Research*, 27, 1623–8.

Gabbett, T.J. and Jenkins, D.G. (2011). Relationship between training load and injury in professional rugby league players. *Journal of Science and Medicine in Sport*, 14, 204–9.

Gabbett, T.J. and Seibold, A. (2013). Relationship between tests of physical qualities, team selection, and physical match performance in semi-professional rugby league players. *Journal of Strength and Conditioning Research*, 27, 3259–65.

Gabbett, T., Kelly, J., Ralph, S., *et al.* (2009). Physiological and anthropometric characteristics of junior elite and sub-elite rugby league players, with special reference to starters and non-starters. *Journal of Science and Medicine in Sport*, 12, 215–22.

Gabbett, T., Jenkins, D., and Abernethy, B. (2010a). Physical collisions and injury during professional rugby league skills training. *Journal of Science and Medicine in Sport*, 13, 578–83.

Gabbett, T.J., Jenkins, D.G., and Abernethy, B. (2010b). Physiological and skill demands of 'on-side' and 'off-side' games. *Journal of Strength and Conditioning Research*, 24, 2979–83.

Gabbett, T.J., Jenkins, D.G., and Abernethy, B. (2011a). Correlates of tackling ability in high-performance rugby league players. *Journal of Strength and Conditioning Research*, 25, 72–9.

Gabbett, T.J., Jenkins, D.G., and Abernethy, B. (2011b). Physical collisions and injury in professional rugby league match-play. *Journal of Science and Medicine in Sport*, 14, 210–5.

Gabbett, T.J., Jenkins, D.G., and Abernethy, B. (2011c). Relationships between physiological, anthropometric, and skill qualities and playing performance in professional rugby league players. *Journal of Sports Sciences*, 29, 1655–64.

Gabbett, T.J., Jenkins, D.G., and Abernethy, B. (2011d). Relative importance of physiological, anthropometric, and skill qualities to team selection in professional rugby league. *Journal of Sports Sciences*, 29, 1453–61.

Gabbett, T.J., Jenkins, D.G., and Abernethy, B. (2012a). Influence of wrestling on the physiological and skill demands of small-sided games. *Journal of Strength and Conditioning Research*, 26, 113–20.

Gabbett, T.J., Jenkins, D.G., and Abernethy, B. (2012b). Physical demands of professional rugby league training and competition using microtechnology. *Journal of Science and Medicine in Sport*, 15, 80–6.

Gabbett, T.J., Ullah, S., and Finch, C.F. (2012c). Identifying risk factors for contact injury in professional rugby league players – application of a frailty model for recurrent injury. *Journal of Science and Medicine in Sport*, 15, 496–504.

Gabbett, T.J., Polley, C. Dwyer, D.B., *et al.* (2014). Influence of field position and phase of play on the physical demands of match-play in professional rugby league forwards. *Journal of Science and Medicine in Sport*, 17, 556–61.

Gabbett, T.J., Stein, J.G., Kemp, J.G., *et al.* (2013). Relationship between tests of physical qualities and physical match performance in elite rugby league players. *Journal of Strength and Conditioning Research*, 27, 1539–45.

Gamble, P. (2004). A skill-based conditioning games approach to metabolic conditioning for elite rugby football players. *Journal of Strength and Conditioning Research*, 18, 491–7.

Gissane, C., Jennings, D., Jennings, S., *et al.* (2001a). Physical collisions and injury rates in professional super league rugby. *Cleveland Medical Journal*, 4, 147–55.

Gissane, C., White, J., Kerr, K., *et al.* (2001b). Physical collisions in professional super league. The demands of different player positions. *Cleveland Medical Journal*, 4, 137–46.

Higham, D.G., Pyne, D.B., Anson, J.M., *et al.* (2012). Movement patterns in rugby sevens: effects of tournament level, fatigue and substitute players. *Journal of Science and Medicine in Sport*, 15, 277–82.

Hill-Haas, S.V., Coutts, A.J., Rowsell, G.J., *et al.* (2009). Generic versus small-sided game training in soccer. *International Journal of Sports Medicine*, 30, 636–42.

Impellizzeri, F.M., Marcora, S.M., Castagna, C., *et al.* (2006). Physiological and performance effects of generic versus specific aerobic training in soccer players. *International Journal of Sports Medicine*, 27, 483–92.

Johnston, R.D. and Gabbett, T.J. (2011). Repeated-sprint and effort ability in rugby league players. *Journal of Strength and Conditioning Research*, 25, 2789–95.

Kennett, D.C., Kempton, T., and Coutts, A.J. (2012). Factors affecting exercise intensity in rugby-specific small-sided games. *Journal of Strength and Conditioning Research*, 26, 2037–42.

Krustrup, P., Mohr, M., Ellingsgaard, H., and Bangsbo, J. (2005). Physical demands during an elite female soccer game: importance of training status. *Medicine and Science in Sports and Exercise*, 37, 1242–8.

Meir, R., Arthur, D., and Forrest, M. (1993). Time and motion analysis of professional rugby league: a case study. *Strength and Conditioning Coach*, 1, 24–9.

McLean, B.D., Coutts, A.J., Kelly, V., *et al.* (2010). Neuromuscular, endocrine, and perceptual fatigue responses during different length between-match microcycles in professional rugby league players. *International Journal of Sports Physiology and Performance*, 5, 367–83.

McLean, D.A. (1992). Analysis of the physical demands of international rugby union. *Journal of Sports Sciences*, 10, 285–96.

Morton, R.H. (1997). Modelling training and overtraining. *Journal of Sports Sciences*, 15, 335–40.

Noakes, T.D., St Clair Gibson, A., and Lambert, E.V. (2005). From catastrophe to complexity: a novel model of integrative central neural regulation of effort and fatigue during exercise in humans: summary and conclusions. *British Journal of Sports Medicine*, 39, 120–4.

Quarrie, K.L., Hopkins, W.G., Anthony, M.J., *et al.* (2013). Positional demands of international rugby union: evaluation of player actions and movements. *Journal of Science and Medicine in Sport*, 16, 353–9.

Rampinini, E., Bishop, D., Marcora, S.M., *et al.* (2007a). Validity of simple field tests as indicators of match-related physical performance in top-level soccer players. *International Journal of Sports Medicine*, 28, 228–35.

Rampinini, E., Impellizzeri, F.M., Castagna, C., *et al.* (2007b). Factors influencing the physiological responses to small-sided soccer games. *Journal of Sports Sciences*, 25, 659–66.

Scrimgeour, A.G., Noakes, T.D., Adams, B., *et al.* (1986). The influence of weekly training distance on fractional utilization of maximum aerobic capacity in marathon and ultra-marathon runners. *European Journal of Applied Physiology*, 55, 202–9.

Spencer, M., Lawrence, S., Rechichi, C., *et al.* (2004). Time-motion analysis of elite field hockey, with special reference to repeated-sprint activity. *Journal of Sports Sciences*, 22, 843–50.

Suarez-Arrones, L., Nunez, F.J., Portillo, J., *et al.* (2012). Match running performance and exercise intensity in elite female Rugby Sevens. *Journal of Strength and Conditioning Research*, 26, 1858–62.

Sykes, D., Twist, C., Nicholas, C., *et al.* (2011). Changes in locomotive rates during senior elite rugby league matches. *Journal of Sports Sciences*, 29, 1263–71.

Varley, M.C., Gabbett, T.J., and Aughey, R.J. (2013). Activity profiles of professional soccer, rugby league, and Australian football match-play. *Journal of Sports Sciences*, doi:10 .1080/02640414.2013.823227.

Waldron, M., Twist, C., Highton, J., *et al.* (2011). Movement and physiological match demands of elite rugby league using portable global positioning systems. *Journal of Sports Sciences*, 29, 1223–30.

2

STRENGTH AND POWER TRAINING FOR RUGBY

Daniel Travis McMaster, Michael R. McGuigan, and Nicholas D. Gill

2.1 An introduction to strength and power

Muscular strength and power are critical components that contribute to success in sports such as rugby union and rugby league (Baker and Newton 2008a; Comfort *et al.* 2011; Crewther *et al.* 2011), specifically in tasks such as scrummaging, mauling, and tackling. The one-repetition maximum (1RM) bench press, back squat, and power clean are the most common exercises that have been used for the assessment of maximum strength in highly trained rugby athletes (Argus *et al.* 2009; Baker and Newton 2006; Hansen *et al.* 2011b; Comfort 2012). Concentric power (peak and mean power) and jump height are the two most commonly reported performance variables within rugby (Baker 2001b; Bevan *et al.* 2010; Cronin and Hansen 2005). Peak power can be defined as the maximum instantaneous value achieved during the concentric phase at a given load; whereas mean power is calculated as the area under the concentric portion of a power-time curve using a given load (Sapega and Drillings 1983). The load that maximises an athlete's power output is often referred to as the Pmax load; this can be expressed as mean or peak power and is often predicted based on a polynomial equation applied to the individual power-load curve (Baker and Newton 2007; Harris *et al.* 2007; Bevan *et al.* 2010; McGuigan *et al.* 2009).

Maximum strength and ballistic capabilities such as force-velocity–power are crucial to competing in rugby union and rugby league at the elite level. Rugby is typified by combination of match specific force (e.g. scrummaging, mauling, rucking, and lifting), power (e.g. tackling, fending, jumping, decelerating, accelerating, and changing directions) and velocity (e.g. sprinting, kick-chasing, counter-attacking, line-breaking, line defence, kicking, and passing) governed actions. In general, the forwards perform more force-dominant tasks, such as driving, tackling, rucking, mauling, and wrestling. In contrast, the backs perform more velocity-dominant tasks, such as maximum sprinting and kicking; whilst some positions (e.g. rugby union back row forwards) tend to perform a combination of force, velocity, and power specific tasks (Quarrie *et al.* 2013).

Training programmes in rugby emphasise hypertrophy, strength, and power development, as being a strong and muscular athlete is beneficial to maximising force production and absorbing impacts (Appleby *et al.* 2012; Argus *et al.* 2010; Baker 2001b; Baker and Newton 2008a; Corcoran 2010; Coutts *et al.* 2007; Hansen *et al.* 2011b). Given the spectrum of strength and power demands between the tight-five, loose forwards, and inside and outside backs in rugby union, it would be advantageous to determine whether certain types of strength and ballistic training affect different parts of the force–velocity continuum. Positional specific development tends to be less of a concern in rugby league due to the homogeneity between positions.

A specific training stimulus or dosage causes a neuromuscular and morphological response, which in turn leads to adaptations over time (Folland and Williams 2007; Appleby *et al.* 2012). The type of training stimulus will cause specific neuromuscular and morphological changes and affect change in strength and power of the training-specific movements (e.g. squat, press, pull, and jump) (Folland and Williams 2007). Exposure to a new training stimulus will initially (two to four weeks) cause a number of neuromuscular changes, such as increases in muscle fibre recruitment, coordination, and firing frequency with minimal changes in morphology (Hakkinen 1994; Folland and Williams 2007). These neuromuscular changes might lead to improvements in dynamic force (i.e. strength) and power production (Folland and Williams 2007; Hakkinen 1994). A number of different morphological adaptations can occur after this initial period (after week three): an increase in muscle cross-sectional area, musculotendinous stiffness/thickness, hypertrophy, and changes in muscle fibre pennation angles that should further develop maximum strength and ballistic qualities (e.g. power production) (Folland and Williams 2007; Fry 2004; Hakkinen 1994; Blazevich and Sharp 2005).

In professional and semi-professional rugby, a training year is divided into a six-to twelve-week off-season, a three to six-week pre-season and a twenty-to thirty-week in-season in southern and northern hemispheres. There are a number of overlapping competitions in the southern and northern hemispheres that a single professional rugby union player might be involved in. Professional rugby league competitions in the northern and southern hemispheres are less complex. Both rugby code competition periods are equally as long (8–10 months/30–40 games) and physically demanding, often resulting in diminished performance and/or injuries. Training programmes implemented in rugby need to embrace a shifting focus that varies with such factors as the yearly training plan, positional demands, and individual strengths and weaknesses of the athletes. Programmes might place an isolated or mixed emphasis on hypertrophy, strength, and ballistic power development in accordance with the training phase (e.g. off-season, pre-season, in-season) and individual athlete needs.

2.2 Assessment strategies

When creating strength and power profiles, practitioners must carefully consider the benefits and limitations of the following:

- various measurement systems (e.g. force plates, videos, jump mats, optical sensors, linear position transducers, and accelerometers)

- attachment sites of the measurement system
- testing apparatus (bar type [free weight vs. fixed])
- movement patterns (e.g. jump, throw, squat, clean, pull, press, direction of movement, contraction type, movement depth)
- loading parameters (e.g. single load, absolute load, relative load, incremental loading)
- warm-up strategies (e.g. cycling, dynamic, static, post-activation potentiation, motivation)
- rest periods
- performance variables (e.g. displacement, velocity, force, power, strength)
- data processing techniques (e.g. sampling frequency, filtering, and smoothing options)

2.2.1 Maximum strength assessments

A number of dynamic and isometric assessments have been utilized to create strength profiles and to monitor changes over time in highly trained rugby athletes (Comfort *et al.* 2011; Hoffman and Kang 2003). These assessments provide general information regarding the strength qualities of players that might not entirely represent rugby specific qualities. The various maximum dynamic strength (McGuigan and Winchester 2008; Argus *et al.* 2011) and isometric strength (Blazevich *et al.* 2002; McGuigan and Winchester 2008) testing methods are reliable (ICC > 0.91; CV < 4.5%) for assessing these respective capabilities.

Strength and conditioning practitioners for rugby most often utilize the bench press, back squat, and clean to assess maximum strength (Argus *et al.* 2009; Baker and Newton 2006; Cronin and Hansen 2005; Comfort 2012). The required squat depths (i.e. quarter, half, parallel, and full) and knee angles (70 to 110°) vary between investigators/practitioners, which in turn affects the 1RM result (Blazevich *et al.* 2002; Harris *et al.* 2000; McGuigan and Winchester 2008; Argus *et al.* 2009). The technical requirements of the bench press are more consistent, as a bar-to-chest depth is generally used, as is required by the International Powerlifting Federation (IPF 2012) and applied researchers (McGuigan and Winchester 2008; Coutts *et al.* 2007). A number of different warm-up strategies can be implemented, such as dynamic stretching, cycle ergometry (5–10 min) (Blazevich *et al.* 2002; Nibali *et al.* 2013), potentiation exercises, and motivation to maximise strength (Cormie *et al.* 2006; Samuel *et al.* 2008). The isometric mid-thigh pull and squat are also often implemented in the laboratory setting to assess maximum strength. Maximum isometric strength tests are less accessible and therefore less popular than the 1RM, as a force measurement system such as a force plate is required to assess strength qualities, such as peak force (West *et al.* 2011). The isometric squat (90 to 140°) and isometric mid-thigh pull (120 to 145°) knee angles, contraction durations (3–6 s), inter-trial rest intervals (2–5 min), and force plate sampling frequencies (200 to 1,000 Hz) vary between investigations

(Blazevich *et al.* 2002; McGuigan and Winchester 2008; West *et al.* 2011). These dynamic and isometric strength tests provide a non-specific measurement of rugby specific strength, but may not necessarily provide a true representation of the required rugby specific strength qualities (Comfort *et al.* 2011; Quarrie and Wilson 2000). Scrummaging and tackling specific force have also been assessed in rugby union and league (Preatoni *et al.* 2013; Quarrie and Wilson 2000; Usman *et al.* 2010; Pain *et al.* 2008). Given the methodological differences, comparisons of the same strength measure between applied researchers and strength and conditioning coaches is difficult. Strength and conditioning practitioners need to be aware of the benefits and limitations of the different assessment methods currently available, as these can potentially affect the outcome measures.

2.2.2 Power assessments

The explosive qualities of rugby players are generally quantified and assessed via position transducer and force plate technologies during explosive squatting, jumping, pulling, pressing, and throwing movements (Baker 2001b; Harris *et al.* 2007; McGuigan *et al.* 2009; Argus *et al.* 2013; Nibali *et al.* 2013; McMaster *et al.* 2013a). Movement patterns with a flight phase, such as jumping and throwing, allow the athlete to accelerate throughout the entire range of motion resulting in greater velocity and power outputs than traditional non-ballistic movements (Baker and Newton, 2005, Cronin *et al.*, 2001). Vertical jumps and bench throws have been implemented to create force-velocity-power profiles incorporating a variety of loads for the purpose of assessing and monitoring ballistic performance (Argus *et al.* 2011; Bevan *et al.* 2010; Baker 2013).

When implementing vertical jump and bench throw profiling protocols, the Sports Scientist and Strength and Conditioning coach must carefully consider the same assessment strategy factors as are listed in section 2.2 of this chapter. A number of different vertical jump and bench throw testing protocols have been implemented to reliably (ICC $\geq$ 0.83; CV $\leq$ 8.5%) assess displacement, velocity, force, and power across the various absolute and relative loads using the previously mentioned measurement systems (Argus *et al.* 2013; Baker *et al.* 2001a; Bevan *et al.* 2010; Cormack *et al.* 2008b; Cronin *et al.* 2004; Hansen *et al.* 2011a). It is clear that reliable and valid measures of the ballistic capacities of these athletes are important. Current physical performance assessments are utilized to create standards and develop athlete profiles to better inform programming. Athlete performance profiles can be further improved by assessing rugby specific tasks covering the entire force-velocity-power spectrum, such as passing, throwing and kicking velocities, fending and tackling power outputs, and scrummaging, mauling, and blocking forces. A key purpose of any athlete assessment is to obtain insight into the training needs of the athlete. Therefore, all these factors need to be taken into consideration to ensure that any testing provides information that can be of practical use and potentially improve performance of the athletes.

2.3 Normative data

2.3.1 Maximum strength

Maximal strength values are dependent on a number of factors, including age, training history, playing position, and physical characteristics. The 1RM bench press, back squat, and power clean in highly trained rugby players can typically range from 110 to 190 kg, 140 to 250 kg, and 100 to 140 kg, respectively (Argus *et al.* 2009, 2013; Baker and Newton 2008b; Crewther *et al.* 2010; Harris *et al.* 2008; Comfort 2012). In rugby union, forwards typically have superior maximum upper and lower body strength qualities in comparison to backs due to body mass, increased strength demands of scrumming, mauling, and tackling from a stationary position (Crewther *et al.* 2009). Mean and peak forces of 1,400 to 2,000 N have been reported in rugby players during the isometric back squat and 2,100 to 3,500 N during the mid-thigh pull (McGuigan and Winchester 2008; Quarrie and Wilson 2000; West *et al.* 2011). It should be noted that the large ranges in maximum dynamic and isometric strength might be a result of the various testing methods and large variations in somatotype within and between codes. The heterogeneity of these rugby–football code populations can be off set by normalising maximum strength to body mass and represented as a strength per kilogram (kg) of body mass ratio to allow for an unbiased comparison between players (Atkins 2004; Crewther *et al.* 2011). Allometric scaling has also been used to take into account the body size of individuals (Crewther *et al.* 2011). The isometric and dynamic strength tests can be used to assess and monitor maximum strength adaptations as well as effectively inform weight-room specific programming. However, these may not necessarily provide a true representation of the required rugby specific isometric/dynamic strength qualities (Comfort *et al.* 2011; Quarrie and Wilson 2000). Rugby specific strength tests have been developed to quantify individual tackling capabilities (Usman *et al.* 2010) and scrum forces (Quarrie and Wilson 2000); however, their diagnostic value to strength and conditioning practice remains inconclusive.

2.3.2 Power capabilities

Maximal peak power has been reported across a range of bench throw (20–60% 1RM; 35–70 kg) (Baker and Newton 2006; Bevan *et al.* 2010; Baker 2001b; Argus *et al.* 2013; McMaster *et al.* 2013a) and vertical jump loads (0–45% 1RM) (Cronin *et al.* 2004; Argus *et al.* 2011; Bevan *et al.* 2010), which is dependent on the measurement system and the group or individual being assessed. The maximal peak power in highly trained rugby players can range between 800 to 1,500 W during the bench throw using relative loads between 20 and 60 per cent 1RM (40–80 kg) (Baker and Newton 2008b; Bevan *et al.* 2010; Argus *et al.* 2013; McMaster *et al.* 2013a) and between 5,000 and 9,000 W during the vertical jump using loads between zero/body mass and 45 per cent 1RM (0–100 kg) (Comfort *et al.* 2011; Argus *et al.* 2011; Bevan *et al.* 2010; Harris *et al.* 2007; McGuigan *et al.* 2009). Large variations in peak power can be attributed to the wide range in physical characteristics between the various rugby position specific demands. Individual tackling forces of 1,400 N (non-dominant shoulder) to 2,100 N (dominant shoulder) and scrum forces between 1,000 to 1,700 N have been reported in highly trained rugby union players (Usman *et al.* 2010; Quarrie and Wilson 2000; Preatoni *et al.* 2013). It is important for practitioners to establish their own normative data/benchmarks for the group of athletes they are working with due to the large effect of different measurement methods and other factors that can influence the results in any test of power capacities.

2.4 Training applications: development, retention, decay

The training volume (dose) required to develop, retain, and decay strength and ballistic/power capabilities can be classified as high, moderate, and low, respectively (McMaster *et al.* 2013b; Cronin and Sleivert 2005; Cormie *et al.* 2011). The literature currently recommends that three to five sets of two to six repetitions at 85 to 98% 1RM be prescribed to improve strength; and three to five sets of two to six repetitions at zero to 60% of 1RM to improve ballistic (power) capacities (Baker and Newton, 2005, 2007; McMaster *et al.* 2013b). Numerous periodized loading schemes, such as linear, non-linear, undulating, conjugate, and block training have been prescribed to continually develop strength and power overtime (Baker 1998, 2001b, 2007; Issurin 2008; Prestes *et al.* 2009).

Strength and power maintenance have been investigated to a lesser extent in rugby, but generally the intensity and session volume are held constant and the weekly training frequency is reduced by 33 to 66% (Tan 1999; Baker 1998, 2001b). In rugby, the demands of a match and lengthy competition can have acute and accumulative effects on strength and power (McLean *et al.* 2010; Argus *et al.* 2009). This accumulation of fatigue might lead to performance decrements if suitable monitoring methods and recovery modalities are not in place (Twist and Highton 2013). Training programmes have been implemented successfully to prevent decay and even improve strength and power performance throughout the competitive season in elite rugby players (Baker 1998, 2001b). During detraining, the weekly rates of decay in power and strength are of great interest, as they allow practitioners to determine the minimum and maximum durations that training can be ceased before another training stimulus is required. This, in turn, might allow practitioners to periodize training programmes more effectively. A residual effect is the maximum detraining duration in which an athlete can retain their strength or power, whereas the decay rate is a measure of the speed at which power and strength is lost over time. It has also been suggested that maximal strength can be retained for up to 30 ± 5 days post-training and that maximal speed can only be retained for 5 ± 3 days post-training (Issurin 2008). This highlights the need to reconsider current periodisation strategies in the rugby context (Issurin 2008). Maximal speed and maximal power production utilize similar energy requirements and neuromuscular activation processes (e.g. motor unit recruitment/firing frequencies), therefore should have similar adaptations to detraining. Currently, there is limited research

TABLE 2.1 Dose-response guidelines for strength and power development in rugby code athletes (McMaster *et al.* 2013b)

| Quality | Volume and intensity | | | | Percent increase per session(s) | | | |
	MP per session	Sets per MP	Reps	%1RM	1	5	10	20
Strength	2–5	3–6	1–6	80–100	0.5	2.5	5.0	10.0
Power (force)	2–5	3–6	2–6	85–98	0.1	0.5	1.0	2.0
Power (velocity)	2–5	3–6	2–6	20–60	0.2	1.0	2.0	4.0

MP = movement pattern; *Reps* = repetitions; *%1RM* = percentage of one-repetition maximum utilized

investigating these aspects in elite rugby union players. Table 2.1 shows the proposed dose-response guidelines for power and strength development in contact sports such as rugby.

2.4.1 Maximum strength

The required dose to develop maximal strength can be described as moderate frequency, with two to four weekly sessions per muscle group required. Each session is to include three to five movement patterns per session (each pattern containing three to six sets of one to six repetitions each) performed at high intensity (80–100% 1RM) (McMaster *et al.* 2013b; Peterson *et al.* 2005). Rugby players that resistance train each muscle group two to three times per week should expect monthly strength increases of 4 to 8% if periodized correctly, although there will be large individual differences (Argus *et al.* 2010; Appleby *et al.* 2012; Hansen *et al.* 2011b; Harris *et al.* 2000; McMaster *et al.* 2013b). Strength and conditioning researchers and practitioners often implement a range of different hypertrophy, strength, and power loading schemes to increase maximum strength qualities, including conjugate-mixed method (Argus *et al.* 2010; Harris *et al.* 2000; Hoffman *et al.* 2009), stepwise-blocks (Stone *et al.* 1999), linear (Coutts *et al.* 2007), non-linear (Hoffman *et al.* 2009), cluster sets (Hansen *et al.* 2011b), heavy load-high force (Harris *et al.* 2000), and power specific training (Harris *et al.* 2000; McBride *et al.* 2002). Regardless of the method of periodisation utilized, it appears that maximum strength can be improved with as little as 10–20 strength training sessions (Argus *et al.* 2010; Hansen *et al.* 2011b). If volume and intensity are constant, then the magnitude of change in strength is dependent on the total number of training sessions (duration x frequency) performed (Tan 1999). Strength adaptation rates are also dependent on training age and experience because as these two variables increase, strength adaptation rates diminish (Baker and Newton 2006; Folland and Williams 2007; Issurin 2008; Rhea and Alderman 2004). The magnitude of strength improvement tends to be greater in weaker, less experienced players (Appleby *et al.* 2012; Baker and Newton 2008a; Baker 2013). Longitudinal studies tracking changes in strength in elite rugby players have found moderate improvements during the first twelve months and diminished returns thereafter (Baker and Newton 2006; Appleby *et al.* 2012; Baker 2013). The retention of strength qualities is of great importance for preventing injuries and maintaining consistent performance throughout the season, particularly where the competition periods are lengthy (18 to 24 weeks).

Based on the current research, it appears that maximum strength can be maintained with as little as one resistance training session per week if session intensity and volume are maintained (Argus *et al.* 2009; Hoffman and Kang 2003). There is little detraining data in elite rugby, but researchers studying other elite athletes and resistance-trained individuals have reported that maximum strength can be maintained for up to four weeks with more substantial losses occurring thereafter (Hakkinen 1994; McMaster *et al.* 2013b; Izquierdo *et al.* 2007). It is also suggested that strength plays an important role in increasing ballistic (power) capabilities regardless of somatotype, as stronger athletes often have more developed morphological qualities and potentially greater neuromuscular capacity (Argus *et al.* 2009; Baker and Newton 2008b; Cormie *et al.* 2010).

2.4.2 Power capabilities

The required dose to develop power can be described as high, with three to five weekly sessions per muscle group required. Each session is to include three to five movement patterns (with each pattern containing three to six sets of two to six repetitions each) at a low-moderate intensity (at or below 60% 1RM) (Baker and Newton 2006; Cormie *et al.* 2011; Kawamori and Haff 2004). Although substantial individual differences exist, power increases between 3 to 12% have been reported after four to eight weeks of ballistic training and maximum strength combined with ballistic training (Lockie *et al.* 2012; Hansen *et al.* 2011b; Harris *et al.* 2000, McBride *et al.* 2002; Hoffman *et al.* 2005). These low-volume, low-intensity training loads are utilized to optimize upper and lower body power due to the high movement velocities and high power outputs generated with these training loads (Baker and Newton 2005, 2007). It should be noted that a number of researchers recommend using hypertrophy (three to five movement patterns per session with three to four sets of six to ten repetitions each, performed at 70–85% 1RM per movement pattern) and/ or maximum strength training loads to improve power through an increase in the force component (Folland and Williams 2007; McBride *et al.* 2002; Wilson *et al.* 1993). To a lesser extent, power improvements ranging from 1 to 5% have also been reported after four to twelve weeks of hypertrophy/maximum strength training (Hoffman *et al.* 2004, 2009, 2005; Hansen *et al.* 2011b). The basis for the prescription of heavy loads is related to hypertrophic adaptations and motor unit recruitment, in that near maximal force production is needed to recruit and fully activate the Type II muscle fibres (Wilson *et al.* 1993). Current ballistic intensity prescription guidelines span the entire loading spectrum (0–98% 1RM) depending on the performance variable of interest (e.g. force, power, or velocity) (Figure 2.1).

Long-term power adaptations are also affected by training age and experience following the concept of diminishing returns (Baker and Newton, 2006; Folland

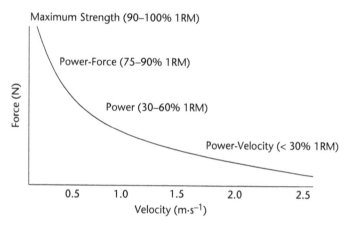

FIGURE 2.1   Force-power-velocity continuum (McMaster 2012, with permission)

and Williams 2007; Issurin 2008). The longitudinal tracking of power in elite rugby league players showed a large increase in power (15%) after the first two years and a small decrease in power between the second and fourth year (-3%), which supports the concept of diminishing returns in elite athletes (Baker and Newton, 2006). Similar to maximal strength, power retention in rugby players can be achieved with as little as one to two weekly training sessions, providing session intensity and volume are maintained over time (Baker 2001a, 2001b, 2013; Appleby *et al.* 2012). It has been demonstrated that muscular power can be maintained and, under the right training stimulus, even improved throughout a competitive rugby season (Baker 2001b; Cormack *et al.* 2008a; Argus *et al.* 2009).

The detraining effects on ballistic (power) capabilities in rugby are scarce. However, some inferences can be drawn from previous research using elite athletes. Vertical jump performance can be maintained for up to eight weeks of resistance detraining, if a ballistic stimulus (e.g. a field session, plyometrics, sprint training) is provided as part of the training dosage (Gabbett 2006). It is believed that a training stimulus must be provided every five to eight days to retain power capabilities (Issurin 2008). There is also evidence to suggest that high velocity qualities (body weight/unloaded ballistic movements, e.g. jump squats) may decrease at a greater rate than high force qualities (loaded ballistic movements, e.g. loaded jump squats) based on the purported neuromuscular and morphological adaptations due to detraining (Hakkinen 1994; Folland and Williams 2007; McMaster *et al.* 2013b). Further investigations looking at weekly/bi-weekly strength, speed, and ballistic performance changes over these off-season/detraining periods are recommended to effectively quantify decay rates and residual effects in rugby.

2.5 Summary

Strength and power assessment, development, and retention in elite rugby athletes are crucial considerations for practitioners. The strength and conditioning practitioner must carefully consider the benefits and limitations of the various measurement systems, testing apparatus, movement patterns, loading parameters, warm-up strategies, rest periods, and the performance variables of interest currently available. Assessment selections must reflect the required rugby strength and power demands and be of practical/meaningful benefit to the athlete's development. The dosage required to develop strength is described as high frequency, moderate volume, and high intensity; whereas the required dose to develop ballistic-power capabilities can be described as high frequency, low volume, and low–moderate intensity. Maximum strength training loads can also be employed to improve power through an increase in force production.

Case study: resistance training programme design and implementation for rugby

Introduction

The complexity of the rugby calendar in both hemispheres (e.g. numerous competitions, long seasons, and club and representative duties) makes training- and playing-load monitoring difficult, yet vitally important. A number of factors must be considered, such as playing position, training age, game exposure, strengths and weaknesses, injury history, and alterations in recent training load. All of these factors should be used to formulate the specific and individual plan for the player from a training (e.g. content and load) and game exposure perspective. Two practical case study training examples are provided below.

Player A

The coaching staff and national squad of selectors have indicated that Player A, a tight-head prop, needs to improve his explosiveness off the line in defence (acceleration), be more dynamic in the collision, and be quicker in 'the hit' during the scrum. His strength and power assessments from May indicate that he is extremely strong (e.g. 1RM squat = 240 kg), but possesses average to below average explosive capabilities during the 50 kg squat jump (peak power = 4,300 W), bodyweight squat jump (peak power = 4,700 W), drop jump (reactive strength), and sprint acceleration (t_{10m} = 1.90 s) relative to his position. During the four weeks prior to May testing, Player A had been performing base strength squats, deadlifts, and snatch pulls (6, 5, 4, and 3 repetitions per lift) early each week (e.g. Monday/Tuesday), followed by a power day consisting of the full snatch, blue band resisted box squats, and power cleans (4 sets of 3 repetitions) later in the week (e.g. Thursday/Friday).

The directive from the coaches, selectors, and his test results were aligned, so an adjustment to his lower body lifting programme was made. His first session each week consisted of heavy squats, snatch pulls, and barbell step-ups (5 sets of 3 repetitions), and his second session consisted of the same power session with the addition of a 50 kg jump squat (4 sets of 3 repetitions). This training routine was performed for two months (dependent on game time, travel, and recovery) and the changes that

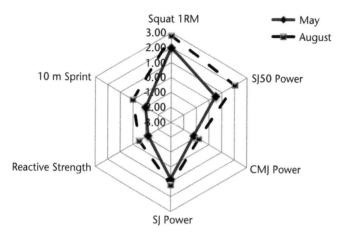

FIGURE 2.2 Player A (prop) performance profile. All values are represented as standardised z-scores relative to playing position (front-row): one-repetition maximum parallel back squat (Squat 1RM); peak concentric power produced during a static squat jump with an external load of 50 kg (SJ 50 Power); peak concentric power produced during a body weight static squat jump (SJ Power); peak concentric power produced during a body weight countermovement jump (CMJ Power); reactive strength is a ratio between jump height and contact time during a 50 cm drop jump measured via a force plate (reactive strength); 10 metre sprint time from a split stance starting 50 cm behind the first set of infrared timing lights (10 m sprint).

occurred can be seen in Figure 2.2, represented as standardised z-scores. A z-score provides a ranking of each player's performance on a given test (e.g. 1RM squat) relative to the mean and standard deviation of the squad or position (Pettitt, 2010). For example, a z-score of zero is equal to the mean, a z-score of 1.0 is one standard deviation above the mean and a z-score of -2.0 is two standard deviations below the mean. Essentially Player A increased his strength (1RM squat = 280 kg), power capabilities during the 50 kg squat jump (5,300 W), and sprint acceleration (t_{10m} = 1.85 s) with minimal changes in bodyweight squat, countermovement, and drop jump performance. It would appear that the addition of heavy barbell step-up and loaded jump squats simply improved his maximum strength, loaded power, and acceleration capabilities but had little effect on his light load velocity and power capabilities.

Player B

Player B is an outside back who has played a lot of rugby in the past three months. The coaching staff and selectors have indicated that he seems to have lost his ability to beat an opposition defender in a one-on-one situation. His strength and power assessments from May indicate that his maximum strength is good (1RM squat = 190 kg), but his power capability during the 50 kg squat jump (3,500 W) is poor. Likewise, his vertical jump power output (5,700 W), reactive strength (1.50 Units), and sprint ability (t_{30m} = 3.97 s) were below the back-line average. The observations of his on-field performance were consistent with his performance profile. In the four weeks prior to May testing, Player B had been performing heavy clean pulls, backs squats, barbell step-ups (4 sets of 3 repetitions), Nordic hamstring drops (3 sets of 6 repetitions), weighted calf raises, and lunges (3 sets of 10 repetitions) early each week (e.g. Monday/Tuesday), followed by a power day consisting of the full snatch, 50 kg jump squats, and power cleans (4 sets of 3 repetitions) later in the week (e.g. Thursday/Friday).

The directive from the coaches and his testing results were aligned, so an adjustment to his weekly programme was made. His first session each week consisted of the following strength and power complexes: heavy squats with box jumps, heavy clean pulls with hurdle jumps (continuous) and heavy barbell step-up with assisted over speed jumps (3 sets of 4 repetitions for the heavy lifts supplemented with 6 jumps), Nordic hamstring drops (3 sets of 8 repetitions), and weighted calf raises (3 sets of 10 repetitions). In the second session, he completed the same power-based session with the addition of agility ladder work/change in direction tasks (10 repetitions), hurdle jumps, assisted jumps, and resisted jumps (3 sets of 4 repetitions). A one versus one speed-evasion drill (6 sets of 30 metres) was also performed after on-field training sessions twice per week. This training routine was performed for two months (dependent on game time, travel, and recovery) and the changes that occurred can be seen in Figure 2.3. Essentially, player B increased his bodyweight

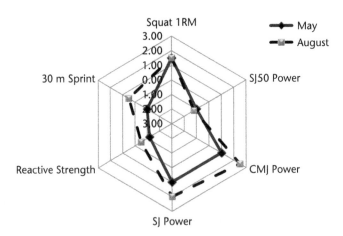

FIGURE 2.3 Player B (outside back) performance profile. All values are represented as standardised z-scores relative to playing position (backline). One-repetition maximum parallel back squat (Squat 1RM); peak concentric power produced during a static squat jump with an external load of 50 kg (SJ 50 Power); peak concentric power produced during a body weight static squat jump (SJ Power); peak concentric power produced during a body weight counter-movement jump (CMJ Power); reactive strength is a ratio between jump height and contact time during a 50 cm drop jump measured via a force plate (reactive strength); 30 metre sprint time from a split stance starting 50 cm behind the first set of infrared timing lights (30 m sprint).

vertical jump power capabilities (7,000 W) and sprint ability (t_{30m} = 3.85 s) with minimal shifts in maximum strength and loaded squat jump power.

The two cases presented above indicate the use of physical performance profiles to effectively monitor maximum strength, power, and sprint ability in elite rugby players. It is clear from the two examples that players A and B adapted to the small variations in training that were targeted by coaching staff observations of diminished on-field performance tasks and reinforced by the physical performance assessments.

References

Appleby, B., Newton, R., and Cormie, P. (2012). Changes in strength over a 2-year period in professional rugby union players. *Journal of Strength and Conditioning Research*, 26, 2538–46.

Argus, C., Gill, N., Keogh, J., *et al.* (2013). Assessing the variation in the load that produces maximal upper-body power. *Journal of Strength and Conditioning Research*, 28, 240–4.

Argus, C.K., Gill, N., Keogh, J., *et al.* (2010). Effects of a short-term pre-season training programme on the body composition and anaerobic performance of professional rugby union players. *Journal of Sports Sciences*, 28, 679–86.

Argus, C.K., Gill, N.D., Keogh, J.W., *et al.* (2011). Assessing lower body peak power in elite rugby-union players. *Journal of Strength and Conditioning Research*, 25, 1616–21.

Argus, C.K., Gill, N.D., Keogh, J.W., *et al.* (2009). Changes in strength, power, and steroid hormones during a professional rugby union competition. *Journal of Strength and Conditioning Research*, 23, 1583–92.

Atkins, S.J. (2004). Normalizing expressions of strength in elite rugby league players. *Journal of Strength and Conditioning Research*, 18, 53–8.

Baker, D. (1998). Applying the in-season periodization of strength and power training to football. *Strength and Conditioning Journal*, 20, 18–27.

Baker, D. (2001a). Acute and long-term power responses to power training: observations on the training of an elite power athlete. *Strength and Conditioning Journal*, 23, 47–56.

Baker, D. (2001b). The effects of an in-season of concurrent training on the maintenance of maximal strength and power in professional and college aged rugby league football players. *Journal of Strength and Conditioning Research*, 15, 172–7.

Baker, D. (2007). Cycle-length variants in periodized strength/power training. *Strength and Conditioning Journal*, 29, 10–7.

Baker, D. and Newton, R.U. (2005). Methods to increase the effectiveness of maximal power training for the upper body. *Strength and Conditioning Journal*, 27, 24–32.

Baker, D.G. and Newton, R.U. (2006). Adaptations in upper-body maximal strength and power output resulting from long-term resistance training in experienced strength-power athletes. *Journal of Strength and Conditioning Research*, 20, 541–6.

Baker, D. and Newton, R. (2007). Change in power output across a high-repetition set of bench throws and jump squats in highly trained athletes. *Journal of Strength and Conditioning Research*, 21, 1007–11.

Baker, D. and Newton, R. (2008a). Observation of 4-year adaptations in lower body maximal strength and power output in professional rugby league players. *Journal of Australian Strength and Conditioning*, 16, 3–10.

Baker, D.G. and Newton, R.U. (2008b). Comparison of lower body strength, power, acceleration, speed, agility, and sprint momentum to describe and compare playing rank among professional rugby league players. *Journal of Strength and Conditioning Research*, 22, 153–8.

Baker, D., Nance, S. and Moore, M. (2001a). The load that maximizes the average mechanical power output during explosive bench press throws in highly trained athletes. *Journal of Strength and Conditioning Research*, 15, 20–4.

Baker, D.G. (2013). 10-year changes in upper body strength and power in elite professional rugby league players—the effect of training age, stage, and content. *Journal of Strength and Conditioning Research*, 27, 285–92.

Bevan, H.R., Bunce, P.J., Owen, N.J., *et al.* (2010). Optimal loading for the development of peak power output in professional rugby players. *Journal of Strength and Conditioning Research*, 24, 43–7.

Blazevich, A.J., Gill, N., and Newton, R.U. (2002). Reliability and validity of two isometric squat tests. *Journal of Strength and Conditioning Research*, 16, 298–304.

Blazevich, A.J. and Sharp, N.C. (2005). Understanding muscle architectural adaptation: macro and micro level research. *Cells Tissues Organs*, 181, 1–10.

Comfort, P. (2012). Within and between session reliability of power, force, and rate of force development during the power clean. *Journal of Strength and Conditioning Research* 27, 1210–4.

Comfort, P., Graham-Smith, P., Matthews, M., *et al.* (2011). Strength and power characteristics of English elite rugby league players. *Journal of Strength and Conditioning Research*, 25, 1374–84.

Corcoran, G. (2010). Analysis of the anatomical, functional, physiological, and morphological requirements of athletes in rugby union. *Journal of Australian Strength and Conditioning*, 18, 24–8.

Cormack, S. J., Newton, R. U., McGuigan, M.R., *et al.* (2008a). Neuromuscular and endocrine responses of elite players during an Australian rules football season. *International Journal of Sports Physiology and Performance*, 3, 439–53.

Cormack, S. J., Newton, R.U., McGuigan, M.R., *et al.* (2008b). Reliability of measures obtained during single and repeated countermovement jumps. *International Journal of Sports Physiology and Performance*, 3, 131–44.

Cormie, P., Deane, R. S., Triplett, N.T, *et al.* (2006). Acute effects of whole-body vibration on muscle activity, strength, and power. *Journal of Strength and Conditioning Research*, 20, 257–61.

Cormie, P., McGuigan, M., and Newton, R. (2011). Developing maximal neuromuscular power: Part 2—training considerations for improving maximal power production. *Sports Medicine*, 41, 125–46.

Cormie, P., McGuigan, M.R., and Newton, R.U. (2010). Influence of strength on magnitude and mechanisms of adaptation to power training. *Medicine and Science in Sports and Exercise*, 42, 1566–81.

Coutts, A., Reaburn, P., Piva, T., *et al.* (2007). Changes in selected biochemical, muscular strength, power, and endurance measures during deliberate overreaching and tapering in rugby league players. *International Journal of Sports Medicine*, 28, 116–24.

Crewther, B.T., Cook, C.J., Lowe, T.E., *et al.* (2010). The effects of short-cycle sprints on power, strength, and salivary hormones in elite rugby players. *Journal of Strength and Conditioning Research*, 25, 32–9.

Crewther, B.T., Lowe, T., Weatherby, R.P., *et al.* (2009). Prior sprint cycling did not enhance training adaptation, but resting salivary hormones were related to workout power and strength. *European Journal of Applied Physiology*, 105, 919–27.

Crewther, B.T., McGuigan, M.R., and Gill, N.D. (2011). The ratio and allometric scaling of speed, power, and strength in elite male rugby union players. *Journal of Strength and Conditioning Research*, 25, 1968–75.

Cronin, J., McNair, P., and Marshall, R. (2001). Developing explosive power: a comparison of technique and training. *Journal of Science and Medicine in Sport*, 4, 59–70.

Cronin, J. and Sleivert, G. (2005). Challenges in understanding the influence of maximal power training on improving athletic performance. *Sports Medicine*, 35, 213–34.

Cronin, J.B. and Hansen, K.T. (2005). Strength and power predictors of sports speed. *Journal of Strength and Conditioning Research*, 19, 349–57.

Cronin, J.B., Hing, R.D., and McNair, P.J. (2004). Reliability and validity of a linear position transducer for measuring jump performance. *Journal of Strength and Conditioning Research*, 18, 590–3.

Folland, J. and Williams, A. (2007). The adaptations to strength training: morphological and neurological contributions to increased strength. *Sports Medicine*, 37, 145–68.

Fry, A.C. (2004). The role of resistance exercise intensity on muscle fibre adaptations. *Sports Medicine*, 34, 663–79.

Gabbett, T. (2006). Performance changes following a field conditioning program in junior and senior rugby league players. *Journal of Strength and Conditioning Research*, 20, 215–21.

Hakkinen, K. (1994). Neuromuscular adaptation during strength training, aging, detraining, and immobilization. *Physical and Rehabilitation Medicine*, 6, 161–98.

Hansen, K., Cronin, J., and Newton, M. (2011a). The reliability of linear position transducer and force plate measurement of explosive force-time variables during a loaded jump squat in elite athletes. *Journal of Strength and Conditioning Research*, 25, 1447–56.

Hansen, K., Cronin, J., Pickering, S., et al. (2011b). Does cluster loading enhance lower body power development in preseason preparation of elite rugby union players? *Journal of Strength and Conditioning Research*, 25, 2118–26.

Harris, G.R., Stone, M.H., O'Bryant, H.S., et al. (2000). Short-term performance effects of high power, high force, or combined weight-training methods. *Journal of Strength and Conditioning Research*, 14, 14–20.

Harris, N.K., Cronin, J.B., and Hopkins, W.G. (2007). Power outputs of a machine squat-jump across a spectrum of loads. *Journal of Strength and Conditioning Research*, 21, 1260–4.

Harris, N.K., Cronin, J.B., and Hopkins, W.G., et al. (2008a). Relationship between sprint times and the strength/power outputs of a machine squat jump. *Journal of Strength and Conditioning Research*, 22, 691–8.

Hoffman, J., Cooper, J., Wendell, M. et al. (2004). Comparison of Olympic vs traditional power lifting training programs in football players. *Journal of Strength and Conditioning Research*, 18, 129–35.

Hoffman, J., Ratamess, N., Klatt, M., et al. (2009). Comparison between different off-season resistance training programs in division III American college football players. *Journal of Strength and Conditioning Research*, 23, 11–9.

Hoffman, J.R. and Kang, J. (2003). Strength changes during an in-season resistance training program for football. *Journal of Strength and Conditioning Research*, 17, 109–14.

Hoffman, J.R., Ratamess, N.A., Cooper, J.J., et al. (2005). Comparison of loaded and unloaded jump squat training on strength/power performance in college football players. *Journal of Strength and Conditioning Research*, 19, 810–5.

IPF. (2012). International Powerlifting Federation: Technical Rules Book.

Issurin, V. (2008). Block periodization versus traditional training theory: a review. *Journal of Sports Medicine and Physical Fitness*, 48, 65–75.

Izquierdo, M., Ibanez, J., Gonzalez-Badillo, J.J., et al. (2007). Detraining and tapering effects on hormonal responses and strength performance. *Journal of Strength and Conditioning Research*, 21, 768–75.

Kawamori, N. and Haff, G.G. (2004). The optimal training load for development of muscular power. *Journal of Strength and Conditioning Research*, 18, 675–84.

Lockie, R.G., Murphy, A.J., Schultz, A.B., et al. (2012). The effects of different speed training protocols on sprint acceleration kinematics and muscle strength and power in field sport athletes. *Journal of Strength and Conditioning Research*, 26, 1539–50.

McBride, J. M., Triplett-McBride, T., Davie, A. *et al.* (2002). The effect of heavy vs. light-load jump squats on the development of strength, power, and speed. *Journal of Strength and Conditioning Research*, 16, 75–82.

McGuigan, M. and Winchester, J. (2008). The relationship between isometric and dynamic strength in college football players. *Journal of Sports Science and Medicine*, 7, 101–5.

McGuigan, M.R., Cormack, S., and Newton, R.U. (2009). Long-term power performance of elite Australian rules football players. *Journal of Strength and Conditioning Research*, 23, 26–32.

McLean, B.D., Coutts, A.J., Kelly, V., *et al.* (2010). Neuromuscular, endocrine, and percep-tual fatigue responses during different length between-match microcycles in professional rugby league players. *International Journal of Sports Physiology and Performance*, 5, 367–83.

McMaster, D.T., Gill, N., McGuigan, M., *et al.* (2013a). Force-velocity-power assessment in semi-professional rugby union players. *Journal of Strength and Conditioning Research*, doi: 10.1519/JSC.0b013e3182a1da46

McMaster, D.T., Gill, N., Cronin, J., *et al.* (2013b). The development, retention, and decay rates of strength and power in elite rugby union, rugby league, and American football. *Sports Medicine*, 43, 367–84.

Nibali, M.L., Chapman, D.W., Roberg, R.A., *et al.* (2013). A rationale for assessing the lower-body power profile in team sport athletes. *Journal of Strength and Conditioning Research*, 27, 388–97.

Pain, M.T., Tsui, F., and Cove, S. (2008). In vivo determination of the effect of shoulder pads on tackling forces in rugby. *Journal of Sports Science*, 26, 855–62.

Peterson, M.D., Rhea, M. R., and Alvar, B.A. (2005). Applications of the dose-response for muscular strength development: a review of meta-analytic efficacy and reliability for designing training prescription. *Journal of Strength and Conditioning Research*, 19, 950–8.

Pettitt, R.W. (2010). The standard difference score: a new statistic for evaluating strength and conditioning programs. *Journal of Strength and Conditioning Research*, 24, 287–91.

Preatoni, E., Stokes, K., England, M., *et al.* (2013). The influence of playing level on the bio-mechanical demands experienced by rugby union forwards during machine scrummaging. *Scandinavian Journal of Medicine and Science in Sports*, 23, e178–84.

Prestes, J., De Lima, C., Frollini, A.B., *et al.* (2009). Comparison of linear and reverse linear periodization effects on maximal strength and body composition. *Journal of Strength and Conditioning Research*, 23, 266–74.

Quarrie, K.L., Hopkins, W.G., Anthony, M.J., *et al.* (2013). Positional demands of international rugby union: evaluation of player actions and movements. *Journal of Science and Medicine in Sport*, 16, 353–9.

Quarrie, K.L. and Wilson, B.D. (2000). Force production in the rugby union scrum. *Journal of Sports Science*, 18, 237–46.

Rhea, M. R. and Alderman, B.L. (2004). A meta-analysis of periodized versus nonperiodized strength and power training programs. *Research Quarterly*, 75, 413–22.

Samuel, M.N., Holcomb, W.R., Guadagnoli, M.A., *et al.* (2008). Acute effects of static and ballistic stretching on measures of strength and power. *Journal of Strength and Conditioning Research*, 22, 1422–8.

Sapega, A. and Drillings, G. (1983). The definition and assessment of muscular power. *Journal of Orthopaedic and Sports Physical Therapy*, 5, 7–9.

Stone, M., Sanborn, K., Smith, L., *et al.* (1999). Effects of in-season (5 weeks) creatine and pyruvate supplementation on anaerobic performance and body composition in American football players. *International Journal of Sport Nutrition*, 9, 146–65.

Tan, B. (1999). Manipulating resistance training program variables to optimize maximum strength in men: A review. *Journal of Strength and Conditioning Research*, 13, 289–304.

Twist, C. and Highton, J. (2013). Monitoring fatigue and recovery in rugby league players. *International Journal of Sports Physiology and Performance*, 8, 467–74.

Usman, J., McIntosh, A., and Best, J. (2010). The investigation of shoulder forces in rugby union. *Journal of Science and Medicine in Sport*, 13, 63.

West, D.J., Owen, N.J., Jones, M.R., *et al.* (2011). Relationships between force-time characteristics of the isometric midthigh pull and dynamic performance in professional rugby league players. *Journal of Strength and Conditioning Research*, 25, 3070–5.

Wilson, G.J., Newton, R.U., Murphy, A.J., *et al.* (1993). The optimal training load for the development of dynamic athletic performance. *Medicine and Science in Sport and Exercise*, 25, 1279–86.

3

PERIODIZATION AND PLANNING OF TRAINING FOR RUGBY

Dave Sykes

3.1 Introduction

Periodization involves the division of an entire seasonal programme into smaller periods of training units (Issurin 2010) in order to provide a framework for planned and systematic variation of training (Gamble 2006). A key goal of periodization is to prevent stagnation (Plisk and Stone 2003), but it should also reduce the potential for overtraining, maintain performance throughout a season, and ensure players peak at the appropriate times of the year (Stone *et al.* 1999). Focusing solely on senior elite professional players, this chapter will describe the optimal methods for periodizing rugby training across the year.

Rugby requires the development and maintenance of multiple physical qualities (Chadd 2010) over an extended competitive season (Gamble 2006). Perhaps the most appropriate model is the classical periodization model, which divides the annual year into the following macrocycles: preparation (pre-season), competition (in-season), and transition (off-season; Bompa 1999) (Figure 3.1).

When planning the training programme, several factors need to be considered, such as the perceived importance of matches, difficulty of matches, and the extent of disruption caused by travel (Kelly and Coutts 2007). Therefore, the annual periodized plan should include details of all training camps, along with domestic and international fixtures. International travel to matches, tournaments, and training camps outside of the players' country of residence can be particularly disruptive when transmeridian travel across several time zones is required, resulting in players suffering from 'jet lag' (see Chapter 10). An annual periodized programme should also take into account the technical proficiency and physical maturation of the players in the squad. For example, the physiological, pre-habilitation, and movement proficiency goals for a pre-adolescent with no resistance training background will be very different from those of an experienced senior player.

Month	Sep	Oct	Nov	Dec	Jan	Feb	Mar	Apr	May	Jun	Jul	Aug
Macrocycle	Off-season		Pre-season			In-season						
Mesocycle	Rest / Off-season	Off-season	General prep	Specific prep	Specific prep / Pre-comp	Pre-comp / Early	Early	Mid	Mid	Late	Late / Play-offs	Play-offs
Club fixtures					F F	F L L L	L L L L L	C L L	L L C	L C L L	L L	P P P P
International fixtures	I	I I I										
Match difficulty					3 6	4 9 6 7	9 6 6 3 2	9 8 3	4 7 9	6 9 8 2	4 5 1	9 9 9 9
Travel	2	2 2 2			2 1	0 0 0 2	1 1 0 1 2	1 1 2	1 0 1	0 1 1 0	1 0 1	

FIGURE 3.1 Overview of an example annual periodized plan for a northern hemisphere rugby club playing their domestic season in summer

Note: F = Friendly; L = League; C = Cup; I = International; Match difficulty (1–10; 1 = easiest, 10 = most difficult); Travel (0 = home; 1 = away; 2 = away with substantial travel)

TABLE 3.1 Typical training schedule for a seven-day microcycle during the off-season

Time of day	Day						
	Mon	Tue	Wed	Thu	Fri	Sat	Sun
Morning	Whole body strength endurance gym session	Swimming	Off	Whole body strength endurance gym session	Off	Off	Road Cycling
Afternoon	Off	Off	Off	Field-based interval running session	Off	Off	Off

3.2 Off-season

Whilst traditionally the off-season has been a period of complete rest, this phase is now used to prepare players for the forthcoming pre-season. After an initial two-week break that allows players to have a vacation, low-to-moderate intensity training generally recommences to prevent substantial detraining. At the same time, training should be appreciably different from pre- and in-season to prevent tedium. Whilst it might be argued that a degree of flexibility can aid adherence to training over the off-season, it is perhaps useful for players to have some form of weekly routine. Therefore, a seven-day microcycle is used so that training activities are performed on the same day each week, enabling players to plan social and family commitments around their weekly training schedule. Table 3.1 provides a typical weekly training schedule for a rugby player during the off-season after the initial two-week vacation.

3.2.1 Gym-based training

Given that there are a greater number of muscular strains and joint sprains observed during the pre-season than at other times during the year in sub-elite (Gabbett 2004; Gabbett and Domrow 2007) and elite (Killen et al. 2010) players, training during the off-season should prepare players to reduce this risk of injury. It is well documented that substantial bilateral asymmetries in concentric (Knapik et al. 1991; Orchard et al. 1997) and eccentric (Fousekis et al. 2011) muscular strength place athletes at a greater risk of muscular injuries. Therefore, unilateral exercises (e.g., single-leg squats) should be incorporated into the off-season macrocycle to attenuate asymmetrical imbalances (Table 3.2). Baker and Newton (2004) postulated that large anterior to posterior strength imbalances (e.g., of the shoulder internal and external rotators) could also increase the risk of muscle strains or tendon impingement (e.g., bicep or rotator cuff). Indeed, McDonough and Funk (2013) observed that poor internal shoulder rotation range of movement (which can be caused by anterior to posterior muscular imbalances) was predictive of shoulder injuries in rugby league players. Baker and Newton (2004) suggest rugby players should be capable of lifting similar loads in a chin-up (combined body mass and external load) and flat barbell bench press. It is therefore important to allocate equal time to developing upper body 'pushing' and 'pulling' strength over the off-season to prevent anterior to posterior strength imbalances from developing. Finally, given the high degree of abdominal and trunk muscle activation required during loaded bilateral lower body exercises (e.g., back squats; Hamlyn *et al.* 2007), isometric strength of the trunk and abdominal muscles should be developed during the off-season.

In order to reduce the monotony of training, gym-based training is usually conducted unsupervised, away from the training facility (Gamble 2006), with less emphasis on technically demanding exercises that might require corrective feedback. From personal experience, it is advisable to select exercises that do not heavily feature during the pre- or competitive-season to avoid the tedium of performing the same exercises for extended periods of time. Therefore, whilst deadlifts with submaximal loads could be used as a means for developing isometric core strength during the off-season (Hamlyn *et al.* 2007), isolated isometric exercises under unstable conditions (Anderson and Behm 2005; Vera-Garcia *et al.* 2000) provide an alternative method of achieving the same goal whilst adding exercise variety to the overall annual plan. It is also advisable to select unilateral upper body exercises (e.g., dumbbell shoulder press) or even asymmetrical unilateral upper body exercises (e.g., alternate dumbbell shoulder press; Behm *et al.* 2005). These exercises are extremely effective for developing the shoulder stabilisers (Saeterbakken and Fimland 2013) and produce greater activation of the abdominal and trunk muscles compared to performing the equivalent exercises using a barbell (Saeterbakken and Fimland 2012).

Poor range of movement in the hip and knee flexors and extensors predisposes team sport players to muscular strains (Bradley and Portas 2007). Therefore, it is pertinent to maintain or improve lower body flexibility during the off-season to further reduce the likelihood of soft tissue injuries during the pre-season. Eccentric resistance training through a full range of movement is an effective method of increasing lower

TABLE 3.2 A sample gym programme in week one of the off-season

Day one		Day two	
Exercise	*Sets × Reps*	*Exercise*	*Sets × Reps*
Single-leg squats with band assistance	3 × 10 EL	Single-leg stiff-leg Deadlifts	3 × 10 EL
Single-arm dumbbell row with neutral grip	3 × 10 EA	Chin-ups with wide pronated grip	3 × 10
Seated dumbbell shoulder press (without back support)	3 × 10	Alternate flat dumbbell bench press	3 × 10 EA
Isometric side bridge	3 × 15 s ES	Isometric flat Swiss ball prone bridge	3 × 15 seconds
Swiss ball Supermans	3 × 10		
Standing cable external shoulder rotations	3 × 10 EA	Standing dumbbell front raises	3 × 10

Note: EL = Each leg; ES = Each side; EA = Each arm

limb flexibility (O'Sullivan *et al.* 2012). Whilst eccentrically-biased exercise is likely to cause muscle soreness in the days after training in players who are unaccustomed (Howatson *et al.* 2007), lower training intensities in the off-season are unlikely to have a detrimental impact on subsequent training sessions at this stage of the year.

In order to develop a strength endurance base that enables players to endure repeated mechanical stress in training during pre-season (Chadd 2010), it is recommended that reverse block linear periodization be used (Rhea *et al.* 2003). This approach facilitates a gradual increase in set volume and a corresponding decrease in intensity every three to five microcycles.

3.2.2 Field-based training

The primary goal of field training in the off-season is to maintain aerobic capacity to reduce the likelihood of injuries during the subsequent general preparatory mesocycle (Killen *et al.* 2010). Additionally, aerobic exercise will reduce the extent to which players must restrict calorie intake to prevent excessive increases in body fat over the off-season (Siff 2002). Most practitioners advise players to engage in low impact recreational activities (e.g., road cycling or swimming) over the off-season (Siff 2002). These are generally performed twice per week for 40–60 minutes at 70–80 per cent maximum heart rate. Players might also be advised to perform a short (20–30 minute) low-to-moderate volume field running session per week, as this is more specific to the type of training that will be performed during pre-season. However, this training should be restricted to longer duration (30 s) intervals at or just below maximal aerobic speed with a 1:1 work to rest ratio (Billat *et al.* 2000). Maximal speed, agility, or plyometrics should not be performed during the off-season (Gamble 2006).

3.2.3 Rehabilitation

The off-season enables players requiring minor surgical procedures to address persistent injuries that are not severe enough to prevent them from participating in matches during the competitive season, but ultimately require treatment. Therefore, the later part of the off-season can be used for rehabilitating minor injuries, especially where a period of immobilization is advisable immediately post-operation. Regardless of the injury, the aim of the latter stage of the rehabilitation period should be to integrate players back into full training through gradual linear increases in load-volume. During this period, the player should be closely monitored by the physiotherapist to evaluate how the injury site is responding to increases in training load-volumes and the diversification of activities.

3.2.4 Musculoskeletal screenings

Prior to pre-season training commencing, musculoskeletal screenings should be conducted by the physiotherapist to identify players predisposed to injuries due to movement restrictions (Bradley and Portas 2007). This information allows the design of a pre-habilitation programme that specifically addresses the musculoskeletal issues and informs the appropriate selection of resistance training exercises by the strength and conditioning coach. For example, a player with poor calf flexibility resulting in restricted anterior knee displacement when squatting will be unable to perform a loaded squat without excessive anterior torso lean at the bottom of the movement (Durall and Manske 2005), which substantially increases hip torque and loading of the lower back (Fry *et al.* 2003). The annual periodized programme should be modified for that particular individual (i.e., until their calf flexibility has been improved) to reduce the likelihood of lower back injuries from performing loaded squats (Yule 2007).

3.2.5 Player profiling

Traditionally player profiling has been conducted immediately prior to pre-season to assess players' current physical status and the effectiveness of pre-season training. However, given that at the start of pre-season a number of players might be in the latter stages of injury rehabilitation and that players are more susceptible to injury during early pre-season (Killen *et al.* 2010), maximal tests at this stage of the season should be used cautiously. Additionally, exhaustive testing in-season is impractical due to scheduled fixtures. Coupled with musculoskeletal screenings and body composition evaluations, submaximal assessments at the start of pre-season provide a pragmatic approach that enables longitudinal monitoring of fitness for all players.

3.3 Pre-season

Depending on players' involvement in international fixtures, the pre-season is typically ten to fourteen weeks in duration. This is divided into three sub-phases (known as mesocycles): general preparation, specific preparation, and pre-competition. Each mesocycle is divided into smaller microcycles, which are traditionally seven days in length to reflect a standard calendar week (Issurin 2010). As there are no fixtures during the pre-season, it might be more appropriate for microcycles to be nine days in duration to allow a three peak microcycle (see Figure 3.2). This is conducted cyclically whilst allowing adequate recovery between high load-volume training sessions. Consequently, rest days are not constrained to weekends and the calendar day in which activities are performed will change weekly.

3.3.1 General preparation

General preparation is the first mesocycle within the pre-season macrocycle. This phase is typically three to four weeks in duration and comprises two to three consecutive nine-day microcycles.

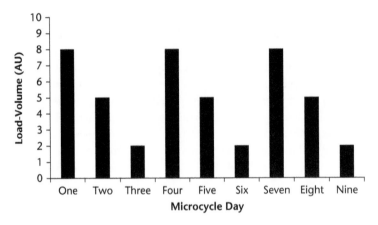

FIGURE 3.2 Load-volume for a nine-day three peak microcycle

3.3.1.1 Resistance training

Rugby is a contact sport where increases in body mass are beneficial for generating momentum in collisions (Baker and Newton 2008; Waldron *et al.* 2014). Moreover, muscular cross-sectional area is highly correlated with maximal strength (Maughan *et al.* 1983). Multi-joint exercises that utilize large muscle groups (e.g. sumo deadlifts, bilateral squats, stiff-leg deadlifts, and chin-ups) should be selected to ensure that an acute anabolic hormonal response is generated (Hansen *et al.* 2001). Compound multi-joint free weights exercises will also allow continued development of isometric core strength by increasing the intensity of abdominal and trunk muscle activation beyond that observed in the isolated isometric core exercises performed during the off-season (Comfort *et al.* 2011; Hamlyn *et al.* 2007; Nuzzo *et al.* 2008). A 1:1 ratio of 'push' to 'pull' upper body exercises should be continued to maintain anterior to posterior muscular balance. Olympic lifts can also be revisited to refine players' technique so that these exercises can be safely and effectively utilized in subsequent phases of the annual programme.

Whilst evidence suggests non-linear periodization is more effective than linear periodization for developing muscular cross-sectional area (Simão *et al.* 2012) and maximal strength (Miranda *et al.* 2011), these findings have yet to be confirmed in elite athletes. Disparities between non-linear periodization models also make comparisons between studies difficult. For example, non-linear periodization could involve daily (Baker 2007), weekly (Apel *et al.* 2011), or bi-weekly (Baker 2007) undulations in intensity and volume. The optimal method of periodization for developing maximal strength and hypertrophy in elite athletes is also unclear (Painter *et al.* 2012). However, on the basis of preliminary findings from studies conducted with recreational athletes, the intensity (as a percentage of maximum for each lift) should be varied across the mesocycle in a non-linear manner (Gamble 2006). From personal observations, a high proportion of rugby teams utilize weekly undulating periodization during pre-season, with no more than 10% variation in

TABLE 3.3 Example gym programmes for the general preparation mesocycle

Session 1a (morning)		Session 1b (afternoon)	
Exercise	*Sets × Reps*	*Exercise*	*Sets × Reps*
Clean first pull	3 × 8	Overhead squats	3 × 8
Incline dumbbell bench press	3 × 8	Scoop Romanian deadlift	3 × 8
Chin-ups with pronated grip	3 × 8	Flat dumbbell chest fly	3 × 8
		Barbell rollouts	3 × 8

Session 2		Session 3	
Exercise	*Sets × Reps*	*Exercise*	*Sets × Reps*
Front squat	3 × 8	Hang shrug with snatch grip	3 × 8
Stiff-leg deadlifts	3 × 8	Sumo deadlift	3 × 8
Bent-over barbell row	3 × 8	Eccentric Nordic curls	3 × 8
Upright row	3 × 8	Decline barbell bench press	3 × 8
Seated dumbbell shoulder press (with back support)	3 × 8	Chin-ups with supinated grip	3 × 8
Flat isometric side bridge	3 × 20 s ES	External dumbbell rotations	3 × 8 EA

Note: ES = Each side; EA = Each arm

intensity within each mesocycle. During the general preparation phase loads of 75–85% 1RM should therefore be selected in a non-linear fashion to elicit a hypertrophic response (Wernbom *et al.* 2007).

Based on whole body workouts, it is recommended that resistance training be conducted two to three times per week for optimal muscular hypertrophy (Wernbom *et al.* 2007). Therefore, four gym sessions spread over three days have been included in the example nine-day microcycle (Table 3.3). Resistance training should be scheduled prior to field-based training (Table 3.4) to maximise hypertrophic gains during this phase (Gotto *et al.* 2005).

3.3.1.2 Field-based training

A 3:1 step-loading paradigm incorporating a subtle linear increase in load-volume for three consecutive microcycles prior to an unloading microcycle (Turner 2011) should be used throughout the pre-season phase. This reduces the likelihood of injuries from sudden increases in training load-volumes or cumulative fatigue. In addition to performing skill-based training, one session per microcycle should be dedicated to rugby-specific endurance. During this mesocycle there should be a steady shift towards shorter (10–15 s) intervals up to 120% of maximal aerobic speed with a 1:1 work-to-rest ratio (Dupont *et al.* 2002, 2004). In addition, time should be allocated during skill-based sessions to practice tackle, hit-up, and ball-steal techniques. At this stage of the season the emphasis is primarily on developing

TABLE 3.4 A typical schedule for a nine-day microcycle during the general and specific preparation mesocycles

Time of day	Day								
	One	Two	Three	Four	Five	Six	Seven	Eight	Nine
Morning	Whole body gym session	Skill-based field session (contact drills)	Off	Whole body gym session	Skill-based field session (handling drills)	Off	Whole body gym session	Skill-based field session	Off
Afternoon	Whole body gym session	Off	Off	Field-based conditioning session	Off	Off	Field-based conditioning session*	Off	Off

* Only performed during specific preparation mesocycle

the skill, so contact drills are performed separately from conditioning-based running drills (Gabbett 2008). Warm-ups can also be used to re-introduce low intensity plyometric exercises and refine linear sprinting technique through technique drills and submaximal sprint efforts (Wathen *et al.* 2000).

3.3.2 Specific preparation

Depending on the length of the playing season and number of pre-season friendlies arranged, the specific preparation mesocycle is generally six to eight weeks in duration.

3.3.2.1 Resistance training

Muscle power (specifically strength-speed) is known to discriminate between professional and semi-professional rugby union (Argus *et al.* 2012) and rugby league (Baker and Newton 2008) players. Additionally, peak power during ballistic exercises with heavier loads is highly correlated to maximal strength (Baker and Nance 1999; Baker 2001). Therefore, it is important to develop both of these qualities during the pre-season, incorporating ballistic exercises (e.g. jump squats, bench throws; Baker 2001), Olympic lifts (Hori *et al.* 2005), and powerlifting exercises with bands (Wallace *et al.* 2006) or chains (Baker and Newton 2009) into the programme. In addition, bilateral multi-joint exercises (e.g. back squat, stiff-leg deadlift, and barbell bench press; Fleck and Kraemer 1997) should be performed on stable surfaces to maximise peak force and rate of force development (McBride *et al.* 2006) and hence augment the necessary neural adaptations required for the development of maximal strength.

Weekly undulating periodization should be used to vary training loads for strength-orientated exercises. However, during the specific preparation phase loads of >85% 1RM should be utilized in order to emphasise maximal strength development rather than hypertrophy (Campos *et al.* 2002). Maximal strength and power training is likely to be more effective when performed prior to field-based training (Leveritt and Abernethy 1999) and neuromuscular adaptations might be greater when conducted in the morning (Sedliak *et al.* 2009). Therefore, scheduling resistance training in the morning prior to field-based training in the afternoon could result in improved adaptations. Utilizing split-day routines also appears to be more effective than one session for developing maximal strength (Häkkinen and Kallinen 1994). However, when both power and strength exercises are performed during the same training session, power-orientated exercises should be performed prior to maximal strength exercises (Table 3.5).

3.3.2.2 Field-based training

At this stage of the pre-season, training shifts towards activities that closely replicate the demands of competitive matches. Although Plisk and Gambetta (1997) suggest conditioning drills should be modelled upon competitive match demands, activities

TABLE 3.5 An example resistance programme during the specific preparation mesocycle

Exercise	Set × Reps	Intensity (%1RM)
Hang power cleans[P]	4 × 4	90
Back squat[S]	4 × 4	90
Wide grip chin-ups with pronated grip[S]	4 × 4	90
Flat barbell bench press[S]	4 × 4	90

P = power-orientated exercise; S = strength-orientated exercise

that are based on average match data from the entire game are unlikely to adequately prepare players for the most intensive periods of match-play (Austin *et al.* 2011a, b). Therefore, conditioning drills should replicate the most intense high intensity effort bout observed in a match (Austin *et al.* 2011a, b) or the most demanding five-minute period of a match (Di Mascio and Bradley 2013). Incorporating contact into drills will also better reflect the demands of competitive matches (Gabbett *et al.* 2012; Johnston *et al.* 2014). Throughout the mesocycle there should also be a shift towards full contact conditioning games as these replicate the locomotive and contact demands of competitive rugby league matches (Gabbett *et al.* 2012) and offer the benefit of practicing technical skills under fatigue and developing decision making and communication skills (Gamble 2004; 2006). A comprehensive overview of conditioning for rugby can be found in Chapter 1.

3.3.3 Pre-competition

As the season approaches focus shifts towards tactical awareness with a greater number of team practice sessions to prepare players for the forthcoming fixtures (Hedrick 2002). Accordingly, coaches will normally arrange two to three non-competitive matches seven days apart to allow them to experiment with team formations and tactics. Consequently, the specific preparation mesocycle consists of two to three seven-day microcycles based on the turnaround between matches. Essentially this short mesocycle provides an opportunity to establish a training routine for the season.

3.4 In-season

Whilst Taplin (2005) advocates breaking the competitive season into early, mid, and late competition mesocycles, it seems logical to include a fourth mesocycle encompassing the play-offs and major finals. As a result, each mesocycle comprises five to eight microcycles, with the length of each microcycle dependent on the turnaround between matches. In-season, coaches must balance adequate recovery with physically demanding training to avoid residual fatigue that has a negative effect on match performance (Gamble 2006). Therefore, high load-volume training sessions should be conducted in the middle of the week and training load-volumes tapered

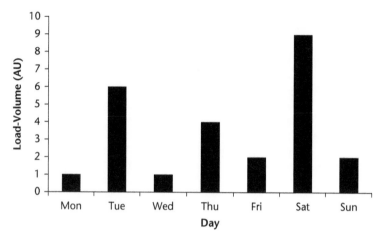

FIGURE 3.3   Load-volume of field sessions throughout a seven-day microcycle with games on consecutive Saturdays

towards the end of the week to avoid residual fatigue ahead of the preceding game (Figure 3.3).

Additional time must be allocated to tactical preparation ahead of matches and correction of rugby-specific technical skills (Baker 1998). For professional players, additional time should be allocated to conduct media interviews, support community projects, and attend commercial, sponsorship, and fund raising activities.

3.4.1 Resistance training

Given that the competitive rugby season is 20–30 weeks in duration, coupled with the increased focus on technical skill and recovery, strategies to maintain maximal strength and power in-season are important. Although complex training is a popular method of training maximal strength and power simultaneously (Young *et al.* 1998), logistics dictate that it is very difficult to utilize this training modality with large squads (Jeffreys 2008). In particular, the optimal rest between exercises is highly dependent on the intensity of the pre-load exercise and exercise selected (Baker 2003; Kilduff *et al.* 2007), whilst responses will also vary greatly between individuals (Comyns *et al.* 2006). An alternative approach is to utilize concurrent training whereby players perform resistance training twice per week. The first workout early in the week emphasises maximal strength/hypertrophy maintenance (Table 3.6), and a second session two to three days later emphasises power development (Baker 1998).

Baker (2007) advocates the use of wave-like periodization that involves linear weekly increases in intensity (as a percentage of 1RM) for three to four weeks. This pattern is then repeated over a similar time frame but at a slightly higher starting intensity (Figure 3.4). Increases in intensity occur irrespective of intensity and

TABLE 3.6 A typical schedule for a seven-day microcycle during the competition macrocycle

Time of day	Day						
	Mon	Tue	Wed	Thu	Fri	Sat	Sun
Morning	Off	Max strength/ hypertrophy maintenance	Off	Power maintenance	Pre-match video	Travel	Injury assessment/ recovery session
Afternoon	Off	Conditioning-based field session	Off	Skill-based field session	Tactical field session	Match	Post-match video

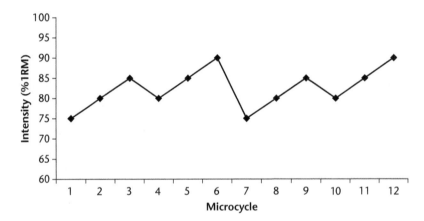

FIGURE 3.4 Intensity of resistance exercises throughout two consecutive mesocycles (each consisting of six microcycles) for maximal strength exercises

volume, being manipulated in a non-linear manner within the week due to maximal strength and power training being conducted on separate days (Baker 2007). Moreover, Baker (1998) promotes an active recovery week after every two consecutive six-week mesocycles in-season, which would result in a recovery week subsequent to the late competition mesocycle. Baker (2001) observed that maximal upper body strength and maximal upper and lower body power could be maintained across a competitive 29-week season using this approach.

3.4.2 Field-based training

Together with the stimulus of regular matches, one conditioning-based training session per week appears adequate for maintaining fitness at a level similar to the end of pre-season (Mohr and Krustrup 2014). Given that a decline in fitness has been observed from the middle to the end of the season in team sports (Mohr and Krustrup 2014), it is important to maintain field-based conditioning even towards the end of the competition macrocycle. When a reduction in fitness occurs towards the end of the season, it is likely because of teams 'over-tapering', leading to matches of greater importance. Whilst there will be large inter-individual differences in the rate and magnitude of recovery after matches (see Chapter 5), typically players will take two to three days to recover post-match (McLean *et al.* 2010). Therefore, in order to allow recovery from the previous game and reduce residual fatigue leading into the subsequent match, it is recommended that the field conditioning session should be performed towards the middle of the microcycle, with at least two days of recovery from the previous match and three days of recovery prior to the next match. This not only means reducing the distance covered during training sessions (particularly at high speeds), but also having a concomitant reduction in the number and intensity of contacts given their propensity to increase muscle damage and soreness (Twist *et al.* 2012). Field sessions the day before matches (which are typically limited to technical content) should ideally be kept to about 30–40 minutes and should include lower running speeds and should be unopposed or against passive opponents.

Additional match-related conditioning might be necessary to maintain 'match fitness' in those individuals who are not regularly selected. To replicate match demands as closely as possible, training should be moderate to high load-volume and movement specific and, where possible, involve decision making. Therefore, when there is a large number of players who do not participate in a competitive match, conditioning games might be the most effective conditioning modality (Gamble 2004). However, when training numbers are small, game-related circuits (e.g. Singh *et al.* 2010) and field-based match simulation protocols (e.g. Roberts *et al.* 2010; Sykes *et al.* 2013) provide a useful means of replicating the demands of competitive games.

3.5 Conclusion

The annual periodized plan for rugby should be divided into three broad macrocycles: off-season, pre-season, and in-season. The off-season provides a mental break from the monotony of organized training, prevents substantial detraining, and prepares players for the forthcoming pre-season. The pre-season emphasizes physical development with a gradual shift from general to sport-specific field conditioning and from hypertrophy to maximal strength and power training. Consequently, the pre-season is divided into general, specific, and pre-competition mesocycles to reflect the shift in emphasis as the competitive season approaches. Given the prolonged duration, coupled with the increased focus on technical skill and recovery, the in-season is about maintenance (rather than development) of physical qualities. The annual periodized plan should provide a progressive and systematic guideline for training that enables the player to perform optimally on a week-to-week basis. However, individual training programmes should be adaptable to account for minor injuries that prevent a player from performing certain exercises or due to individual responses to training or matches. Matches can also be rescheduled due to adverse weather conditions or at the request of television networks. Therefore, it is important for practitioners to be flexible despite working to a predetermined annual plan.

References

Anderson, K. and Behm, D.G. (2005). Trunk muscle activity increases with unstable squat movements. *Canadian Journal of Applied Physiology*, 30, 33–45.

Apel, J.M., Lacey, R.M., and Kell, R.T. (2011). A comparison of traditional and weekly undulating periodized strength training programs with total volume and intensity equated. *Journal of Strength and Conditioning Research*, 25, 694–703.

Argus, C.K., Gill, N.D., and Keogh, J.W. (2012). Characterization of the differences in strength and power between different levels in competition in rugby union athletes. *Journal of Strength and Conditioning Research*, 26, 2698–704.

Austin, D., Gabbett, T., and Jenkins, D. (2011a). Repeated high-intensity exercise in professional rugby union. *Journal of Sports Sciences*, 29, 1105–12.

Austin, D.J., Gabbett, T.J., and Jenkins, D.J. (2011b). Repeated high-intensity exercise in professional rugby union. *Journal of Strength and Conditioning Research*, 25, 1898–904.

Baker, D. (1998). Applying the in-season periodization of strength and power training to football. *Strength and Conditioning*, 20, 18–24.

Baker, D. (2001). The effects of an in-season of concurrent training on the maintenance of maximal strength and power in professional and college-aged rugby league football players. *Journal of Strength and Conditioning Research*, 15, 172–7.

Baker, D. (2003). Acute effect of alternating heavy and light resistances on power output during upper-body complex power training. *Journal of Strength and Conditioning Research*, 17, 493–7.

Baker, D. (2007). Cycle-length variants in periodized strength/power training. *Strength and Conditioning Journal*, 29, 10–7.

Baker, D. and Nance, S. (1999). The relation between strength and power in professional rugby league players. *Journal of Strength and Conditioning Research*, 13, 224–9.

Baker, D. and Newton, R.U. (2004). An analysis of the ratio and relationship between upper body pressing and pulling strength. *Journal of Strength and Conditioning Research*, 18, 594–8.

Baker, D. and Newton, R.U. (2008). Comparison of lower body strength, power, acceleration, speed, agility, and sprint momentum to describe and compare playing rank among professional rugby league players. *Journal of Strength and Conditioning Research*, 22, 153–8.

Baker, D.G. and Newton, R.U. (2009). Effect of kinetically altering a repetition via the use of a chain resistance on velocity during the bench press. *Journal of Strength and Conditioning Research*, 23, 1941–6.

Behm, D.G., Leonard, A.M., Young, W.B., et al. (2005). Trunk muscle electromyographic activity with unstable and unilateral exercises. *Journal of Strength and Conditioning Research*, 19, 193–201.

Billat, V., Slawinski, J., Bocquet, V., et al. (2000). Intermittent runs at the velocity associated with maximal oxygen uptake enables subjects to remain at maximal oxygen uptake for a longer time than intense but submaximal runs. *European Journal of Applied Physiology*, 81, 188–96.

Bompa, T. (1999). *Theory and methodology of training*, 4th ed. Champaign, IL: Human Kinetics.

Bradley, P.S. and Portas, M.D. (2007). The relationship between preseason range of motion and muscle strain injury in elite soccer players. *Journal of Strength and Conditioning Research*, 21, 1155–9.

Campos, G.E.R., Luecke, T.J., Wendeln, H.K., *et al.* (2002). Muscular adaptations in response to three different resistance-training regimens: specificity of repetition maximum training zones. *European Journal of Applied Physiology*, 88, 50–60.

Chadd, N. (2010). An approach to the periodization of training during the in-season for team sports. *Professional Strength and Conditioning*, 18, 5–10.

Comfort, P., Pearson, S.J., and Mather, D. (2011). An electromyographical comparison of trunk muscle activity during isometric trunk and dynamic strengthening exercises. *Journal of Strength and Conditioning Research*, 25, 149–54.

Comyns, T.M., Harrison, A.J., Hennessy, L.K., *et al.* (2006). The optimal complex training rest interval for athletes from anaerobic sports. *Journal of Strength and Conditioning Research*, 20, 471–6.

Di Mascio, M. and Bradley, P.S. (2013). Evaluation of the most intense high-intensity running period in English FA premier league soccer matches. *Journal of Strength and Conditioning Research*, 27, 909–15.

Dupont, G., Blondel, N., Lensel, G., *et al.* (2002). Critical velocity and time spent at a high level of VO_2 for short intermittent runs at supramaximal velocities. *Canadian Journal of Applied Physiology*, 27, 103–15.

Dupont, G., Akakpo, K., and Berthoin, S. (2004). The effect of in-season, high intensity interval training in soccer players. *Journal of Strength and Conditioning Research*, 18, 584–9.

Durall, C.J. and Manske, R.C. (2005). Avoiding lumbar spine injury during resistance training. *Strength and Conditioning Journal*, 27, 64–72.

Fleck, S.J. and Kraemer, W.J. (1997). *Designing resistance training programs*, 2nd ed, Champaign, IL: Human Kinetics.

Fousekis, K., Tsepis, E., Poulmedis, P., *et al.* (2011). Intrinsic risk factors of non-contact quadriceps and hamstring strains in soccer: a prospective study of 100 professional players, *British Journal of Sports Medicine*; 45: 709–14.

Fry, A.C., Smith, C., and Schilling, B.K. (2003). Effect of knee position on hip and knee torques during the barbell squat. *Journal of Strength and Conditioning Research*, 17, 629–33.

Gabbett, T.J. (2004). Influence of training and match intensity on injuries in rugby league. *Journal of Sports Sciences*, 22, 409–17.

Gabbett, T.J. (2008). Influence of fatigue on tackling technique in rugby league players. *Journal of Strength and Conditioning Research*, 22, 625–32.

Gabbett, T.J. and Domrow, N. (2007). Relationships between training load, injury, and fitness in sub-elite collision sport athletes. *Journal of Sports Sciences*, 25, 1507–19.

Gabbett, T.J., Jenkins, D.G., and Abernethy, B. (2012). Physical demands of professional rugby league training and competition using microtechnology. *Journal Science and Medicine in Sport*, 15, 80–6.

Gamble, P. (2004). A skill-based conditioning games approach to metabolic conditioning for elite rugby football players, *Journal of Strength and Conditioning Research*, 18, 491–7.

Gamble, P. (2006). Periodization of training for team sports athletes. *Strength and Conditioning Journal*, 28, 56–66.

Gotto, K., Higashiyama, M., Ishii, N., *et al.* (2005). Prior endurance exercises attenuates growth hormone response to subsequent resistance exercise. *European Journal of Applied Physiology*, 94, 333–8.

Häkkinen, K. and Kallinen, M. (1994). Distribution of strength training volume into one or two daily sessions and neuromuscular adaptations in female athletes. *Electromyography and Clinical Neurophysiology*, 34, 117–24.

Hamlyn, N., Behm, D.G., and Young, W.B. (2007). Trunk muscle activation during dynamic weight-training exercises and isometric instability activities. *Journal of Strength and Conditioning Research*, 21, 1108–12.

Hansen, S., Kvorning, T., Kjaer, M., *et al.* (2001). The effect of short-term strength training on human skeletal muscle: the importance of physiologically elevated hormone levels. *Scandinavian Journal of Medicine and Science in Sports*, 11, 347–54.

Hedrick, A. (2002). Designing effective resistance training programs. *Strength and Conditioning Journal*, 24, 7–15.

Hori, N., Newton, R.U., Nosaka, K., *et al.* (2005). Weightlifting exercises enhance athletic performance that requires high-load speed-strength. *Strength and Conditioning Journal*, 27, 50–5.

Howatson, G., van Someren, K.A., and Hortobágyi, T. (2007). Repeated bout effect after maximal eccentric exercise. *International Journal of Sports Medicine*, 28, 557–63.

Issurin, V.B. (2010). New horizons for the methodology and physiology of training periodization. *Sports Medicine*, 40, 189–206.

Jeffreys, I. (2008). A review of post activation potentiation and its application in strength and conditioning. *Professional Strength and Conditioning*, 12, 17–25.

Johnston, R.D., Gabbett, T.J., Seibold, A.J., *et al.* (2014). Influence of physical contact on pacing strategies during game-based activities. *International Journal of Sports Physiology and Performance*, 9, 811–6.

Kelly, V.G. and Coutts, A.J. (2007). Planning and monitoring training loads during the competition phase in team sports. *Strength and Conditioning Journal*, 29, 32–7.

Kilduff, L.P., Bevan, H., Owen, N., *et al.* (2007). Optimal loading for peak power output during the hang power clean in professional rugby players. *International Journal of Sports Physiology and Performance*, 2, 260–9.

Killen, N.M., Gabbett, T.J., and Jenkins, D.G. (2010). Training loads and incidence of injury during the preseason in professional rugby league players. *Journal of Strength and Conditioning Research*, 24, 2079–84.

Knapik, J.J., Bauman, C.L., Jones, B.H., *et al.* (1991). Preseason strength and flexibility imbalances associated with athletic injuries in female collegiate athletes. *American Journal of Sports Medicine*, 19, 76–81.

Leveritt, M. and Abernethy, P.J. (1999). Acute effects of high-intensity endurance exercise on subsequent resistance activity. *Journal of Strength and Conditioning Research*, 13, 47–51.

Maughan, R.J., Watson, J.S., and Weir, J. (1983). Strength and cross-sectional area of human skeletal muscle. *Journal of Physiology*, 338, 37–49.

McBride, J.M., Cormie, P., and Deane, R. (2006). Isometric squat force output and muscle activity in stable and unstable conditions. *Journal of Strength and Conditioning Research*, 20, 915–8.

McDonough, A. and Funk, L. (2013). Can glenohumeral joint isokinetic strength and range of movement predict injury in professional rugby league? *Physical Therapy in Sport*, 15, 91–6.

McLean, B.D., Coutts, A.J., Kelly, V., *et al.* (2010). Neuromuscular, endocrine, and perceptual fatigue responses during different length between-match microcycles in professional rugby league players. *International Journal of Sports Physiology and Performance*, 5, 367–83.

Miranda, F., Simão, R., Rhea, M., *et al.* (2011). Effects of linear vs. daily undulatory periodized resistance training on maximal and submaximal strength gains. *Journal of Strength and Conditioning Research*, 25, 1824–30.

Mohr, M. and Krustrup, P. (2014). Yo-Yo intermittent recovery test performances within an entire football league during a full season. *Journal of Sports Sciences*, 32, 315–27.

Nuzzo, J.I., McCaulley, G.O., Cormie, P., *et al.* (2008). Trunk muscle activity during stability ball and free weight exercises, *Journal of Strength and Conditioning Research*, 22, 95–102.

Orchard, J., Marsden, J., Lord, S., *et al.* (1997). Preseason hamstring muscle weakness associated with hamstring muscle injury in Australian footballers. *American Journal of Sports Medicine*, 25, 81–5.

O'Sullivan, K., McAuliffe, S., and DeBurca, N. (2012). The effects of eccentric training on lower limb flexibility: a systematic review. *British Journal of Sports Medicine*, 46, 838–45.

Painter, K.B., Haff, G.G., Ramsey, M.W., *et al.* (2012). Strength gains: block versus daily undulating periodization weight training among track and field athletes. *International Journal of Sports Physiology and Performance*, 7, 161–9.

Plisk, S.S. and Gambetta, V. (1997). Tactical metabolic training: Part 1. *Strength and Conditioning Journal*, 19, 44–53.

Plisk, S.S. and Stone, M.H. (2003). Periodization strategies. *Strength and Conditioning Journal*, 25, 19–37.

Rhea, M.R., Phillips, W.T., Burkett, L.N., *et al.* (2003). A comparison of linear and daily undulating periodized programs with equated volume and intensity for local muscular endurance. *Journal of Strength and Conditioning Research*, 17, 82–7.

Roberts, S.P., Stokes, K.A., Weston, L., *et al.* (2010). The Bath University rugby shuttle test (BURST): a pilot study. *International Journal of Sports Physiology and Performance*, 5, 64–74.

Saeterbakken, A.H. and Fimland, M.S. (2012). Muscle activity of the core during bilateral, unilateral, seated, and standing resistance exercise. *European Journal of Applied Physiology*, 24, 1671–8.

Saeterbakken, A.H. and Fimland, M.S. (2013). Effects of body position and loading modality on muscle activity and strength in shoulder presses. *Journal of Strength and Conditioning Research*, 27, 1824–31.

Sedliak, M., Finni T., Cheng, S., *et al.* (2009). Effect of time-of-day specific strength training on muscular hypertrophy in men. *Journal of Strength and Conditioning Research*, 23, 2451–7.

Siff, M.C. (2002). Functional training revisited. *Strength and Conditioning Journal*, 24, 495–504.

Simão, R., Spineti J., De Salles, B.F., *et al.* (2012). Comparison between nonlinear and linear periodized resistance training: hypertrophic and strength effects. *Journal of Strength and Conditioning Research*, 26, 1389–95.

Singh, T.K.R., Guelfi, K.J., Landers, G., *et al.* (2010). Reliability of a contact and non-contact simulated team game circuit. *Journal of Sports Science and Medicine*, 9, 638–42.

Stone, M.H., O'Bryant, H.S., Schilling, B.K., *et al.* (1999). Periodization: effects of manipulating volume and intensity. Part 1. *Strength and Conditioning Journal*, 21, 56–62.

Sykes, D., Nicholas, C., Lamb, K., *et al.* (2013). An evaluation of the external validity and reliability of a rugby league match simulation protocol. *Journal of Sports Sciences*, 31, 48–57.

Taplin, I. (2005). *The RFU guide for coaches: Fitness and conditioning*, London: A and C Black Publishers Ltd.

Turner, A. (2011). The science and practice of periodization: a brief review. *Strength and Conditioning Journal*, 33, 34–46.

Twist, C., Waldron, M., Highton, J., *et al.* (2012). Neuromuscular, biochemical, and perceptual post-match fatigue in professional rugby league forwards and backs. *Journal of Sports Sciences*, 30, 359–67.

Vera-Garcia, F.S., Grenier, F.S., and McGill, S. (2000). Abdominal muscle response during curl-ups on both stable and labile surfaces. *Physical Therapy*, 80, 564–9.

Wallace, B.J., Winchester, J.B., and McGuigan, M.R. (2006). Effects of elastic bands on force and power characteristics during the back squat. *Journal of Strength and Conditioning Research*, 20, 268–72.

Waldron, M., Worsfold, P.R., Twist, C., *et al.* (2014). The relationship between physical abilities, ball-carrying, and tackling among elite youth rugby league players. *Journal of Sports Sciences*, 32, 542–9.

Wathen, D., Baechle, T.R., and Earle, R.W. (2000). Training variation: Periodization, in Baechle T.R. and Earle R. W. (ed), *Essentials of strength training and conditioning*, Champaign, IL: Human Kinetics.

Wernbom, M., Augustsson, J., and Thomeé, R. (2007). The influence of frequency, intensity, volume and mode of strength training on whole muscle cross-sectional area in humans. *Sports Medicine*, 37, 225–63.

Young, W.B., Jenner, A., and Griffiths, K. (1998). Acute enhancement of power performance from heavy load squats. *Journal of Strength and Conditioning Research*, 12, 82–4.

Yule, S. (2007). The back squat. *Professional Strength and Conditioning*, 8, 20–3.

4

MONITORING THE MATCH AND TRAINING DEMANDS OF RUGBY

Mark Waldron, Paul Worsfold, and Craig Twist

4.1 Introduction

Quantification of both internal and external load enables rugby practitioners to modify the demands of training in accordance with their periodized programmes. In addition, load measurements enable prescription of exercise thresholds in relation to injury prevalence and avoidance (Gabbett 2004a, b). Heart rate (HR) and rating of perceived exertion (RPE) have prevailed for monitoring internal training load in the field, owing to their low cost, and practicality. Such methods include session-RPE (s-RPE; Foster *et al.* 2001) and the summated HR method (Edwards 1993), which are now commonplace in rugby research and applied practice. The introduction of video and Global Positioning Systems (GPS) in elite team sport has also advanced our understanding of training load, turning attention to the external demands of rugby players. It is the aim of this chapter to provide critical review of such methods, with reference to their relationship with training practices in rugby league and union.

4.2 Monitoring the external demands of training and competition in rugby

The temporal running patterns of rugby match-play are intermittent in nature, whereby clustered periods of repeated maximal exertions, such as tackling, accelerating, and sprinting, separate prolonged periods of low intensity activity (Austin *et al.* 2011b; Gabbett *et al.* 2012b). Rugby is also a 'collision sport', which describes the coming together of players from opposing sides either as the 'tackling' or the 'tackled' counterpart. Such demands place stress on both aerobic and anaerobic metabolism (Coutts *et al.* 2003) as well as increasing the risk of muscle damage and injury (Twist *et al.* 2012). Accordingly, to better prepare players for competition, it has become increasingly important to understand the external demands of the training and match environment.

4.2.1 The use of time–motion analysis in rugby

Manual time–motion analysis (TMA) requires visual interpretation of the player's gait pattern, sub-categorized into incremental movement classifications of: standing, walking, jogging, striding, sprinting, and backward and lateral movements (McLean 1992; Deutsch *et al.* 2007; King *et al.* 2009; Austin *et al.* 2011a, b). The player's movement is then manually timed, with speed (and thus distance) estimated based upon pre-determined values associated with each movement classification (see Reilly and Thomas 1976). Alternatively, the distance of the player can be estimated based on their movement between pre-identified visual cues around the pitch-side and timed with a stopwatch (with speed=distance/time). Quantifying movement can be incorporated into conditioning practices, enabling rugby coaches to prepare players for the external demands that they are likely to experience in a match. Whilst such methods are cost effective and can be reliably administered (Krustrup and Bangsbo 2001), they are labour-intensive for the user and generate relatively simplistic data.

4.2.2 The use of multiple camera systems in rugby

Semi-automated computerised tracking of players has become a preferred approach to the capture of time–motion characteristics in rugby. Semi-automated tracking uses visual image recognition software to identify features unique to an individual (Carling *et al.* 2008; Di Salvo *et al.* 2007). Examples of such features might be colour, shape, or size of the participant (Carling *et al.* 2008). Cameras are situated in specific areas around the perimeter of the playing surface and synchronously digitized in order to calculate the distance and speed of players' movements. The use of such systems is apparent only within elite sporting contexts, largely owing to their high cost and logistical impracticality, therefore limiting their use in training scenarios.

Multiple camera systems, such as Prozone, are thought to provide a valid measurement of distance and speed in team sport, with reports of only 0.4% error in comparison to running speeds assessed via timing gates (Bradley *et al.* 2007; Di Salvo *et al.* 2006). However, Randers *et al.* (2010) reported disparity between GPS (5 Hz and 1 Hz) and a multiple camera system, with coefficient of variation (CV) values ranging from 7–12% for total distance covered during the match. Interestingly, there were large differences between systems with regards to distance covered in separate locomotive categories. For example, the multiple camera systems recorded a greater distance in high intensity running compared to the GPS (5 Hz) by 0.63 km and the manual gait TMA by 0.81 km. Such findings prohibit comparisons between studies using different modes of TMA.

Figueroa *et al.* (2006) highlighted issues with lighting of the playing surface and sharp changes in motion velocity, which cause difficulty in using multiple camera systems in sports where players maintain close proximity (i.e. collisions). Consequently, such systems require frequent (3–42% of the time) human intervention to reconfigure the tracking of players (Di Salvo *et al.* 2009). Whilst the limitations of multiple camera systems should be recognised, the sampling rate of 7.5 to 25 Hz (with the option to increase) remains far superior to alternative measures of TMA. This has important implications for the recognition of accelerations/decelerations in team sport that impose a large metabolic demand on players (Osgnach *et al.* 2010).

Sykes and colleagues were the first to use multiple camera systems to monitor movement demands (Sykes *et al.* 2009) and to show signs of fatigue via variations in the running performance of rugby players across progressive match periods (Sykes *et al.* 2011). In rugby union, multiple camera systems have been used to quantify differences in the match running patterns of positional groups (Roberts *et al.* 2008; Lacome *et al.* 2014). Lacome *et al.* (2014) reported ~ 65% of exercise periods during the match lasted <4 s, ~40% of which were classified as medium intensity. Periods of high-intensity static activity or sprints were interspersed with exercise and recovery periods that varied in intensity and duration, meaning there was no change between the first and second half. Roberts and colleagues reaffirmed these findings, as well as the findings of Duthie *et al.* (2005) that distance covered and high-intensity running remained unchanged between the first and second half of matches. Such findings are at odds with those of other team sports, where a decline in running distance is observed in the late periods of a match (Mohr *et al.* 2003; Sykes *et al.* 2011) and are believed to relate to 'static' exertions that characterise rugby performance. Indeed, static exertions, such as rucking, scrummaging, and mauling in rugby union and collisions in rugby league comprise a substantial part of rugby match-play and come with an increased metabolic cost (Johnston and Gabbett 2011), yet are not reflected by external movement demand. The metabolic and mechanical stresses imposed by periods of static exertion and collisions are still poorly understood and further research in this area would be useful to enhance rugby practice.

4.2.3 The use of global positioning systems (GPS) devices in rugby

The use of portable GPS devices in team sports is now common practice (for detailed reviews see: Aughey 2011; Cummins *et al.* 2013). Portable GPS devices are fitted to the player within a custom harness/vest, positioning the receiver in the region of the thoracic spine. A portable GPS system functions using twenty-seven satellites that orbit around the earth. The GPS device is programmed to receive a radio signal, emitted from an orbiting satellite at the speed of light (Larsson 2003). An atomic clock is fitted within each orbiting satellite and time-matched to a clock held within the portable receiver. The time taken for the signal to travel between each instrument can subsequently be determined. The product of the known speed of the signal and the lag in time between the two synchronized clocks determines the distance travelled between the satellite and the receiver. So called 'pseudo-ranges/distances' can be projected spherically from the connecting satellite, placing the receiver within an encapsulated radius. Using further satellites in concert (a minimum of four), the exact position and subsequent navigation of an object on the earth's surface can be established. The intersection between the projected spherical surfaces, combined with logical assumption that the receiver is positioned on the earth's surface, provides an indication of the position on earth.

Using GPS devices to monitor rugby players during competition have helped to better inform training practices. Indeed, the performance of players during training can be monitored using the same GPS devices used during competition – a capability that is not permitted when using multiple camera systems. Gabbett *et al.* (2012b) reported the disparities in distance covered, and repeated high intensity efforts performed during typical training sessions when compared to matches. Furthermore, whilst traditional aerobic conditioning (i.e. interval or continuous running without the ball) induced higher relative distances, there were few instances of repeated maximal efforts and no collisions recorded. These data help question the specificity and, in turn, the appropriateness of training and conditioning practices designed to stress the appropriate metabolic pathways and to reproduce the kinematic patterns observed during match-play.

4.2.3.1 Validity and reliability of measurements using GPS

Whilst GPS systems are valid (i.e. <5.5% overestimation) when measuring linear distances at slow movement velocities (Jennings *et al.* 2010; Portas *et al.* 2010), accuracy is reduced as movement velocity increases (Jennings *et al.* 2010; Waldron *et al.* 2011a). GPS systems also provide an acceptable assessment of the total distance covered over prolonged multidirectional circuits that replicate the movements encountered during rugby (Jennings *et al.* 2010; Portas *et al.* 2010; Coutts and Duffield 2010). The measurement accuracy of 1, 5, and 10 Hz GPS systems is improved as discrete distances increase during jogging, striding, and sprinting (Jennings *et al.* 2010; Waldron *et al.* 2011a; Varley *et al.* 2012). GPS devices with higher sampling frequencies are also more accurate than those operating at 1 Hz (Jennings *et al.* 2010; Portas *et al.* 2010; Varley *et al.* 2012). However, a recently introduced 15 Hz system compares less favourably in terms of validity and inter-unit reliability to a 10 Hz system from the same manufacturer (Johnston *et al.* 2014). Practitioners should also be mindful that both 1 and 5 Hz GPS systems are known to provide different measures of total distance, high-intensity running distance, and sprint running when compared against camera-based TMA systems (Randers *et al.* 2010). However, all four systems seem capable of identifying reductions in high-intensity running performance between the first and second half of matches.

The inter-unit reliability appears acceptable for the measurement of individuals performing either linear or curvilinear movements (CV <6%; Gray *et al.* 2010). However, the inter-unit reliability for measuring distances during multidirectional circuits is more variable (CV 3.6–30.4%), and seems to be dependent on the speed of movement, the sampling frequency of the GPS device, and the GPS model used (Coutts and Duffield 2010; Castellano *et al.* 2011). Consequently, players should wear the same GPS units during all sessions that researchers/practitioners wish to analyse. Intra-unit reliability appears to be independent of sampling frequency for both linear (CV 4.4–5.3%) and multidirectional movements (3.9–7.7% for 1 Hz GPS devices and 3.4–6.7% for 5 Hz GPS devices; Portas *et al.* 2010). Over longer multidirectional, team sport circuits, intra-unit reliability for distance covered in locomotive categories is also comparable between units (CV 2.0–4.9%; Portas *et al.* 2010). In addition, the intra-unit reliability for measuring sprint performance over distances <30 m is good (CV 0.78–2.3%), with longer sprint distances appearing more favourable (Coutts and Duffield 2010; Waldron *et al.* 2011a).

4.2.3.2 Measurement of relative distance

Whilst total distance is perhaps the most common variable measured (Cummins *et al.* 2013), the different positional demands and playing time associated with rugby means this measure is best expressed as the distance covered per minute of match or training time (i.e. m·min^{-1}). Indeed, the stark differences between rugby union and rugby league players are best realised when the data are expressed in such a manner. For example, elite rugby union forwards tend to cover greater absolute distance (5,850 m vs. 4,181 m), yet less relative distance (64.6 m·min^{-1} vs. 95.2 m·min^{-1}), in competitive matches compared to rugby league forwards (McLellan *et al.* 2011; Waldron *et al.* 2011b; Cahill *et al.* 2013). Rugby union forwards spending more time on the pitch, yet being engaged in more static actions, could explain this.

4.2.3.3 Categorization of movement activity using speed zones

In its simplest form, movement demands for rugby league have been classified into low-intensity activity (<14 km·h^{-1}) and high-intensity running (>14.1 km·h^{-1}) (Gabbett *et al.* 2012b; Waldron *et al.* 2013). Using larger speed zones permits more variation in speed and is therefore likely to be more reliable (Jennings *et al.* 2010). Conversely, studies examining rugby league (McLellan *et al.* 2011; Waldron *et al.* 2011b; Austin and Kelly 2014) and rugby union (Cunniffe *et al.* 2009; Cahill *et al.* 2013) have used multiple zones to classify player movements. Such detail in classifying the physical demands imposed on players is useful for practitioners hoping to replicate these movements when designing training practices. However, it is problematic that studies show no consistency in their classification of speed zones, which also makes comparison between studies, codes, and sports difficult. A further issue also lies in the use of arbitrary (e.g. McLellan *et al.* 2011; Waldron *et al.* 2011b) compared to individualized (e.g. Cahill *et al.* 2013) speed zones. Absolute thresholds are typically based on values previously reported in the literature and are independent of the athlete's individual capacity. Such issues might be overcome using individualized speed zones based on an objective measure, such as peak running speed (Cahill *et al.* 2013), maximal aerobic power (Lacome *et al.* 2014; Waldron *et al.* 2014), or ventilatory (Abt and Lovell 2009) or lactate threshold (Lacome *et al.* 2014). However, there exists no consensus on the most appropriate measure to normalize speeds zones for rugby players. That the majority of studies adopt arbitrary speeds zones also supports the difficulty in employing this approach in an applied setting.

4.2.3.4 Measurement of accelerations and decelerations

Higher sampling frequencies of GPS units have seen accelerations and decelerations emerging as another measure to quantify the demands in rugby (Higham *et al.* 2012). Accelerating and decelerating are associated with increased metabolic load during running (Osgnach *et al.* 2010), contribute to increased fatigue (Akenhead *et al.* 2013), and are correlated with markers of muscle damage observed after a game (Young *et al.* 2012). However, despite the increased reporting of these data using GPS, they possess poor inter- and intra-unit reliability (Waldron *et al.* 2011a; Buchheit *et al.* 2013). Moreover, current 15 Hz GPS units typically report interpolated values, essentially upgrading a 5–10 Hz raw GPS signal (Aughey 2011; Johnston *et al.* 2014). Whilst it is thought that the addition of intermediary data points (interpolation) is supplemented by the GPS-accelerometer (Aughey 2011), observations from our laboratory indicate the adoption of a linear interpolation technique in some devices (Spi-Pro X, GPSports Canberra, Australia). Such processes alter the nature of accelerations and decelerations that are likely to influence the interpretation of match or training load. Practitioners must therefore be careful when selecting GPS devices to measure accelerations and decelerations and ensure that the data provided are meaningful.

4.3.4.5 Measurement of repeated efforts using GPS

Repeated sprint activity has been defined as the occurrence of three or more sprints, separated by <21 s of moderate to low intensity exercise (Spencer *et al.* 2004). Repeated-efforts differ from traditional analyses of repeated sprints, by utilizing the integration of portable GPS with micro electrical mechanical systems (MEMS). Custom algorithms permit the identification of clustered 'collisions' detected via large decelerations that are registered by the in-built, tri-axial accelerometer (Gabbett 2012). A repeated-effort is therefore representative of a period in which the most demanding aspects of rugby, such as contacts and moments of deceleration occur (Gabbett *et al.* 2012b). Given the known relationship between simulated collisions and/or decelerations and indications of acute fatigue and muscle damage (Pointon and Duffield 2012), there is a clear rationale for the use of MEMS to describe external load during match and training activities.

4.3.4.6 Measurement of body load and collisions using GPS

The integrated tri-axial accelerometers with GPS units might be used to generate a measurement known as 'body load'. This is derived from the square root of the sum of the squared instantaneous rate of change in acceleration in each of the three orthogonal axes (anterioposterior [x], mediolateral [y], and vertical [z]). A loading factor can then be applied to instances that occur within one of six zones of progressively larger magnitude (ranging 5 to 10 g), multiplied by the body mass of the player and summated to generate the final body load score (arbitrary units; AU). Body load is moderately associated (r = 0.45 to 0.63) with perceived exertion during a variety of training scenarios in rugby league players (Lovell *et al.* 2013). The utilization of MEMS to monitor body load should be considered as one of the largest advancements in the monitoring of rugby players since this enables a greater understanding of the potential mechanical stress experienced by an individual. Further research is required to better understand the relationship between measurements of external load and the long-term recovery of rugby players.

Manufacturers purport that GPS enables quantification (both number and magnitude) of collisions during training and matches (Gabbett 2012). This is useful given the influence of these actions on the playing demands (Johnston and Gabbett 2011; Gabbett *et al.* 2012a), recovery (Twist *et al.* 2012), and injury potential (Gabbett *et al.* 2010; Gabbett *et al.* 2011). GPS units using only accelerometer data have used six zones representing very light (<5–6 g), light (6.1–6.5 g), moderate (6.5–7.0 g), heavy (7.1–8.0 g), very heavy (8.1–10 g), and severe (>10 g) to quantify impacts in rugby union (Cunniffe *et al.* 2009) and league (McLellan *et al.* 2011) matches. The additions of gyroscopes and magnetometers alongside the accelerometer enable GPS devices to quantify movement direction, and have been used to quantify mild, moderate, and heavy collisions in rugby league (Gabbett *et al.* 2010; Gabbett *et al.* 2012b).

Whilst such information is relevant to the applied practitioner, some caution is needed to ensure that data are meaningful. For example, McLellan *et al.* (2011) observed an average of ~25 impacts when coded from video that contrasted to an average ~464 impacts (moderate to severe) recorded using a 5 Hz GPS with 100 Hz tri-axial accelerometer. However, Gabbett *et al.* (2012) reported more favourable relationships (r = 0.96) between the number of collisions measured using a GPS compared to video analysis, suggesting the addition of the magnetometer and gyroscope alongside the tri-axial accelerometer improved the ability to detect the number of impacts. This notwithstanding, the subjective nature of video analysis to quantify the magnitude of collisions means that further work is required using more objective measures. The use of GPS alongside video might prove useful when trying to provide additional information on the type of collision for conditioning, injury evaluation, or tactical purposes. However, the added time and practitioner input means that this is unattractive.

4.3 Monitoring the internal demands of training and competition in rugby

Quantifying the physiological responses (internal demands) of players alongside external demands enables practitioners to establish the extent of training stimulus that is elicited during different coaching sessions. The integration of heart rate (HR) telemetry in portable GPS devices has enabled the monitoring of global training and match demand, with value corresponding to ~75 to 86% of maximum values reported in adult rugby league (Waldron *et al.* 2011b; Coutts *et al.* 2003) and rugby union (Cunniffe *et al.* 2009) players.

The use of HR to interpret physiological load in the match and training environment is one of the most common methods of inferring global internal load (Viru and Viru 2001). Certain non-intrusive measures based upon average HR recordings, such as the training impulse method (TRIMP), have been devised in order to establish exercise load (Bannister 1991). However, TRIMP scores are likely to underestimate the physiological load of intermittent exercise bouts when predicted from the HR–blood lactate concentration during continuous exercise (Akubat and Abt 2011). The 'summated heart rate' method provides an arbitrary unit of exercise load and preferentially weights the time spent within higher intensity thresholds. This accounts for the variability, and often disproportionate, time spent within different thresholds of maximal HR intensity during stochastic sports, and is calculated as:

$$(\text{Duration in zone } 1 \times 1) + (\text{Duration in zone } 2 \times 2) + (\text{Duration in zone } 3 \times 3)$$
$$+ (\text{Duration in zone } 4 \times 4) + (\text{Duration in zone } 5 \times 5)$$

Where zone $1 = 50$ to 60% of HR_{max}, zone $2 = 60$ to 70% HR_{max}, zone $3 = 70$ to 80% HR_{max}, zone $4 = 80$ to 90% HR_{max}, and zone $5 = 90$ to 100% HR_{max} (Edwards 1993).

This method has been used to evaluate internal load during training (Coutts *et al.* 2009; Impellizzeri *et al.* 2004) and to quantify 'match load' (Waldron *et al.* 2011b). Notwithstanding some of the associated limitations of HR as a marker of physiological load, owing to factors such as dehydration and circadian rhythm (Achten and Jeukendrup 2003); under controlled conditions, such measures offer a practical field-based tool for the detection of internal load.

An alternative method of determining 'load' has been the session-Rating of Perceived Exertion (s-RPE), which is the product of intensity (0–10 scale) and the duration of exercise. Initially posited by Foster *et al.* (2001), this method of quantifying exercise intensity in team sports (Impellizerri *et al.* 2004; Coutts *et al.* 2009) relates favourably with HR and various external markers during rugby training and matches (Waldron *et al.* 2011b; Lovell *et al.* 2013; Weaving *et al.* 2014). That s-RPE can be used either indoors or outdoors to quantify training load for resistance training (Day *et al.* 2004), conditioning, and skills (Lovell *et al.* 2013; Weaving *et al.* 2014) also heightens its appeal as a measurement tool. However, in selecting s-RPE, practitioners should be mindful that its relationship with other markers of training load is influenced by the type of exercise performed (Lovell *et al.* 2013; Weaving *et al.* 2014). For example, relationships between s-RPE and distance (m) were moderate ($r = 0.45 \pm 0.16$) for skills training compared to very large ($r = 0.75 \pm 0.23$) for small-sided games (Lovell *et al.* 2013). A greater proportion of the variance in training load during rugby skills, speed, wrestling, and resistance training can also be explained when a combination of internal and external measures are used (Weaving *et al.* 2014). Based on these observations, it is recommended that rugby practitioners consider the content of the session when selecting the training load measure, and that it might be preferable to use internal and external measures in combination rather than in isolation to better estimate the training dose.

A recent approach has been to estimate the metabolic 'internal' cost of activities performed during matches based upon players' 'external' movement profiles. Conventional assessments of energy expenditure based on HR recordings (Coutts *et al.* 2003) do not appropriately account for the energy cost associated with high intensity bouts that tax the non-oxidative energy pathways (Osgnach *et al.* 2010). Estimating energy expenditure based on the movement profiles of team sports players addresses this problem and circumvents the issues associated with direct assessment of oxygen uptake during matches. Osgnach and co-authors recognized the limitations of conventional assessments of energy expenditure in a team sports environment, particularly in relation to the assessment of 'key' moments of acceleration and deceleration. Based on the model of di Prampero *et al.* (2005), this technique assumes that accelerations (athlete leaning forward) performed on a flat surface induce an equivalent energy cost (EC) to running uphill at constant speed. Accordingly, the magnitude of acceleration can be related to the degree of an inclination, called the equivalent slope (ES). Since previous investigations have established the EC of uphill running (Minetti *et al.* 2002), one is able to factor the equivalent high-intensity accelerations performed during matches into the energetic estimation of running at a given speed (see Osgnach *et al.* 2010). Metabolic power ($W \cdot kg^{-1}$) is simply the product of energy cost ($J \cdot kg^{-1} \cdot m^{-1}$) and the velocity ($m \cdot s^{-1}$) of the player at a given instance. Using this technique, Kempton *et al.* (2014) reported an estimated energy expenditure of $25.7–43.5$ $kJ \cdot kg^{-1}$ in elite rugby league players during match play.

Such models have recently been incorporated into the software of portable GPS devices, thus permitting a real-time estimation of energy expenditure during training and matches. Notwithstanding some of the limitations with identifying velocity changes (accelerations/decelerations) with GPS devices, this approach denotes a clear progression in the application of motion analysis technology to a team sport environment and is likely to be adopted in the rugby codes. Importantly, this method offers team sports practitioners a way of quantifying global training load using a metric (i.e. energy) that more appropriately describes the physiological stimulus of an exercise bout. In addition, data obtained in the field can be directly compared (i.e., using the same units) with laboratory tests or ergometer-based training.

4.4 Conclusion

An accurate assessment of training load ensures a player is responding to training, assists in the modification of training load, and minimises the risk of injury. However, despite the availability of a plethora of methods to quantify the training and match demands of rugby, no single criterion measure exists. This is complicated by the multi-component nature of rugby that comprises a range of external and internal demands contributing to overall training load. When selecting a method to quantify player load, practitioners must consider the mode of training, practicality, reliability, and validity of the measures used. Moreover, data must be meaningful in terms of informing coaching or research practice. The practitioner should also consider employing a combination of external and internal measures to provide a more appropriate assessment of training load.

References

Abt, G. and Lovell, R. (2009). The use of individualized speed and intensity thresholds for determining the distance run at high-intensity in professional soccer. *Journal of Sports Sciences*, 27, 893–98.

Achten, J. and Jeukendrup, A.E. (2003). Heart rate monitoring: applications and limitations. *Sports Medicine*, 33, 517–38.

Akenhead, R., Hayes, P.R., Thompson, K.G., *et al.* (2013). Diminutions of acceleration and deceleration output during professional football match play. *Journal of Science and Medicine in Sports*, 16, 556–61.

Akubat, I. and Abt, G. (2011). Intermittent exercise alters the heart rate-blood lactate relationship used for calculating the training impulse (TRIMP) in team sport players. *Journal of Science and Medicine in Sports*, 14, 249–53.

Aughey, R. (2011). Applications of GPS technologies to field sports. *International Journal of Sports Physiology and Performance*, 6, 295–310.

Austin, D., Gabbett, T., and Jenkins, D. (2011a). Repeated high-intensity exercise in professional rugby union. *Journal of Sports Sciences*, 29, 1105–12.

Austin, D., Gabbett, T., and Jenkins, D. (2011b). The physical demands of Super 14 rugby union. *Journal of Science and Medicine in Sport*, 14, 259–63.

Austin, D.J. and Kelly, S.J. (2014). Professional rugby league positional match-play analysis through the use of global positioning system. *Journal of Strength and Conditioning Research*, 28, 187–93.

Bannister, E.W. (1991). Modeling elite athletic performance. *Physiological testing of elite athletes*, Champaign, IL: Human Kinetics.

Bradley, P.S., Wooster, B., O'Donoghue, P., *et al.* (2007). The reliability of Prozone match-viewer: a video-based technical performance analysis system. *International Journal of Performance Analysis in Sport*, 7, 117–29.

Buchheit, M., Al Haddad, H., Simpson, B.M., *et al.* (2013). Monitoring accelerations with GPS in football: time to slow down? *International Journal of Sports Physiology and Performance*, 9, 442–5.

Cahill, N., Lamb, K., Worsfold, P., *et al.* (2013). The movement characteristics of English Premiership rugby union players. *Journal of Sports Sciences*, 31, 229–37.

Carling, C., Bloomfield, J., Nelsen, L., *et al.* (2008). The role of motion analysis in elite soccer. *Sports Medicine*, 38, 839–62.

Castellano, J., Casamichana, D., Calleja-González, J., *et al.* (2011). Reliability and accuracy of 10 Hz GPS devices for short-distance exercise. *Journal of Science and Medicine in Sports*, 10, 233–4.

Coutts, A.J. and Duffield, R. (2010). Validity and reliability of GPS devices for measuring movement demands of team sports. *Journal of Science and Medicine in Sports*, 13, 133–5.

Coutts, A.J., Rampinini, E., Marcora, S.M., *et al.* (2009). Heart rate and blood lactate correlates of perceived exertion during small-sided soccer games. *Journal of Science and Medicine in Sport*, 12, 79–84.

Coutts, A., Reaburn, P., and Grant, A. (2003). Hearth rate, blood lactate concentration, and estimated energy expenditure in a semi-professional rugby league team during a match: case study. *Journal of Sports Sciences*, 21, 97–103.

Cummins, C., Orr, R., O'Connor, H., *et al.* (2013). Global positioning systems (GPS) and microtechnology sensors in team sports: a systematic review. *Sports Medicine*, 43, 1025–42.

Cunniffe, B., Proctor, W., Barker, J.S., *et al.* (2009). An evaluation of the physiological demands of elite rugby union using global positioning system tracking system. *Journal of Strength and Conditioning Research*, 23, 1195–203.

Day, M.L., McGuigan, M.R., Brice, G., *et al.* (2004). Monitoring exercise intensity during resistance training using the session RPE scale. *Journal of Strength and Conditioning Research*, 18, 353–8.

Deutsch, M.U., Kearney, G.A., and Rehrer, NJ. (2007). Time–motion analysis of professional rugby union players during match-play. *Journal of Sport Sciences*, 25, 461–72.

di Prampero, P.E., Fusi, S., Sepulcri, L., *et al.* (2005). Sprint running: a new energetic approach. *Journal of Experimental Biology*, 2809–16.

Di Salvo, V., Baron, R., Tschan, H., *et al.* (2007). Performance characteristics according to playing position in elite soccer. *International Journal of Sports Medicine*, 28, 222–7.

Di Salvo, V., Collins, A., McNeill, B., *et al.* (2006). Validation of Prozone: A new video-based performance analysis system. *International Journal of Performance Analysis in Sport*, 6, 108–109.

Di Salvo, V., Gregson, W., Atkinson, G., *et al.* (2009). Analysis of high-intensity activity in Premier League soccer. *International Journal of Sports Medicine*, 30, 205–12.

Duthie, G., Pyne, D., and Hooper, S. (2005). Time motion analysis of 2001 and 2002 Super 12 rugby. *Journal of Sports Sciences*, 23, 523–30.

Edwards, S. (1993). *The heart rate monitor book*. Sacramento, CA: Fleet Feet Press.

Foster, C., Florhaug, J.A., Franklin, J., *et al.* (2001). A new approach to monitoring exercise training. *Journal of Strength and Conditioning Research*, 15, 109–15.

Figueroa, P.J., Leite, N.J., and Barros, R.M.L. (2006). Background recovering in outdoor image sequences: An example of soccer players segmentation. *Image and Vision Computing*, 24, 363–74.

Gabbett, T.J. (2004a). Reductions in pre-season training loads reduce training injury rates in rugby league players. *British Journal of Sports Medicine*, 38, 743–9.

Gabbett, T.J. (2004b). Influence of training and match intensity on injuries in rugby league. *Journal of Sports Sciences*, 22, 409–17.

Gabbett, T.J. (2012). Quantifying the physical demands of collision sports: does microsensor technology measure what it claims to measure? *Journal of Strength and Conditioning Research*, 27, 2319–22.

Gabbett, T.J., Jenkins, D.G., and Abernethy, B. (2010). Physical collisions and injury during professional rugby league skills training. *Journal of Science and Medicine in Sport*, 13, 578–83.

Gabbett, T.J., Jenkins, D.G., and Abernethy, B. (2011). Physical collisions and injury in professional rugby league match-play. *Journal of Science and Medicine in Sport*, 14, 210–5.

Gabbett, T.J., Jenkins, D.G., and Abernethy, B. (2012a). Influence of wrestling on the physiological and skill demands of small-sided games. *Journal of Strength and Conditioning Research*, 26, 113–20.

Gabbett, T.J., Jenkins, D.G., and Abernethy, B. (2012b). Physical demands of professional rugby league training and competition using microtechnology. *Journal of Science and Medicine in Sports*, 15, 80–6.

Gray, A.J., Jenkins, D., Andrews, M.H., *et al.* (2010). Validity and reliability of GPS for measuring distance travelled in field-based team sports. *Journal of Sports Sciences*, 28, 1319–25.

Higham, D.G., Pyne, D.B., Anson, J.M., *et al.* (2012). Movement patterns in rugby sevens: effects of tournament level, fatigue, and substitute players. *Journal of Science and Medicine in Sport*, 15, 277–82.

Impellizzeri, F.M., Rampinini, E., Coutts, A.J., *et al.* (2004). Use of RPE-based training load in soccer. *Medicine and Science in Sports and Exercise*, 36, 1042–47.

Jennings, D., Cormack, S., Coutts, A.J., *et al.* (2010). The validity and reliability of GPS units for measuring distance in team sport specific running patterns. *International Journal of Sports Physiology and Performance*, 5, 328–41.

Johnston, R.D. and Gabbett, T.J. (2011). Repeated-sprint and effort ability in rugby league players. *Journal of Strength and Conditioning Research*, 25, 2789–95.

Johnston, R.J., Watsford, M.L., Kelly, S.J., *et al.* (2014). The validity and reliability of 10 Hz and 15 Hz GPS units for assessing athlete movement demands. *Journal of Strength and Conditioning Research*, 28, 1649–55.

Kempton, T., Sirotic, A.C., Rampinini, E., *et al.* (2014). Metabolic power demands of rugby league match-play. *International Journal of Sports Physiology and Performance*. In Press.

King, T., Jenkins, D., and Gabbett, T.J. (2009). A time–motion analysis of professional rugby league match-play. *Journal of Sports Sciences*, 27, 213–9.

Krustrup, P. and Bangsbo, J. (2001). Physiological demands of top-class soccer refereeing in relation to physical capacity: Effect of intense intermittent exercise training. *Journal of Sports Sciences*, 19, 881–91.

Lacome, M., Piscione, J., Hager, J-P., *et al.* (2014). A new approach to quantifying physical demand in rugby union. *Journal of Sports Sciences*, 32, 290–300.

Larsson, P. (2003). Global positioning system and sport-specific testing. *Sports Medicine*, 33, 1093–101.

Lovell, T.W., Sirotic, A., Impellizzeri, F., *et al.* (2013). Factors affecting perception of effort (session rating of perceived exertion) during rugby league training. *International Journal of Sports Physiology and Performance*, 8, 62–9.

McLean, D.A. (1992). Analysis of the physical demands of international rugby union. *Journal of Sports Sciences*, 10, 285–96.

McLellan, C.P., Lovell, D.I., and Gass, G.C. (2011). Biochemical and endocrine responses to impact and collision during elite rugby league match play. *Journal of Strength and Conditioning Research*, 25, 1553–62.

Minetti, A., Moia, C., Roi, G.S., *et al.* (2002). Energy cost of walking and running at extreme uphill and downhill slopes. *Journal of Applied Physiology*, 93, 1039–46.

Mohr, M., Krustrup, P., and Bangsbo, J. (2003). Match performance of high-standard soccer players with special reference to development of fatigue. *Journal of Sports Sciences*, 21, 519–28.

Osgnach, C., Poser, S., Bernardini, R., *et al.* (2010). Energy cost and metabolic power in elite soccer: A new match analysis approach. *Medicine and Science in Sports and Exercise*, 42, 170–8.

Petersen, C., Pyne, D., Portus, M., *et al.* (2009). Validity and reliability of GPS units to monitor cricket-specific movement patterns. *International Journal of Sports Physiology and Performance*, 4, 381–93.

Pointon, M. and Duffield, R. (2012). Cold water immersion recovery following simulated collision sport exercise. *Medicine and Science in Sports and Exercise*, 44, 206–16.

Portas, M.D., Harley, J.A., Barnes, C.A., *et al.* (2010). The validity and reliability of 1-Hz and 5-Hz global positioning systems for linear, multidirectional, and soccer-specific activities. *International Journal of Sports Physiology and Performance*, 5, 448–58.

Randers, M. B., Mujika, I., Hewitt, A., *et al.* (2010). Application of four different football match analysis systems: a comparative study. *Journal of Sports Sciences*, 28, 171–82.

Reilly, T. and Thomas, V. (1976). A motion analysis of work rate in different positional roles in pro football match-play. *Journal of Human Movement Studies*, 2, 87–97.

Roberts, S.P., Trewartha, G., Higgitt, R.J., *et al.* (2008). The physical demands of elite English rugby union. *Journal of Sports Sciences*, 26, 825–33.

Spencer, M., Lawrence, S., Rechichi, C., *et al.* (2004). Time–motion analysis of elite field hockey, with special reference to repeated-sprint activity. *Journal of Sports Sciences*, 22, 843–50.

Sykes, D., Twist, C., Hall, S., *et al.* (2009). Semi-automated time–motion analysis of senior elite rugby league. *International Journal of Performance Analysis in Sport*, 9, 47–59.

Sykes, D., Twist, C., Nicholas, C., *et al.* (2011). Changes in locomotive rates during senior elite rugby league matches. *Journal of Sports Sciences*, 29, 1263–71.

Twist, C., Waldron, M., Highton, J., *et al.* (2012). Neuromuscular, biochemical, and perceptual post-match fatigue in professional rugby league forwards and backs. *Journal of Sports Science*, 30, 359–67.

Varley, M.C., Fairweather, I.H., and Aughey, R.J. (2012). Validity and reliability of GPS for measuring instantaneous velocity during acceleration, deceleration, and constant motion. *Journal of Sports Science*, 30, 121–27.

Viru, A. and Viru, M. (2001). *Biochemical monitoring of sport training*. Champaign, IL: Human Kinetics Publishers. 87–104.

Waldron, M., Twist, C., Highton, J., *et al.* (2011a). Movement and physiological match demands of elite rugby league using portable global positioning systems. *Journal of Sports Science*, 29, 1223–30.

Waldron, M., Worsfold, P., Twist, C., *et al.* (2011b). Concurrent validity and test-retest reliability of a global positioning system (GPS) and timing gates to assess sprint performance variables. *Journal of Sports Science*, 29, 1613–19.

Waldron, M., Highton, J., and Twist, C. (2013). The reliability of a rugby league movement simulation protocol (RLMSP-i) designed to replicate the performance of interchanged players. *International Journal of Sports Physiology and Performance*, 8, 483–9.

Waldron, M., Worsfold, P., Twist, C., *et al.* (2014). A three-season comparison of match performances among selected and unselected elite youth rugby league players. *Journal of Sports Sciences*, 32, 1110–9.

Weaving, D., Marshall, P., Earle, K., *et al.* (2014). A combination of internal and external training load measures explains the greatest proportion of variance in certain training modes in professional rugby league. *International Journal of Sports Physiology and Performance*. [Epub ahead of print].

Young, W.B., Hepner, J., and Robbins, D.W. (2012). Movement demands in Australian rules football as indicators of muscle damage. *Journal of Strength and Conditioning Research*, 26, 492–6.

5

MONITORING FATIGUE AND RECOVERY IN RUGBY PLAYERS

Craig Twist and Jamie Highton

5.1 The demands of rugby and potential contributors to post-match fatigue

Player fatigue is influenced by the volume of games played per season (Hartwig *et al.* 2009) and the number of days and training load imposed on players between games (McLean *et al.* 2010). In the competitive phase of the season (~30 matches, February to October) there are typically five to nine days between matches (McLean *et al.* 2010). Players will also play in tournaments that involve several games over two weeks (e.g. World Cup) or one to two days (e.g. Sevens World Series) which will be influenced by climatic conditions, jet lag, and travel fatigue (West *et al.* 2013b; McGuckin *et al.* 2014). Potential for decreases in physical performance (Johnston *et al.* 2013a; Johnston *et al.* 2013b) and increased injury potential are therefore possible (Dellal *et al.* 2013). In season, matches are combined with multi-component training sessions where training loads are manipulated depending on the number of days between games (McLean *et al.* 2010).

Fatigue includes sensations of tiredness and associated decrements in muscular performance and function (Abiss and Laursen 2005). This is typically characterized in elite rugby league (McLellan *et al.* 2011a; Twist *et al.* 2012; Johnston *et al.* 2013b; Johnston *et al.* 2014) and rugby union (West *et al.* 2013a) players by reductions in muscle function for up to 36 h after a competitive match. However, elite rugby sevens demonstrate reductions for >120 hours after a two-day tournament (West *et al.* 2013b). Perceived soreness and fatigue increase after a match, with values peaking at 24h (McLean *et al.* 2010; Twist *et al.* 2012) and remaining elevated for up to four days. Changes in psychological well-being have also been reported during intensified periods of training (Coutts *et al.* 2007b, c) and competition (Johnston *et al.* 2013a, b; Johnston *et al.* 2014) for rugby players. Co-existing with increases in immunoendocine and hormonal responses (Cunniffe *et al.* 2010; Twist *et al.* 2012), changes in these indirect markers suggest tissue damage and low-frequency fatigue are common in the days after a game or during intense training and/or competition.

Post-game (i.e. up to 72 h) fatigue and recovery time will depend upon the activity duration, movement demands, and contact loads imposed on the individual (Twist *et al.* 2012; Takarada 2003; Johnston *et al.* 2013b; Johnston *et al.* 2014). Multiple accelerations and decelerations during games (Waldron *et al.* 2011b) and training (Gabbett *et al.* 2012) involve eccentric muscle actions that cause structural damage to skeletal muscle tissue (Howatson and Milak 2009). Blunt force trauma also causes damage given the strong association between the number of collisions and blood markers of tissue damage (e.g. creatine kinase, myoglobin) (Takarada 2003; Twist *et al.* 2012) and greater muscle damage when physical contact is included in training (Johnston *et al.* 2014). Metabolic stress from prolonged (~60–80 min), high-intensity (~80% maximum heart rate) exercise might also contribute to tissue damage and glycogen depletion in some positional groups. Muscle glycogen concentration can also remain 30% lower than pre-match values for two days after prolonged intermittent activity (Bangsbo *et al.* 2006), caused by impaired muscle glycogen resynthesis in type II fibres damaged by eccentric exercise (Asp *et al.* 1998). Furthermore, sleep quality (Skein *et al.* 2013), poor nutritional practices (Walsh *et al.* 2011), and alcohol consumption (Barnes *et al.* 2012) will also affect recovery after intense activity.

In most cases, symptoms of fatigue after training or a match are recovered in players by 48–72 h (e.g. Twist *et al.*, 2012; West *et al.* 2013a). However, excessive training/match loads and poor management of recovery in the days after are likely to result in players demonstrating more prolonged signs of fatigue. Left unattended, this under-recovery could affect a player's performance capability and health. Figure 5.1 shows a schematic of the factors influencing fatigue and recovery of the rugby player.

5.2 Monitoring fatigue in rugby players

Understanding the fatigue response after games and throughout the season identifies players' recovery and helps determine appropriate training loads to maximise performance (Fowles 2006). This requires suitable monitoring tools to make informed decisions on each player's status.

5.2.1 Questionnaires and subjective assessments of fatigue

Changes in an athlete's psychological state during periods of intense training and underperformance co-exist with changes in physiological and performance changes (Coutts *et al.* 2007a; Gastin *et al.* 2013). Subjective assessments of fatigue are sensitive to changes in training stress (Coutts *et al.* 2007c; Gastin *et al.* 2013) and can outlast reductions in neuromuscular performance and biochemical markers of fatigue in rugby players (Coutts *et al.* 2007b, c; Twist *et al.* 2012). Mental fatigue can also alter an individual's sense of effort that impairs exercise capacity (Marcora *et al.* 2008), and

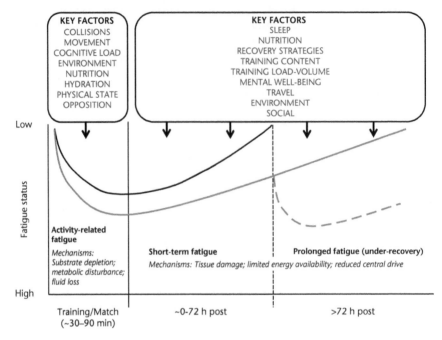

FIGURE 5.1 Factors influencing fatigue and recovery of players during and after rugby-related activity. Black line represents a well-managed player showing a short-term fatigue response to match/training and the typical course of recovery time. Grey line represents a player experiencing higher match/training load followed by greater short-term fatigue response and slower recovery. Dashed line shows fatigue response when under-recovered player is exposed to additional fatiguing activity, leading to increased risk of prolonged and potentially chronic fatigue. Key factors contributing to player fatigue response are indicated above.

appears to be more sensitive to early stages of overreaching than physiological and biochemical changes (Coutts *et al.* 2007a).

Perceptual fatigue measures include Profile of Mood States questionnaire (POMS; Morgan *et al.* 1987), Daily Analysis of Life Demands for Athletes questionnaire (DALDA; Rushall 1990), the Recovery-Stress Questionnaire for athletes (RESTQ-Sport; Kellmann and Kallus 2001), and the Total Quality Recovery scale (TQR; Kenttä and Hassmén 1998). These allow coaches to monitor the complex psychophysiological stresses associated with fatigue and poor recovery, such as muscle soreness, sleep quality, mood disturbances, and attitudes to training. A concern here is the subjectivity of these measures (Meuseen *et al.* 2006; Nédélec *et al.* 2012), and the scope for athletes to manipulate responses to facilitate a favourable outcome. Moreover, where questionnaires are completed daily and are lengthy, player compliance is a concern (Beedie *et al.* 2000). Shorter and simpler questionnaires (e.g. McLean *et al.* 2010; Gastin *et al.* 2013) are common practice in high-performance sports (Taylor *et al.* 2012); although practitioners should note their reduced sensitivity (Robson-Anlsey *et al.* 2009) and rigorously examine their utility before application (Gastin *et al.* 2013).

The use of coach ratings after matches has been used extensively in Australian Rules football to provide subjective evaluations of player performance (Cormack *et al.* 2013; Hunkin *et al.* 2014). These tools show strong associations with measures of fatigue, such that poor performance ratings by coaches coincide with reductions in muscle function and running performance (Cormack *et al.* 2013). These measures might provide a useful tool for identifying underperforming players and are likely to be accepted by coaches given their involvement in the process and that interpretation involves an assessment of player performance.

5.2.2 Heart rate variability (HRV)

Heart rate variability (HRV) measures the time between two beats (R-R interval) providing a non-invasive assessment of autonomic (parasympathetic and sympathetic) responsiveness (Achten and Jeukendrup 2003). HRV gives estimates of the parasympathetic and sympathetic modulation using frequency domain analysis, with the high-frequency band (0.15–0.40 Hz) representative of parasympathetic control and the low frequency band (0.04–0.15 Hz) reflecting sympathetic and parasympathetic control (Malik 1996). The low–high frequency ratio is considered an index of sympathovagal balance, presenting a measure of autonomic cardiovascular control (Bosquet *et al.* 2008). Negative adaptations to training and non-functional over-reaching are associated with reductions in HRV, which are associated with a shift from parasympathetic to sympathetic control of heart rate (Hynynen *et al.* 2006; Bosquet *et al.* 2008). Accordingly, changes in HRV can be used to assess the health and training status of athletes and have been used within elite youth rugby players to report lower cardiac autonomic response for up to four days after a match (Edmonds *et al.* 2013). Such findings are consistent with other studies showing prolonged recovery after a match (McLellan *et al.* 2011a, b; Twist *et al.* 2012; West *et al.* 2013a), and provide additional data that might help coaches to optimize training.

The effect of negative training adaptations on HRV are equivocal; HRV has been noted to increase (Hedelin *et al.* 2000), decrease (Hynynen *et al.* 2006), and remaining unchanged (Bosquet *et al.* 2003) in response to negative training adaptations. Such observations occurred despite athletes still showing symptoms of fatigue and poor performance, and suggest that responses are extremely individualized. Moreover, for HRV to be meaningful in detecting fatigue, it seems necessary to enact a highly standardized protocol that accounts for prior training load, time of day, digestion, and any stimuli that increase sympathetic activity, such as temperature, noise, and caffeine and alcohol intake (Bosquet *et al.* 2008). Where recommendations for weekly and daily measurements of HRV indices are recommended (Plews *et al.* 2013a), such control would be problematic in the chaotic scheduling associated with rugby. For example, only nine players out of a total of twenty-six completed the study by Edmonds *et al.* (2013), with ~33% of those not completing because of 'tardiness'. Practitioners wishing to adopt HRV to monitor training adaptation are recommended to use a minimum of three and five randomly selected valid data points per week in elite and sub-elite athletes, respectively (Plews *et al.* 2013b). Collectively, the practical limitations associated with HRV perhaps detract from its appeal as a suitable measurement tool to assess fatigue status in rugby players.

5.2.3 Blood and salivary borne markers of fatigue and recovery

Whilst resting creatine kinase (CK) concentrations in athletic populations are typically higher than non-athletes because of daily training (Mougios 2007), increases after exercise indicate acute tissue damage. Hunkin *et al.* (2014) proposed that increased CK before a match was likely to represent a state of incomplete recovery from the preceding week and, over time, residual muscle damage. Persistent elevations of CK after absolute rest are also indicative of incomplete recovery or, in severe cases, underlying myopathy (Brancaccio *et al.* 2007). CK is influenced by age, sex, race, muscle mass, physical fitness, and environmental conditions (Brancaccio *et al.*, 2007). Accordingly, these factors should be accounted for when using resting CK to assess the health status and optimize training load of the rugby player. For example, CK monitoring has been recommended with young and inexperienced players and those with lower aerobic running performance to assist in the modulation of training and recovery loads to optimise match preparation and performance (Hunkin *et al.* 2014).

Despite being recommended as a useful measure to monitor acute recovery after matches (McLellan *et al.* 2011b), several issues exist with the validity of CK. CK is strongly related to the number of collisions a player makes (Cunniffe *et al.* 2010; Twist *et al.* 2012), so it is difficult to differentiate between mechanically induced muscle damage and that caused by blunt force trauma. More importantly, plasma CK and more sensitive measures for assessing muscle damage caused by physical contacts (e.g. C-reactive protein) possess a poor temporal relationships with muscle function recovery after exercise-induced muscle damage (Warren *et al.* 1999; Margaritis *et al.* 1999; Singh *et al.* 2011). CK also has extremely large day-to-day (~27%, personal observation) and large individual variability (Hartmann and Mester 2000).

Reductions in glutamine-to-glutamate ratio are reported during intensified periods of rugby training because of lower plasma glutamine and elevated glutamate concentrations (Coutts *et al.* 2007b). Decreases in glutamine could be explained by increased uptake of amino acids for increased gluconeogenesis with glycogen depletion (Halson *et al.* 2003). Whilst reductions in the glutamine to glutamate ratio (<3.58) might provide an index of increased training stress (Smith and Norris 2000), more research is needed to confirm its use as a marker of recovery status.

Salivary (Elloumi *et al.* 2003; McLellen *et al.* 2011a, b; West *et al.* 2013a) and plasma (Cunniffe *et al.* 2010) testosterone (T) and cortisol (C) concentrations (including the T/C ratio) have been studied after elite rugby matches and in the week before a match to establish player recovery from midweek training and readiness to play (Crewther *et al.* 2013; Gaviglio *et al.* 2014). Increases in C immediately after (Elloumi *et al.* 2003; McLellen *et al.* 2011a; West *et al.* 2013a) reflect the physiological (i.e. metabolic demand of exercise, depleted glycogen, tissue damage) and psychological stress (i.e. anticipation, anxiety) of a match or training. Contemporaneous reductions in T and a lowered T/C ratio signals that players experience a catabolic state immediately after a match (Elloumi *et al.* 2003; Cunniffe *et al.* 2010; McLellen *et al.* 2011a, b). However, the catabolic-anabolic state in the days after a rugby match remains unclear. Several studies have reported decreases in the T/C ratio for up to thirty-six hours post match (McLellen *et al.* 2011a, b; West *et al.* 2013a), whereas Elloumi *et al.* (2003) reported values to remain elevated for up to five days. In contrast, Cunniffe *et al.* (2011) examined players after an international rugby match and reported that T/C was lower than pre-game values at 14 hours after a match. This was followed by a rebound anabolic stimulus that saw values increase above pre-game at 36 hours post-match. That T and C represent both physiological and psychological responses to exercise suggests these measures possess high individual variability dependent on the internal and external loads imposed on the player before and during the activity.

Frequent blood and saliva monitoring provides information on the health status of the athletes and mechanistic insights into fatigue (Finaud *et al.* 2006; Alaphillipe *et al.* 2012; Hesiterberg *et al.* 2013). However, these measures are costly, labour-intensive, and practically challenging in the rugby environment. Hesiterberg *et al.* (2013) suggest such data need to be collected frequently with team sport athletes and founded on an extensive database of baseline data to be meaningful. Moreover, poor temporal relationships between bloodborne markers, neuromuscular performance (West *et al.* 2013a), and perceptual measures (Alaphilippe *et al.*, 2012) mean fatigue cannot be judged on a single biochemical, hormonal, or immunological measure alone.

5.2.4 Neuromuscular function

Jump procedures assess stretch-shortening capability of the lower limb musculature and the ability to evaluate muscle fatigue (Komi 2000). They are easy to administer and cause minimal additional fatigue when performed on a regular basis. Whilst the sensitivity of jump procedures to assess neuromuscular fatigue in team sport athletes is questioned (Cormack *et al.* 2008a; Krustrup *et al.* 2010), impaired muscle function after matches has been detected using this method in rugby players (McLellan *et al.* 2011a; Twist *et al.* 2012; West *et al.* 2013a, b). Reductions in jump performance also explain increases in low speed running and a decreasing number of accelerations during matches (Cormack *et al.* 2013).

Video analysis provides the criterion method to measure jump performance (Dias *et al.* 2011) but is labour-intensive in an applied setting. Alternatively, a portable force platform measures muscle force, power, rate of force development, and flight time characteristics. Measuring several parameters is particularly useful because peak force recovers faster after a match than peak power and rate of force development in rugby players (McLellan *et al.* 2011a). These data can also be used to calculate the flight time–contraction time ratio, which represents the time from the initiation of the counter-movement until the player leaves the force plate, and is sensitive to fatigue changes after matches (Cormack *et al.* 2008a, b; Cormack *et al.* 2013). Protocols have included single countermovement jumps (McLean *et al.*

2010; McLellan *et al.* 2011a), whilst others have suggested multiple jumps (i.e. 5 repeated countermovement jumps). This is because several variables within this protocol might react differently than a single jump and could be useful in understanding the mechanisms of fatigue (Cormack *et al.* 2008a). Moreover, the reliability of the countermovement jump using a force platform is acceptable, with intra- and inter-day coefficients of variation (CV) of between 1–6% (Cormack *et al.* 2008c). Jump performance can also be assessed using a contact mat or similar system, which are cheaper but provide only measures of flight time, predicted jump height based on vertical displacement, and contact time. This method underestimates jump height when compared to the criterion measure (Dias *et al.* 2011) but has good inter-day reliability (CV = 1.9–6.6%, Moir *et al.* 2008).

Though often ignored, measurements of upper body muscle function are necessary in rugby players to detect fatigue caused by pushing, pulling, and grappling during physical collisions. To date only peak power and peak force during a plyometric push-up have been measured on a portable force platform (ICC = 0.86). This method was able to detect reductions in upper body function of rugby league players because of fatigue caused by intensified competition (Johnston *et al.* 2013a) or an increase in the number of collisions during training (Johnston *et al.* 2014).

The introduction of rotary encoders into the training environment that measure bar velocity during resistance exercises can be employed for monitoring upper and lower body neuromuscular function (Jennings *et al.* 2005; Argus *et al.* 2012). Where players resume resistance training in the days after a match, practitioners could monitor the power output during core exercises (e.g. bench press, squat, and prone pull) to ascertain recovery status and make informed judgments on the necessary training load. These apparatus have acceptable measurement error for the assessment of power output in multi-joint exercises (ICC = 0.97; 95% limits of agreement = -17 ± 96W, Jennings *et al.* 2005), thus providing a worthwhile measurement tool.

Neuromuscular function in rugby players can also been assessed using isometric and isokinetic dynamometry (Duffield *et al.* 2012; Twist and Sykes, 2011). Indeed, lower isometric force immediately after a match is related to a player's mean running speed and total playing time (Duffield *et al.* 2012). Whilst these methods provide reliable measures of muscle function (ICC = >90%; CV = <8%) and are able to provide data on isolated muscle groups, assessment of only single joint movements means these are perhaps limited to a research or clinical setting (Abernethy *et al.* 1995).

Measures of sprint performance are typically impaired after prolonged intermittent activity (Magalhaes *et al.* 2010) and provide insight into movement-specific fatigue. Typical sprint distances during rugby matches are ~10 m (Waldron *et al.* 2011b; Cahill *et al.* 2013), so this seems a logical distance to assess. Over-ground sprinting ability is often assessed using infrared timing gates, which have been shown to provide reliable data over short (10 to 30 m) distances (CV = 1.0–1.5%; Waldron *et al.* 2011a). Alternatively, sprint performance over short distances can be monitored reliably (CV = 0.8–2.1%) during training and matches using global positioning system (GPS) devices (Waldron *et al.* 2011a). Measuring sprint performance during training and matches, rather than in a closed environment, helps the practitioner better understand the impact of fatigue on training quality. Lastly, the use of a cycle ergometer sprint test has been described to examine neuromuscular fatigue after matches in team sport athletes (Wehbe *et al.* 2014). This protocol comprises 2×6 s 'all-out' efforts to provide a measure of peak lower limb power, that is independent of an imposed body mass load and does not involve eccentric loading of the musculature. These are distinct advantages to running and jump protocols, particularly when coaches are keen to limit additional fatigue or minimize injury risk.

5.2.5 Performance tests

Measures of sub-maximal and maximal performance have been used to assess fatigue in team sport athletes (e.g. Coutts *et al.* 2007b, c; Rowsell *et al.* 2009). Increases in RPE are observed with fatigue and exercise-induced muscle damage (Coutts *et al.* 2007a), and can determine an athlete's recovery status. These protocols are easy to administer as part of a warm-up; however, the validity of subjective measures can be influenced when individuals are assessed within large groups. Maximal exercise to exhaustion has been used to assess the fatigue status of rugby league players during a six-week intensified training period. Fatigue in the last two weeks of a six-week intensified rugby training programme was detected with a 5–10 per cent in reduction in peak speed during maximal shuttle running to exhaustion (Coutts *et al.* 2007b). However, the use of maximal tests should be carefully considered given their potential to cause additional fatigue (Nédélec *et al.* 2012). Like many performance tests, these procedures are also criticised for their lack of sport specificity (Meeusen *et al.* 2006). Alternatively, the use of reliable rugby simulation protocols (e.g. Roberts *et al.* 2010; Sykes *et al.* 2013; Waldron *et al.* 2012) provides a model that replicates the movement demands of a match. Here, where other signs of fatigue are detected, practitioners can have a player perform short cycles (~5–10 min) of the simulation protocol whilst assessing his or her movement (GPS) physiological (heart rate) and perceptual measures (RPE) to monitor the player's match performance capacity. Additionally, the simulation could be used to ascertain that an athlete has recovered from a period of intensified training or his or her readiness to resume playing after injury.

5.3 Interpretation of fatigue data

Making an informed decision on whether a player's recovery warrants attention based upon the aforementioned markers can be a difficult task. Indeed, making a judgment on any 'true' change in any maker of post-exercise recovery depends on the reliability associated with each measure. The use of arbitrary cut-off points (e.g., change of 5%) across different measurements to identify a fatigued condition is discouraged, as this might fall within the boundaries of typical variation for some measurements (e.g., jump measurements ~1–6%; Cormack *et al.* 2008a), but not others (e.g., CK ~ 27%; personal observations). Likewise, making judgments on an increase or decrease in any measure, whilst appealing, should be interpreted with caution if its reliability is poor and normative values are unknown. Therefore, we

TABLE 5.1 An overview of tools for measuring fatigue and recovery status in rugby players

Tool	Measures	Change after match	Reliability	Advantages	Disadvantages	Minimum recommendation
Questionnaires	Muscle soreness Fatigue Mood Sleep quality	↑ peak 1-2 d ↑ peak 1-2 d ? ?	Unknown	Easy to use and sensitive to changes in performance	Subjective means players can easily manipulate responses	Record weekly, within 2–3 d post match (depending on training schedule)
Neuromuscular function	CMJ flight time Force Power	↓ peak 1 d → →	Good	Indirect marker of fatigue	Difficult to identify match-specific fatigue	Record weekly, 2–3 d post match (depending on training schedule)
Performance tests	Running velocity RPE Heart rate	↓ ↑ ↔	Good	Identifies performance capability	Time consuming and potential to increase fatigue	Use when other markers suggest fatigue or when returning from injury
Bloodborne markers	Creatine kinase Cytokines (e.g. IL-6) Testosterone: Cortisol Glutamate: Glutamine	↑ peak 1 d ↑ peak 1 d ↓ 0 h, ↑or↓ →	Varied	Underlying mechanisms of fatigue and health status	Costly; poor temporal relationship with performance and perceptual changes	Only use when other markers suggest investigation of health status

h = hour(s); d = day(s); CMJ = countermovement jump; ↓ = decrease; ↑ = increase; ↔ = unchanged propose that identifying a meaningful change in fatigue status should be based on reliability and inter-day variability of the measure (CV) for each individual by simply taking repeated measures of the parameter (e.g. vertical jump height) and calculating the (SD/mean) × 100. Practitioners can be confident that a true change has occurred in the recovery parameter if the change is greater than the CV for that given measurement. Thereafter, a judgment can be made as to the magnitude of the change in that parameter using modified standardized effects, multiplying the CV by 0.3, 0.9, and 1.6 to determine what would be a small, moderate, and large change in the measure of fatigue, respectively (Hopkins *et al.* 2009). However, such an approach to measuring a meaningful change in perceptual fatigue is not appropriate (for example, a calculated small change of 0.3 is not possible when scores are only free to change by increments of 1 as with many recovery questionnaires). The combination of measured changes in neuromuscular function or performance can be employed with perceptual data to determine the fatigue status of a rugby player. For example, typical changes of approximately one to two (on a scale of one to five) in muscle soreness, fatigue, and attitude to training in the 48 hours after a rugby league match have previously been observed (Twist *et al.* 2012). A change of this magnitude, in addition to a meaningful change in neuromuscular function or performance, can be considered to be indicative of fatigue and required the initiation of rest or a given recovery strategy (see Chapter 7) until measures return to values close to baseline.

5.4 Conclusion

The rugby player is exposed to high-volume and high-stress activity that can lead to underperformance. Poor management leads to detrimental consequences for the player, such as performance decrements, increased injury potential, and poor health. Practitioners should employ a range of appropriate measurement tools that allow evaluation of the many facets contributing to player fatigue (see summary in Table 5.1). Selected tests should also be cost effective and easily embedded into the training schedule. Where these tests identify a risk to the player's health status, a more comprehensive understanding of the mechanisms underpinning fatigue should be investigated. Athletes and coaches must also be educated on the rationale for regular monitoring within the programme. This will ensure that data are not misinterpreted and are used to effectively manage the health status and performance potential of the athlete.

References

Abbiss, C.R. and Laursen, P.B. (2005). Models to explain fatigue during prolonged endurance cycling. *Sports Medicine*, 35, 865–98.

Abernethy, P., Wilson, G., and Logan, P. (1995). Strength and power assessment. *Sports Medicine*, 19, 401–17.

Achten, J. and Jeukendrup, A.E. (2003). Heart rate monitoring: applications and limitations. *Sports Medicine*, 33, 517–38.

Alaphilippe, A., Mandigout, S., Ratel, S., *et al.* (2012). Longitudinal follow-up of biochemical markers of fatigue throughout a sporting season in young elite rugby players. *Journal of Strength and Conditioning Research*, 26, 3376–84.

Argus, C.K., Gill, N.D., and Keogh, J.W.L. (2012). Characterization of the differences in strength and power between different levels of competition in rugby union athletes. *Journal of Strength and Conditioning Research*, 26, 2698–704.

Asp, S., Daugaard, J.R., Kristiansen S., *et al.* (1998). Exercise metabolism in human skeletal muscle exposed to prior eccentric exercise. *Journal of Physiology*, 509, 305–13.

Bangsbo, J., Mohr, M., and Krustrup, P. (2006). Physical and metabolic demands of training and match-play in the elite football player. *Journal of Sports Sciences*, 24, 665–74.

Barnes, M.J., Mundel, T., and Stannard, S.R. (2012). The effects of acute alcohol consumption on recovery from a simulated rugby match. *Journal of Sports Sciences*, 30, 295–304.

Beedie, C.J., Terry, P.C., and Lane, A.M. (2000). The profile of mood states and athletic performance: two meta-analyses. *Journal of Applied Sport Psychology*, 12, 49–68.

Bosquet, L., Papelier, Y., Leger, L., *et al.* (2003). Night heart rate variability during overtraining in male endurance athletes. *Journal of Sports Medicine and Physical Fitness*, 43, 506–12.

Bosquet, L., Merkari, S., Arvisais, D., *et al.* (2008). Is heart rate a convenient tool to monitor overreaching? A systematic review of the literature. *British Journal of Sports Medicine*, 42, 709–14.

Brancaccio, P., Maffulli, N., and Limongelli, F.M. (2007). Creatine kinase monitoring in sport medicine. *British Medical Bulletin*, 81/82, 209–30.

Cahill, N., Lamb, K., Worsfold, P., *et al.* (2013). The movement characteristics of English Premiership rugby union players. *Journal of Sports Sciences*, 31, 229–37.

Coutts, A.J., Wallace, L.K., and Slattery, K.M. (2007a). Monitoring changes in performance, physiology, biochemistry, and psychology during overreaching and recovery in triathletes. *International Journal of Sports Medicine*, 28, 125–34.

Coutts, A.J., Reaburn, P., Piva, T.J., *et al.* (2007c). Monitoring for overreaching in rugby league players. *European Journal of Applied Physiology*, 99, 313–24.

Coutts, A.J, Reaburn, P., Piva, T.J., *et al.* (2007d). Changes in selected biochemical, muscular strength, power, and endurance measures during deliberate overreaching and tapering in rugby league players. *International Journal of Sports Medicine*, 28, 116–24.

Cormack, S.J., Newton, R.U., and McGuigan, M.R. (2008a). Neuromuscular and endocrine responses of elite players to an Australian Rules football match. *International Journal of Sports Physiology and Performance*, 3, 359–74.

Cormack, S.J., Newton, R.U., and McGuigan, M.R., *et al.* (2008b). Neuromuscular and endocrine responses of elite players during an Australian Rules football season. *International Journal of Sports Physiology and Performance*, 3, 439–53.

Cormack, S.J., Newton, R.U., and McGuigan, M.R., *et al.* (2008c). Reliability of measures obtained during single and repeated countermovement jumps. *International Journal of Sports Physiology and Performance*, 3, 131–44.

Cormack, S.J., Mooney, M.G., Morgan, W., *et al.* (2013). Influence of neuromuscular fatigue on accelerometer load in elite Australian football players. *International Journal of Sports Physiology and Performance*, 8, 373–8.

Crewther, B.T., Sanctuary, C.E., Kilduff, L.P., *et al.* (2013). The workout responses of salivary-free testosterone and cortisol concentrations and their association with the subsequent competition outcomes in professional rugby league. *Journal of Strength and Conditioning Research*, 27, 471–6.

Cunniffe, B., Hore, A.J., Whitcome, D.M., *et al.* (2010). Time course of changes in immuneoendocrine markers following an international rugby game. *European Journal of Applied Physiology*, 108, 113–22.

Cunniffe, B., Hore, A.J., Whitcome, D.M., *et al.* (2011). Immunoendocrine responses over a three-week international rugby union series. *Journal of Sports Medicine and Physical Fitness*, 51, 329–38.

Dellal, A., Lago-Peñas, C., Rey, E., *et al.* (2013). The effects of a congested fixture period on physical performance, technical activity, and injury rate during matches in a professional soccer team. *British Journal of Sports Medicine*, doi: 10.1136/bjsports-2012-091290

Dias, J.A., Dal Pupo, J., Reis, D.C., *et al.* (2011). Validity of two methods for estimation of vertical jump height. *Journal of Strength and Conditioning Research*, 25, 2034–9.

Duffield, R., Murphy, A., Snape, A., *et al.* (2012). Post-match changes in neuromuscular function and the relationship to match demands in amateur rugby league matches. *Journal of Science and Medicine in Sport*, 15, 238–43.

Edmonds, R.C., Sinclair, W.H., and Leicht, A.S. (2013). Effect of a training week on heart rate variability in elite youth rugby league players. *International Journal of Sports Medicine*, 34, 1087–92.

Elloumi, M., Maso, F., Michaux, O., *et al.* (2003). Behavior of saliva cortisol (C), testosterone (T), and the T/C ratio during a rugby match and during the post-competition recovery days. *European Journal of Applied Physiology*, 90, 23–8.

Finaud, J., Scislowski, V., Lac, G., *et al.* (2006). Antioxidant status and oxidative stress in professional rugby players: evolution throughout a season. *International Journal of Sports Medicine*, 27, 87–93.

Fowles, J.R. (2006). Technical issues in quantifying low-frequency fatigue in athletes. *International Journal of Sports Physiology and Performance*, 1, 169–71.

Gabbett, T.J., Jenkins, D.G., and Abernethy, B. (2012). Physical demands of professional rugby league training and competition using microtechnology. *Journal of Science and Medicince in Sports*, 15, 80–6.

Gastin, P.B., Meyer, D., and Robinson, D. (2013). Perceptions of wellness to monitor adaptive responses to training and competition in elite Australian football. *Journal of Strength and Conditioning Research*, 27, 2518–26.

Gaviglio, C.M., Crewther, B.T., Kilduff, L.P., *et al.* (2014). Relationship between pre-game free testosterone concentrations and outcome in rugby union. *International Journal of Sports Physiology and Performance*, 9, 324–31.

Halson, S.L., Lancaster, G., Jeukendrup, A.E., *et al.* (2003). Immunological responses to overreaching in cyclists. *Medicine and Science in Sports and Exercise*, 35, 854–61.

Hartmann, U. and Mester, J. (2000). Training and overtraining markers in selected sport events. *Medicine and Science in Sports and Exercise*, 32, 209–15.

Hartwig, T.B., Naughton, G., and Searl, J. (2009). Load, stress, and recovery in adolescent rugby union players during a competitive season. *Journal of Sports Sciences*, 27, 1087–94.

Hedelin, R., Wiklund, U., Bjerle, P., *et al.* (2000). Cardiac autonomic imbalance in an overtrained athlete. *Medicine and Science in Sports and Exercise*, 32, 1531–3.

Heisterberg, M.F., Fahrenkrug, J., Krustrup, P., *et al.* (2013). Extensive monitoring through multiple blood samples in professional soccer players. *Journal of Strength and Conditioning Research*, 27, 1260–71.

Hopkins, W.G., Marshall, S. W., Batterham, A.M., and Hanin, J. (2009). Progressive statistics for studies in sports medicine and exercise science. *Medicine and Science in Sports and Exercise*, 41, 3–12.

Howatson, G. and Milak, A. (2009). Exercise-induced muscle damage following a bout of sport specific repeated sprints. *Journal of Strength and Conditioning Research*, 23, 2419–24.

Hunkin, S.L., Fahrner, B., and Gastin, P.B. (2014). Creatine kinase and its relationship with match performance in elite Australian Rules football. *Journal of Science and Medicine in Sport*, 17, 332–6.

Hynynen, E., Uusitalo, A., Konttinen, N., *et al.* (2006). Heart rate variability during night sleep and after awakening in overtrained athletes. *Medicine and Science in Sports and Exercise*, 38, 313–7.

Jennings, C.L., Viljoen, W., Durandt, J., *et al.* (2005). The reliability of the FitroDyne as a measure of muscle power. *Journal of Strength and Conditioning Research*, 19, 859–63.

Johnston, R.D., Gabbett, T.J., and Jenkins, D.G. (2013a). Influence of an intensified competition on fatigue and match performance in junior rugby league players. *Journal of Science and Medicine in Sport*, 16, 460–5.

Johnston, R., Gabbett, T.J., Seibold, A.J., *et al.* (2014). Influence of physical contact on neuromuscular fatigue and markers of muscle damage following small-sided games. *Journal of Science and Medicine in Sport*, 17, 535–40.

Johnston, R., Gibson, N.V., Twist, C., *et al.* (2013b). Physiological responses to an intensified period of rugby league competition. *Journal of Strength and Conditioning Research*. 27, 643–54.

Kellmann, M. and Kallus, K.W. (2001). *The recovery–stress questionnaire for athletes: User manual.* Champaign, IL: Human Kinetics.

Kenttä, G. and Hassmén, P. (1988). Overtraining and recovery: A conceptual model. *Sports Medicine*, 26, 1–16.

Komi, P. (2000). Stretch-shortening cycle: a powerful model to study normal and fatigued muscle. *Journal of Biomechanics*, 33, 1197–206.

Krustrup, P., Zebis, M., Jensen, J.M., *et al.* (2010). Game-induced fatigue patterns in elite female soccer. *Journal of Strength and Conditioning Research*, 24, 437–41.

Magalhães, J., Rebelo, A., Oliveira, E., *et al.* (2010). Impact of Loughborough Intermittent Shuttle Test versus soccer match on physiological, biochemical, and neuromuscular parameters. *European Journal of Applied Physiology*, 108, 39–48.

Malik, M. (1996). Heart rate variability: Standards of measurement, physiological interpretation, and clinical use. Task Force of the European Society of Cardiology and the North American Society of Pacing and Electrophysiology. *Circulation*, 93, 1043–65.

Margaritis, I., Tessier, F., Verdera, F., *et al.* (1999). Muscle enzyme release does not predict muscle function impairment after triathlon. *Journal of Sports Medicine and Physical Fitness*, 39, 133–39.

Marcora, S.M., Bosio, A., and de Morree, H.M. (2008). Locomotor muscle fatigue increase cardiorespiratory responses and reduces performance during intense cycling exercise independently from metabolic stress. *American Journal of Physiology – Regulatory, Integrative and Comparative Physiology*, 294, 874–83.

McGuckin, A., Sinclair, W.H., Sealey, R.M., *et al.*, (2014). The effects of air travel on performance measures of elite Australian rugby league players. *European Journal of Sport Science*, 14, S116–22.

McLean, B.D., Coutts, A.J., Kelly, V., et al. (2010). Neuromuscular, endocrine, and perceptual fatigue responses during different length between-match microcycles in professional rugby league players. *International Journal of Sports Physiology and Performance*, 5, 367–83.

McLellan, P.M., Lovell, D.I., and Gass, G.C. (2011a). Markers of a post-match fatigue in professional rugby league players. *Journal of Strength and Conditioning Research*, 25, 1030–39.

McLellan, P.M., Lovell, D.I., and Gass, G.C. (2011b). Biochemical and endocrine responses to impact and collision during elite rugby league match play. *Journal of Strength and Conditioning Research*, 25, 1553–62.

Meeusen, R., Duclos, M., Gleeson, M., *et al.* (2006). Prevention, diagnosis, and treatment of the Overtraining Syndrome. *European Journal of Sports Science*, 6, 1–14.

Moir, G., Shastri, P., and Connaboy, C. (2008). Intersession reliability of vertical jump height in women and men. *Journal of Strength and Conditioning Research*, 22, 1779–84.

Mougios, V. (2007). Reference intervals for serum creatine kinase in athletes. *British Journal of Sports Medicine*, 41, 674–8.

Morgan, W.P., Brown, D.R., Raglin, J.S., et al. (1987). Psychological monitoring of over-training and staleness. *British Journal of Sports Medicine*, 21, 107–14.

Nédélec, M., McCall, A., Carling, C., et al. (2012). Recovery in soccer: part I – post-match fatigue and time course of recovery. *Sports Medicine*, 42, 997–1015.

Plews, D.J., Laursen, P.B., Stanley, J., et al. (2013a). Training adaptation and heart rate variability in elite endurance athletes: opening the door to effective monitoring. *Sports Medicine*, 43, 773–81.

Plews, D.J., Laursen, P.B., Stanley, et al. (2013b). Monitoring training with heart rate variability: How much compliance is needed for valid assessment? *International Journal of Sports Physiology and Performance*, 9, 783–90.

Roberts, S.P., Stokes, K.A., Weston, L., et al. (2010). The Bath University rugby shuttle test (BURST): A pilot study. *International Journal of Sports Physiology and Performance*, 5, 64–74.

Robson-Ansley, P.J., Gleeson, M., and Ansley, L. (2009). Fatigue management in the preparation of Olympic athletes. *Journal of Sports Sciences*, 27, 1409–20.

Rowsell, G.J., Coutts, A.J., Reaburn, P., et al. (2009). Effects of cold-water immersion on physical performance between successive matches in high-performance junior male soccer players. *Journal of Sports Science*, 27, 565–73.

Rushall, B.S. (1990). A tool for measuring stress tolerance in elite athletes. *Journal of Applied Sports Psychology*, 2, 51–66.

Singh, T.K., Guelfi, K.J., Landers, G., et al. (2011). A comparison of muscle damage, soreness, and performance following a simulated contact and non-contact team sport activity circuit. *Journal of Science and Medicine in Sport*, 14, 441–6.

Smith, D.J. and Norris, S.R. (2000). Changes in glutamine and glutamate concentrations for tracking training tolerance. *Medicine and Science in Sports and Exercise*, 32, 684–9.

Skein, M., Duffield, R., Minett, G.M., et al. (2013). The effect of overnight sleep deprivation following competitive rugby league matches on post-match physiological and perceptual recovery. *International Journal of Sports Physiology of Performance*, 8, 556–64.

Sykes, D., Nicholas, C., Lamb, K., et al. (2013). An evaluation of the external validity and reliability of a rugby league match simulation protocol. *Journal of Sports Science*, 31, 48–57.

Takarada, Y. (2003). Evaluation of muscle damage after a rugby match with special reference to tackle plays. *British Journal of Sports Medicine*, 37, 416–9.

Taylor, K., Chapman, D.W., Cronin, J.B., et al. (2012). Fatigue monitoring in high performance sport: A survey of current trends. *Journal of Australian Strength and Conditioning*, 20, 12–23.

Twist, C. and Sykes, D. (2011). Evidence of exercise-induced muscle damage following a simulated rugby league match. *European Journal of Sports Science*, 11, 401–9.

Twist, C., Waldron, M., Highton, J., et al. (2012). Neuromuscular, biochemical and perceptual post-match fatigue in professional rugby league forwards and backs. *Journal of Sports Science*, 30, 359–67.

Waldron, M., Highton, J., and Twist, C. (2012). The reliability of a rugby league movement-simulation protocol designed to replicate the performance of interchanged players. *International Journal of Sports Physiology and Performance*, 8, 483–9.

Waldron, M., Worsfold, P., Twist, C., et al. (2011a). Concurrent validity and test-retest reliability of a global positioning system (GPS) and timing gates to assess sprint performance variables. *Journal of Sports Science*, 29, 1613–9.

Waldron, M., Twist, C., Highton, J., *et al.* (2011b). Movement and physiological match demands of elite rugby league using portable global positioning systems. *Journal of Sports Science*, 29, 1223–30.

Walsh, M., Cartwright, L., Corish, C., *et al.* (2011). The body composition, nutritional knowledge, attitudes, behaviors, and future education needs of senior schoolboy rugby players in Ireland. *International Journal of Sport Nutrition and Exercise Metabolism*, 21, 365–76.

Warren, G.L., Lowe, D.A., and Armstrong, R.B. (1999). Measurement tools used in the study of eccentric contraction-induced injury. *Sports Medicine*, 27, 43–59.

Wehbe, G., Gabbett, T., and Dwyer, D. (2014). Neuromuscular fatigue monitoring in team sport athletes using a cycle ergometer test. *International Journal of Sports Physiology and Performance*. In Press.

West, D.J., Finn, C.V., Cunningham, D.J., *et al.* (2013a). The neuromuscular function, hormonal, and mood responses to a professional rugby union match. *Journal of Strength and Conditioning Research*, 28, 194–200.

West , D.J , Cook , C.J., Stokes, K.A., *et al.* (2013b). Profiling the time-course changes in neuromuscular function and muscle damage over two consecutive tournament stages in elite rugby sevens players. *Journal of Science and Medicine in Sport*. http://dx.doi.org/10.1016/j.jsams.2013.11.003 [Epub ahead of print].

6

MATCH DAY STRATEGIES TO ENHANCE THE PHYSICAL AND TECHNICAL PERFORMANCE OF RUGBY PLAYERS

Mark Russell, Christian J. Cook, and Liam P. Kilduff

6.1 Introduction

Sports Scientists and Strength and Conditioning coaches associated with professional rugby teams spend the majority of the competitive season trying to ensure that the training and recovery strategies employed by their athletes will ensure optimal performance on the day of competition. However, there are additional opportunities on match days where performance can be optimized with a number of acute physiological and nutritional strategies. Although not mutually exclusive, these strategies can broadly be classified into two categories: 1) those that have primarily focused on enhancing physical performance outcomes, including an appropriately designed warm-up, heat maintenance strategies, post-activation potentiation (PAP), ischemic pre-conditioning (IPC), prior exercise, and hormonal priming; and 2) those that have focused on improved technical (i.e. skill) performance, which primarily includes the nutritional interventions of caffeine, creatine, and carbohydrate ingestion. This chapter aims to explore the potential practical use of these strategies and, where appropriate, to identify factors that modulate the efficacy of such interventions.

6.2 Strategies focused on enhanced physical performance

6.2.1 Warm-up

Warm-up routines are a widely accepted practice prior to nearly every athletic competition and typically include varying intensities of exercise, dynamic stretching, and technical practice in preparation for the subsequent activity. Fradkin *et al.* (2010) reported that 79% of studies investigating the effects of warm-up practices on subsequent physical performance observed improvements. Although a number of non-temperature related mechanisms have been proposed to explain the ergogenic effects of the warm-up (e.g. elevated baseline oxygen consumption, PAP, increased mental preparedness; Bishop 2003a, b), previous research has highlighted the role of increased muscle temperature (T_m) on performance. Strong associations between T_m and power output have been reported, with each 1°C increase in T_m equating to a 4% increase in power output (Sargeant 1987). Increases in T_m of ~3–4°C have been suggested to elicit an optimal warm-up effect (Mohr *et al.* 2004; Faulkner *et al.* 2013). To contextualize this, an active warm-up consisting of moderate intensity exercise (80–100% of the lactate threshold) produces rapid increases in T_m within 3–5min and reaches a relative equilibrium after ~10–20 minutes of exercise. However, few studies have sought to investigate strategies that seek to optimise warm-up practices (Ingham *et al.* 2013). It is therefore plausible that the warm-up strategies employed before rugby match-play also remain to be optimized, especially in relation to the intensity and duration separating the end of the warm-up and subsequent exercise.

The warm-up aims to smooth the transition from a state of rest to a state of exercise without inducing residual fatigue. Therefore, the intensity of the warm-up is a key consideration for the efficacy of this pre-competition strategy. It appears that an athlete's normal warm-up practices, especially in relation to exercise intensity, are typically less than optimal (Cook *et al.* 2013; Ingham *et al.* 2013). For example, increasing the intensity of a prior exercise bout from 300 m of striding (consisting of 6 × 50 m separated by a 45–60 s active recovery) to an equidistant warm-up incorporating 100 m of striding (2 × 50 m separated by a 45–60 s active recovery) and 200 m of race pace running resulted in a ~1% improvement in subsequent 800 m time trial performance (Ingham *et al.* 2013). Similarly, in elite bob-skeleton athletes, increasing the typical warm-up intensity by ~30% resulted in improved mean 20 m resisted sprint performances (Cook *et al.* 2013). It is yet to be determined whether similar benefits also exist when skilled as opposed to physical performance is the focus.

The rules and demands of competitive rugby matches mean that at the end of the warm-up there is a period of time that precedes kick-off when a physical warm-up can no longer be performed. With respect to international rugby matches, this delay might be prolonged by the requirements to undertake additional duties such as meeting with dignitaries and observing national anthems. The time delay between the end of the warm-up and the start of competition influences the efficacy of the warm-up procedures employed and the positive impact on performance (Cook *et al.* 2013; West *et al.* 2013b). Both T_m and T_{core} show substantial decreases during periods of inactivity after a warm-up (Mohr *et al.* 2004; West *et al.* 2013b). Notably, West and colleagues (2013b) demonstrated that a 40% rise in T_{core} gained through the warm-up was lost within 20 minutes of completing the process. Therefore, the timeframe separating the warm-up and the start of exercise must be considered when seeking to optimize the benefits of the preceding activity. It would appear that any longer than twenty minutes of recovery would reduce the effectiveness of the warm-up on subsequent exercise performance.

6.2.2 Heat maintenance strategies

Passive heat maintenance involves the use of an external heat source, such as heated clothing, outdoor survival jackets, and heating pads, which can be applied to the desired muscle groups to maintain post warm-up muscle temperature, and thus the temperature mediated pathways that will aid performance (Kilduff *et al.* 2013a; Cook *et al.* 2013; Kilduff *et al.* 2013b). For example, Cook *et al.* (2013) demonstrated a 65% greater tympanic temperature when an active warm-up was performed with an outdoor survival jacket. These results were also associated with an improvement in 20 m sled sprinting performance, when compared to a control condition. Similarly, a recent study by Kilduff *et al.* (2013b) demonstrated that repeated sprint performance and lower body peak power output were greater when professional rugby league players wore a blizzard survival garment during a 15 minute post-warm-up recovery period, compared to a control condition. The decline in lower body peak power output after the warm-up was related to the decline in T_{core} (r = 0.71; Kilduff *et al.* 2013b). Accordingly, maintaining body temperature during the post warm-up recovery period is vital to prevent decrements in subsequent performance. For athletes who are unable to perform a further active warm-up within the final 20 minutes preceding competition, passive heat maintenance offers an effective and practical method for preserving body temperature, which helps to combat the decrements in performance that might occur through the loss of T_m.

Although the half-time break is often considered crucial for primarily tactical and recovery reasons, it can be viewed as a 10–15 minute period of physiological preparation preceding the second half of a match. With this in mind, a number of studies have investigated strategies that seek to optimize half-time practices with the aim of improving intermittent sports performance in the second half. In soccer, Mohr *et al.* (2004) identified that moderate-intensity running commencing after seven minutes of a half-time recovery period attenuated a 1.5°C reduction in T_m and a 2.4% decrement in mean sprint performance observed in a passive control condition. Additionally, the decrease in T_m at half-time was correlated to the reduction in sprint performance observed during the half-time break (r = 0.60). Beneficial effects of active heat maintenance strategies have also been observed when different modes of exercise have been performed in the latter stages of the half-time period (e.g. intermittent agility exercise, whole body vibration, small-sided games, and lower body resistance exercises; Lovell *et al.* 2013; Zois *et al.* 2013). Interestingly, it appears that skilled performance is also maintained when technically focused half-time activities are performed (Zois *et al.* 2013). Although the evidence supporting the efficacy of active heat maintenance strategies are predominantly derived from soccer-based research, it is plausible that the half-time re-warm-up strategies benefiting soccer players will also be effective for rugby players.

6.2.3 Post-activation potentiation (PAP)

The ability of a muscle group to produce force can be influenced by the contractive history of that given muscle group (Kilduff *et al.* 2008). Although not all studies have demonstrated positive findings, a large body of research has shown that muscle performance can be acutely enhanced after a preloading stimulus due to PAP (Gouvea *et al.* 2013). After a preload stimulus, mechanisms of muscle potentiation and fatigue co-exist, and thus any resulting performance benefits are dependent on the balance between these two factors. Where transient benefits to physical performance have been observed and attributed to PAP, the mechanisms are suggested to relate to an increased sensitivity of the actin-myosin myofilaments to Ca^{2+}, enhanced motor neuron recruitment, and/or a more favourable central input to the motor neuron (Tillin and Bishop 2009). Not all studies have identified positive effects, with several factors modulating an athlete's ability to harness the effects of PAP, including the strength of the participant, volume and type of the preload stimulus, and the duration of recovery between the preload stimulus and subsequent activity.

Previous authors have observed differentiation of the PAP response according to the strength of the participant (Guillich and Schmidtbleicher 1996; Hamada *et al.* 2000; Gourgoulis *et al.* 2003). For example, using one repetition maximum (1RM) squat data and a mean split analysis, Gourgoulis *et al.* (2003) observed a greater countermovement jump height improvement between individuals who were deemed as being either strong or less strong (+4.01% and +0.42%, respectively). Similarly, a greater potentiation response resulted after a heavy preload stimulus (five sets of one repetition at 90% 1RM with two minute recovery) in athletes when compared to recreationally trained individuals (Chiu *et al.* 2003). Moreover, when junior elite rugby league players were differentiated according to their ability to squat against a resistance of twice their body mass, stronger players demonstrated the effects of PAP faster than their weaker counterparts and also demonstrated a greater magnitude of response (Seitz *et al.* 2014). Therefore stronger individuals might be better able to harness the effects of PAP, and correlations between 3RM strength and ΔPAP (i.e. difference between peak power output and baseline power output) would certainly support this supposition (r = 0.489; Kilduff *et al.* 2008).

From a mechanistic perspective, Gullich and Schmidtbleicher (1996) reported greater peak H-reflex responses (Athletes: $1.42 \pm 0.17\%$–42% vs. Students: $1.11 \pm 0.25\%$–11% potentiation) and an enhanced ability to maintain this response (Athletes: 8.1 ± 3.6 vs. Students: 5.9 ± 3.8 minutes) in athletes versus recreational sports students. Additionally, the relationships between the existence of PAP and type II fibre content might also explain this phenomenon (Hamada *et al.* 2000), as stronger individuals would have a higher proportion of fast twitch fibres which are associated with a greater capacity for myosin regulatory light chain phosphorylation (Grange *et al.* 1993). Irrespective of the mechanism(s) responsible, the strength of the rugby player should be considered when examining the suitability of PAP.

The importance of the volume of the preload stimulus was demonstrated by Hamada *et al.* (2003). During a fatiguing protocol of isometric maximal voluntary contractions of the knee extensors (16 × 5 s each separated by 3 s of rest), maximal twitches were evoked before the first contraction, during each 3 s rest period and at intervals during the 5 minute recovery period after the final contraction. A gradual increase of twitch peak torque occurred over the first three contractions, demonstrating a 127% increase from baseline values. However, twitch peak torque progressively decreased for the remainder of the trial with a reduction of 32% below baseline by the sixteenth contraction. This demonstrates that after an initial peak, as the volume of contractions continued to increase, so did fatigue. Interestingly, upon completion of the fatiguing protocol twitch peak torque gradually increased and exceeded baseline values after 30–120 s of recovery (+32%). This demonstrates that the decay of PAP was slower than the decay in fatigue; therefore a net potentiated response was observed during the recovery period.

Although Hamada *et al.* (2003) has provided evidence about the importance of training volume on the PAP response, the exercise modality used is different from what might commonly be employed by practitioners. For example, PAP has traditionally been induced through the use of multiple sets of heavy isotonic resistance exercise. Where a single set of heavy isotonic exercise has been performed, improvements in power production are primarily absent (Baker 2003; Jensen and Ebben 2003; Brandenburg 2005; McBride *et al.* 2005). Consequently, it appears that when trying to harness the effects of PAP, multiple sets of a preload stimulus should be programmed.

The majority of studies examining the PAP phenomenon have employed heavy (75–95% 1RM) resistance exercise as the preload stimulus. However, bearing in mind the practical considerations associated with the pre-competition practices of rugby players, this approach might not be feasible before a game. Therefore, methods of inducing PAP which require less equipment might be better tolerated by players and coaches on the day of competition. Ballistic activities such as weighted jumps are associated with the preferential recruitment of type II motor units (Desmedt and Godaux 1977), and therefore may be utilized as a PAP stimulus. Previous research has also reported that depth jumps are able to increase strength (Masamoto *et al.* 2003) and high velocity performance (Hilfiker *et al.* 2007), whilst the use of isometric maximal voluntary contractions induce PAP (Guillich and Schmidtbleicher 1996; Hamada *et al.* 2003).

Improvements in jumping performance have been observed in the 2-minute period after a preload stimulus that included jumps against a resistance of 2% body mass (via a weighted vest) during a dynamic warm-up (Faigenbaum *et al.* 2006). Similarly, although effects dissipated after 6 minutes, Chen *et al.* (2013) have reported improvements in countermovement jump height after multiple sets of depth jumps. Using 3 × 3 ballistic bench throws at 30% 1RM, West *et al.* (2013a) have reported that improvements in upper body power output occurred after an 8 minute recovery period and that the magnitude of this improvement in power output was similar to that induced by a more traditional heavy resistance exercise bout (i.e. 3 × 3 bench press at 87% 1RM). Therefore, ballistic activities might provide an alternative method of inducing a PAP response that is comparable in magnitude to that induced during heavy resistance exercise but might be preferable to players and staff on the day of a game.

The PAP response is a function of co-existing states of muscle fatigue and potentiation that are simultaneously present after a preload stimulus has been performed. Consequently, the transient effects of these two conditions dictate the extent of the ergogenic effect attributable to PAP; therefore the recovery time separating the preload stimulus and the subsequent activity is crucial. As the decay in the rate of potentiation is less than the rate of decay of fatigue (Hamada *et al.* 2003), optimized recovery between the preload stimulus and the subsequent exercise favours an acute enhancement of subsequent performance.

Recovery periods ranging from 0–24 minutes have previously separated the conditioning exercise and the subsequent explosive activity. However, relatively few studies have attempted to directly examine the optimal intra-complex recovery time. Jensen and Ebben (2003) examined recovery periods of 10 s, 1, 2, 3, and 4 min between the heavy resistance training and subsequent countermovement jumps, whilst Comyns *et al.* (2006) used recovery periods of 0.5, 2, 4, and 6 min. The relatively short recovery periods used in both of these studies might have contributed to the lack of effects on jump performance observed after heavy resistance training.

In a study incorporating professional rugby players and repeated assessments (i.e. baseline, ~15 s, and every 4 minutes) of explosive activity for 24 minutes after the preload stimulus (3 × 3 at 87% 1RM squat), Kilduff *et al.* (2008) identified that power output, peak rate of force development, and countermovement jump height were significantly elevated above baseline values at ~8 minutes of recovery for ~70% of participants. Similar findings have also been confirmed in upper body actions (Bevan *et al.* 2009). Although individual in nature, it appears that in both upper and lower body exercises a recovery period of ~8 minutes is an optimal timeframe separating the conditioning exercise and the subsequent explosive activity when seeking to harness the effects of PAP.

From a practical perspective, given the transient nature of the PAP response and the timeframe separating the end of the warm-up and the start of a rugby match, the benefit to performance could be limited to the initial stages of a player's involvement in subsequent competition. However, it has not yet been determined whether the tactical introduction of substitute players who have performed a preload stimulus (and thus induced a PAP response) can influence team performance at varying stages of a game or whether PAP could be used as part of a half-time strategy.

6.2.4 Ischemic pre-conditioning (IPC)

Ischemic pre-conditioning (IPC) involves the use of repeated bouts of skeletal muscle ischemia induced using a cuff or tourniquet, interspersed with periods of reperfusion to acutely enhance muscle function (Jean-St-Michel *et al.* 2011; Bailey *et al.* 2012). Mechanisms of IPC and enhanced performance relate to an increase in muscle blood flow resulting from changes in the function of intra-muscular ATP-sensitive potassium channels and adenosine concentrations. Increased blood flow improves oxygen delivery and speeds the clearance of various metabolites including the potential up-regulation of intra- and extra-cellular movement (Brooks 2000). In animal models it has also been proposed that IPC might also improve muscle force and contractility via increased efficiency of excitation contraction coupling (Pang *et al*. 1995). Enhanced efficiency of muscle contraction augments mitochondrial capacity, subsequently improving the balance between metabolic accumulation and removal.

In a protocol involving 4 x 5-minute bouts of bilateral occlusion at 220 mmHg, followed by 45 minutes of rest, Bailey *et al*. (2012) reported significant reductions in blood lactate accumulation and a subsequent 34 s improvement in 5,000 m running performance in a group of healthy males. Similarly, a ~1 per cent (equivalent to 0.7s) improvement in 100 m swim time-trial performance was observed 45 minutes after an upper limb IPC protocol that included 4 × 5 minute of occlusion by a cuff inflated to 15 mmHg greater than measured systolic arterial pressure (Jean-St-Michel *et al*. 2011). Therefore, when used in the hour preceding the start of a match, IPC could enhance the performance of rugby players on the day of competition. However, it must be noted that not all studies examining the effects of IPC in intermittent sports players have yielded positive results (Gibson *et al*. 2013).

6.2.5 Morning exercise

Circadian rhythms influence anaerobic performance, with evidence of an early morning nadir and a subsequent peak in the late afternoon. From an applied perspective, the potential influence of early morning physical activity on subsequent competition performed later in the day is interesting as most rugby matches will commence in the afternoon or evening. Testosterone (T) and cortisol (C) have been implicated in mediating performance in elite athletes (Cook and Crewther 2012b), and show circadian rhythmicity with an early morning peak followed by a transient decline through the day. As some exercise is known to raise T, it might prove beneficial to perform such activities on the morning of competition to offset the circadian decline in T that occurs thereafter.

Ekstrand *et al*. (2013) reported that a morning resistance training session improved afternoon throwing performance and that a six-hour window exists whereby performance in afternoon competitions could be influenced. Furthermore, Cook *et al*. (2014) reported that morning strength training was associated with improvements in countermovement jump peak power output, 40-meter sprint times, and 3RM bench and squat performance performed six hours later in rugby union players. Interestingly, Cook and colleagues (2013b) also reported that morning strength training offset the circadian decline in T; however, it is unclear whether these hormonal changes were causal in the improvements observed. Nevertheless, early evidence suggests that a bout of morning exercise might provide a priming effect, which could improve performance later in the day.

6.2.6 Hormonal priming

In addition to the benefits of elevated T on physical performance (e.g., positive cor-relation between baseline T concentrations and ability to produce power), evidence supports a potential link between endogenous T and aspects of athletic behaviour related to motivation and confidence to compete (Cook and Crewther 2012b). For example, free T concentrations have been positively associated with numerous offensive behaviours in Judo, as well success in both physical and non-physical tasks. Athletes are often engaged in pre-match talks with coaches that outline tactical practices (<2 h before to competition) and aim to motivate and instil confidence through the use of verbal persuasion (<1 h before to competition), with these strat-egies being reinforced through the warm-up and the final 20 minutes before com-petition; however, limited information about the effects of such practices is available. Watching successful skill execution by the athlete, reinforced with positive coach feedback promotes the highest pre-game T and best performance ratings (Cook and Crewther 2012b) when performed 75 minutes before a match. Conversely, videos of successful skill execution by an opposing player, accompanied with cautionary coach feedback produced larger C responses and worse performance ratings. Additionally, within 15 minutes of performance testing, Cook and Crewther (2012a) demonstrated that presenting highly trained males with aggressive or intense train-ing videos acutely raised T, which was associated with improved 3RM back squat performance. Therefore, within 75 minutes of a match, watching videos and receiv-ing associated feedback has the potential to influence hormonal and performance responses and might provide a suitable strategy for the preparation of rugby players before competition.

6.3 Strategies focused on enhanced technical performance

Interventions that influence the skills involved in rugby are likely to be of interest to those involved in the physical and technical preparation of rugby players. A growing body of evidence is emerging to support the role of selected nutritional strategies, primarily the consumption of caffeine, creatine, and carbohydrates, to attenuate reductions in skilled performance that might be attributable to fatigue induced by travel (Chapter 10) and/or match-related causes (Chapter 1).

6.3.1 Caffeine

Caffeine, a central nervous system stimulant, has been reported to enhance concen-tration, cognitive function, decision making, and reaction time during non-sports related tasks (Brice and Smith 2001; Haskell et al. 2005; Van Duinen et al. 2005). In a rugby passing accuracy task that incorporated attempts from dominant and non-dominant sides, caffeine (1 and 5 mg·kg^{-1} BM ingested 90 min before skill test-ing) attenuated the decrements associated with sleep deprivation (sleeping for 3–5 h) (Cook et al. 2011). Notably, no significant differences existed between the two doses of caffeine used. Therefore, consuming acute doses of caffeine 90 minutes before kick-off might be beneficial for rugby players, especially in those players who might have experienced disturbed sleep on the night before a match.

Caffeine has also been proposed to attenuate decrements in skilled performance, concentration or cognitive function that can occur during exercise (Foskett *et al.* 2009). For example, the mean performance of rugby passes made over the duration of a simulated match was improved when caffeine was administered (Stuart *et al.* 2005). Therefore, irrespective of whether the fatigue is travel- or match-related in origin, it appears that caffeine can be of benefit to rugby players.

Some debate exists over the time-course of peak systemic concentrations of caffeine and its metabolites after acute ingestion under either fed or fasted states (Skinner *et al.* 2013). Peak concentrations of caffeine and/or its metabolites are generally observed within one to three hours of ingestion. However, the efficacy of drug administration is related to its speed of absorption via the lower gastrointestinal tract (Ryan *et al.* 2013) and the antagonism of receptors in the upper gastrointestinal tract facilitating a central modulation of motor unit activity and adenosine receptor stimulation (Kalmar 2005).

Caffeinated chewing gums are associated with faster absorption times when compared to a traditional pill-based administration method (Kamimori *et al.* 2002). For example, Ryan *et al.* (2013) improved cycling performance when caffeinated gum containing 300 mg of caffeine was provided five minutes before exercise. Interestingly, providing the same dose 60 and 120 minutes before to the start of exercise negated the ergogenic effects observed. Despite very few studies having investigated the effects of this novel method of caffeine delivery, early evidence suggests that caffeinated gum could benefit the performance of rugby players. The speed of action of caffeinated gum means that it could also plausibly be consumed immediately before a game starts, during half-time, or during the match itself.

6.3.2 Creatine

Creatine has been found to ameliorate cognitive deficiencies induced by sleep deprivation (McMorris *et al.* 2006). Despite a tendency towards a dose response being observed, ingesting creatine (50 and 100 mg·kg⁻¹ BM) 90 minutes before performing a simulated rugby passing task attenuated a decline in skilled performance observed in players who had between 3 and 5 h of sleep on the night preceding testing (Cook *et al.* 2011). Therefore, an acute dose of creatine consumed 90 minutes before a match might benefit the skilled performances of rugby players, especially those who are sleep-deprived.

6.3.3 Carbohydrates

As the brain is primarily dependent on blood glucose concentrations for maintenance of optimal functioning (Duelli and Kuschinsky 2001), it is plausible that decision-making processes and the performance of the skills excuted during rugby match-play are also influenced by exogenous carbohydrate supply. Ingesting sucrose in the form of a 6 per cent carbohydrate-electrolyte beverage before (i.e. within 2 h of commencing exercise and within 5min of starting each half) and during (i.e. every 15 min of exercise) simulated soccer-specific exercise attenuated a decline in soccer shooting performance, specifically relating to the speed of the shots taken post-exercise (Russell *et al.* 2012). A considerable body of literature exists demonstrating the efficacy of carbohydrates on skilled actions in soccer (for a review see Russell and Kingsley 2011); however less support exists with regards to rugby-specific skills and the effects of carbohydrates on rugby skills and warrants further investigation.

Swilling carbohydrate solutions around the mouth before expectoration can positively influence the perception of effort during exercise (for a review see Rollo and Williams 2011) and facilitate increased peak power output during the initial stages of repeated sprint tests (Beaven *et al.* 2013). Such responses have been attributed to the excitation of reward and motor control centres in the brain (Chambers *et al.* 2009) and an increased excitability of the corticomotor pathways (Gant *et al.* 2010) via oral receptor stimulation. Although it remains to be determined whether the presence of carbohydrate in the mouth can facilitate improvements in the skilled performances of rugby players, the benefits of mouth swilling observed during exercise provide a rationale for using this strategy on the day of a match.

6.4 Conclusions

To date, the majority of available research would suggest that a well-structured warm-up (with the addition of heat maintenance strategies in the periods between exercise bouts), PAP, IPC, morning exercise, hormonal priming (through the use of videos), and caffeine, creatine, and carbohydrate consumption can improve the performance of sporting actions commonly executed by rugby players. Therefore Sports Scientists and Strength and Conditioning coaches involved in rugby should consider incorporating these strategies into their athletes practices on the day of competition.

Case study: a theoretical method of implementing multiple match-day strategies that enhance the physical and technical performances of rugby players

Introduction

Implementation of appropriately designed warm-ups, heat preservation strategies, post-activation potentiation (PAP), ischemic pre-conditioning (IPC), morning exercise, hormonal priming, and nutritional supplementation regimes (i.e. caffeine, creatine, and carbohydrate ingestion) positively influence physical and/or technical performance measures when used in isolation on the day of exercise. As most rugby matches commence later in the day (i.e. between 15:00 and 19:00h), sufficient time is available to implement a number of these acute interventions and elicit additive effects. Here we propose a theoretical model that incorporates multiple strategies and could contribute to a multifaceted match-day performance enhancement initiative.

Case presentation

Figure 6.1 provides an overview of typical practices adopted by professional rugby players on the day of a match. Generally, within two hours of a game and after travel to the match venue, a technical/tactical meeting between the team and coaching staff will occur. The preparations that follow might then become more individualized to a player's needs and focus on the organization of the playing kit, self-motivation strategies, one-to-one player/coach interactions, and provision of *ad hoc* medical/physiotherapy attention. A team-based pre-match warm-up will then be undertaken and hydro-nutritional strategies that seek to optimize a player's preparedness for subsequent exercise will continue during this period.

The match-day practices of professional rugby teams are very often structured and rigid in nature. It is therefore important that any proposed modification to the pre-match preparation period seeks to complement, rather than replace existing protocols. Therefore, practical guidelines on how to incorporate such strategies might be beneficial for the Sports Scientist and/or Strength and Conditioning coach. A theoretical model of organizing the pre-match period to incorporate both the practices currently employed and the strategies that we propose to acutely enhance performance is outlined in Figure 6.2.

Based on previous evidence relating to physical performance, a morning resistance exercise session performed six hours before a game could offer an effective strategy for optimized afternoon match performances (Cook *et al.* 2014; Ekstrand *et al.* 2013). A 20-minute resistance session that incorporates upper and lower body lifts of varying intensities (3 sets at 50, 70, 90, and 100% of 3RM separated by 90 s of recovery) has been found to be a time-efficient performance-enhancing strategy. Performing this session before travelling to the match venue might offer a practical method of implementing this strategy (Figure 6.2).

Once at the venue, players should consider the ingestion of caffeine, creatine, and carbohydrates, as enhanced physical and technical performance has been reported when these substances are consumed within 100 minutes of subsequent exercise (Cook *et al.* 2011; Russell *et al.* 2012). Thereafter, 60–75 minutes before kick-off, individualized footage of successful player executions supported by affirmative positive cues from a coach might also benefit performance (Cook and Crewther 2012a, b). However, if such videos focus upon the successful skill executions of opposing players whilst cautionary coach feedback is provided, an enhanced stress response can be observed (Cook and Crewther 2012b).

Repeatedly alternating bouts of ischemia (induced through the use of a cuff or tourniquet) and reperfusion, in a process known as IPC, can elicit performance benefits when the intervention is completed within 45 minutes of subsequent

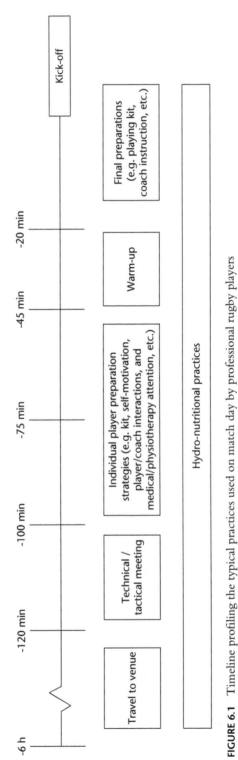

FIGURE 6.1 Timeline profiling the typical practices used on match day by professional rugby players

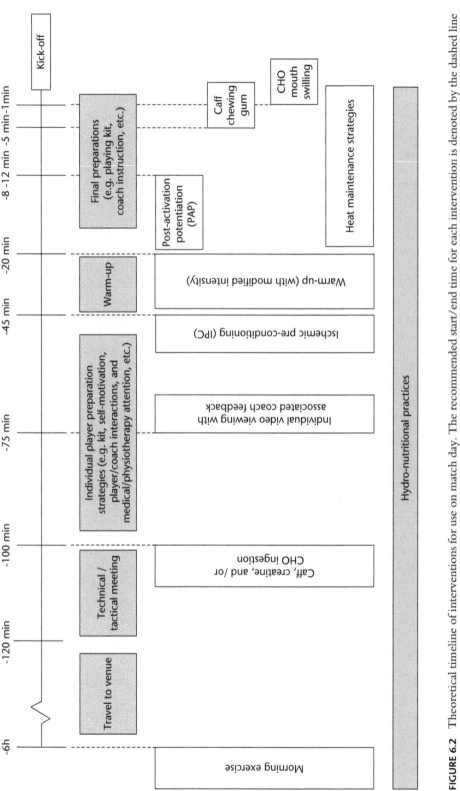

FIGURE 6.2 Theoretical timeline of interventions for use on match day. The recommended start/end time for each intervention is denoted by the dashed line attaching to either the left (start time) or right (end time) side of the box displaying the intervention strategy. Shaded boxes represent current practice whereas open boxes represent modified practice. Caff represents caffeine; CHO represents carbohydrate.

exercise (Jean-St-Michel *et al.* 2011; Bailey *et al.* 2012). Feasibly, IPC could be performed before the warm-up (Figure 6.2) or the warm-up could be modified to incorporate methods of inducing IPC. Similarly, the intensity of 'normal' warm-up practices is usually less than optimal (Cook *et al.* 2013), the Sports Scientist and/or Strength and Conditioning coach responsible for designing the warm-up should carefully consider the intensity of this pre-match strategy. Additionally, no longer than 20 minutes should separate the end of the warm-up and the start of the match (Figure 6.2).

Heated clothing, outdoor survival jackets, and heating pads can be applied to specific areas of the body to minimize muscle temperature loss in the post warm-up period (Kilduff *et al.* 2013a) and might prove especially worthwhile when players are likely to experience prolonged delays before the start of subsequent exercise (e.g. observing national anthems, waiting to be substituted onto the game, and/or between halves of play at half-time; Figure 6.2). Moreover, performing additional exercise in periods separating consecutive bouts might also prove beneficial.

When a suitable recovery time is implemented (i.e. between 8–12 minutes; Figure 6.2) enhanced performance of explosive activities has been observed when preceded by multiple sets of heavy (>75% 1RM) resistance exercise (Gouvea *et al.* 2013). Notably, ballistic activities targeting the musculature of the lower and upper body (e.g. weighted jumps at body mass + 2% and ballistic bench throws at 30% 1RM, respectively) have also been found to induce a PAP response (Faigenbaum *et al.* 2006; West *et al.* 2013a). As some studies have identified comparable PAP responses from ballistic versus traditional heavy resistance exercise (West *et al.* 2013a), ballistic exercises might provide a practical method of inducing PAP and improving subsequent performance during rugby match-play. However, it must be noted that muscular strength is associated with the magnitude of the PAP response; therefore, stronger individuals will likely demonstrate greater effects (Tillin and Bishop 2009).

The presence of caffeine and carbohydrates in the mouth has been found to facilitate motor output and improve subsequent exercise (Beaven *et al.* 2013; Ryan *et al.* 2013a). However, if the duration between the intake of the substance and the subsequent exercise is prolonged, the ergogenic effects of these substances can be lost (Ryan *et al.* 2013). Therefore, within the final five-minute period before kick-off, the provision of caffeinated gum and carbohydrate solutions (for the purposes of mouth swilling) should be considered (Figure 6.2).

Discussion

The support of previous authors for the use of a well structured warm-up means that a method which combines a number of the above strategies for use on the day of competition might be of interest to Sports Scientists and Strength and Conditioning coaches involved with rugby. We have presented a practical model that allows combination of a number of interventions that, individually, have been found to enhance the performance of actions involved in rugby match-play and could theoretically elicit additive effects over the use of such strategies in isolation.

References

Bailey, T.G., Jones, H., Gregson, W., *et al.* (2012). Effect of ischemic preconditioning on lactate accumulation and running performance. *Medicine and Science in Sports and Exercise*, 44, 2084–9.

Baker, D. (2003). Acute effect of alternating heavy and light resistances on power output during upper-body complex power training. *Journal of Strength and Conditioning Research*, 17, 493–7.

Beaven, C.M., Maulder, P., Pooley, A., *et al.* (2013). Effects of caffeine and carbohydrate mouth rinses on repeated sprint performance. *Applied Physiology, Nutrition, and Metabolism*, 38, 633–7.

Bevan, H. R., Owen, N.J. Cunningham, D.J., *et al.* (2009). Complex training in professional rugby players: influence of recovery time on upper-body power output. *Journal of Strength and Conditioning Research*, 23, 1780–5.

Bishop, D. (2003a). Warm up I: potential mechanisms and the effects of passive warm up on exercise performance. *Sports Medicine*, 33, 439–54.

Bishop, D. (2003b). Warm up II: performance changes following active warm up and how to structure the warm up. *Sports Medicine*, 33, 483–98.

Brandenburg, J.P. (2005). The acute effects of prior dynamic resistance exercise using different loads on subsequent upper-body explosive performance in resistance-trained men. *Journal of Strength and Conditioning Research*, 19, 427–32.

Brice, C. and Smith, A. (2001). The effects of caffeine on simulated driving, subjective alertness and sustained attention. *Human Psychopharmacology*, 16, 523–31.

Brooks G.A. (2000). Intra and extra cellular lactate shuttles. *Medicine and Science in Sports and Exercise*, 32, 790–9.

Chambers, E.S., Bridge, M.W., and Jones, D.A. (2009). Carbohydrate sensing in the human mouth: effects on exercise performance and brain activity. *The Journal of Physiology*, 587, 1779–94.

Chen, Z.R., Wang, Y.H. Peng, H.T., *et al.* (2013). The acute effect of drop jump protocols with different volumes and recovery time on countermovement jump performance. *Journal of Strength and Conditioning Research*, 27, 154–8.

Chiu, L.Z., Fry, A.C., Weiss, L.W., *et al.* (2003). Postactivation potentiation response in athletic and recreationally trained individuals. *Journal of Strength and Conditioning Research*, 17, 671–7.

Comyns, T.M., Harrison, A.J., Hennessy, L.K., *et al.* (2006). The optimal complex training rest interval for athletes from anaerobic sports. *Journal of Strength and Conditioning Research*, 20, 471–6.

Cook, C.J. and Crewther, B.T. (2012a). Changes in salivary testosterone concentrations and subsequent voluntary squat performance following the presentation of short video clips. *Hormones and Behavior*, 61, 17–22.

Cook, C.J. and Crewther, B.T. (2012b). The effects of different pre-game motivational interventions on athlete free hormonal state and subsequent performance in professional rugby union matches. *Physiology and Behavior*, 106, 683–8.

Cook, C.J., Crewther, B.T., Kilduff, L.P., *et al.* (2011). Skill execution and sleep deprivation: effects of acute caffeine or creatine supplementation – a randomized placebo-controlled trial. *Journal of the International Society of Sports Nutrition*, 8, 2.

Cook, C., Holdcroft, D., Drawer, S., *et al.* (2013). Designing a warm-up protocol for elite bob-skeleton athletes. *International Journal of Sports Physiology and Performance*, 8, 213–15.

Cook, C.J., Kilduff, L.P., Crewther, B.T., *et al.* (2014). Morning-based strength training improves afternoon physical performance in rugby union players. *Journal of Science and Medicine in Sport*, 17, 317–21.

Desmedt, J.E. and Godaux, E. (1977). Ballistic contractions in man: characteristic recruitment pattern of single motor units of the tibialis anterior muscle. *The Journal of Physiology*, 264, 673–93.

Duelli, R. and Kuschinsky, W. (2001). Brain glucose transporters: relationship to local energy demand. *News in Physiological Sciences*, 16, 71–6.

Ekstrand, L.G., Battaglini, C.L., McMurray, R.G., *et al.* (2013). Assessing explosive power production using the backward overhead shot throw and the effects of morning resistance exercise on afternoon performance. *Journal of Strength and Conditioning Research*, 27, 101–6.

Faigenbaum, A.D., McFarland, J.E., Schwerdtman, J.A., *et al.* (2006). Dynamic warm-up protocols, with and without a weighted vest, and fitness performance in high school female athletes. *Journal of Athletic Training*, 41, 357–63.

Faulkner, S.H., Ferguson, R.A., Gerrett, N., *et al.* (2013). Reducing muscle temperature drop after warm-up improves sprint cycling performance. *Medicine and Science in Sports and Exercise*, 45, 359–65.

Foskett, A., Ali, A., and Gant, N. (2009). Caffeine enhances cognitive function and skill performance during simulated soccer activity. *International Journal of Sport Nutrition and Exercise Metabolism*, 19, 410–23.

Fradkin, A.J., Zazryn, T.R., and Smoliga, J.M., (2010). Effects of warming-up on physical performance: a systematic review with meta-analysis. *Journal of Strength and Conditioning Research*, 24, 140–8.

Gant, N., Stinear, C.M., and Byblow, W.D. (2010). Carbohydrate in the mouth immediately facilitates motor output. *Brain Research*, 1350, 151–8.

Gibson, N., White, J., Neish, M., *et al.* (2013). Effect of ischemic preconditioning on land-based sprinting in team-sport athletes. *International Journal of Sports Physiology and Performance*, 8, 671–6.

Gourgoulis, V., Aggeloussis, N., Kasimatis, P. *et al.* (2003). Effect of a submaximal half-squats warm-up program on vertical jumping ability. *Journal of Strength and Conditioning Research*, 17, 342–4.

Gouvea, A.L., Fernandes, I.A., Cesar, E.P., *et al.* (2013). The effects of rest intervals on jumping performance: a meta-analysis on post-activation potentiation studies. *Journal of Sports Sciences*, 31, 459–67.

Grange, R.W., Vandenboom, R., and Houston, M.E. (1993). Physiological significance of myosin phosphorylation in skeletal muscle. *Canadian Journal of Applied Physiology*, 18, 229–42.

Guillich, A. and Schmidtbleicher, D. (1996). MVC-induced short term potentiation of explosive force. *New Studies Athletics*, 11, 67–81.

Hamada, T., Sale, D.G., MacDougall, J.D., *et al.* (2000). Postactivation potentiation, fiber type, and twitch contraction time in human knee extensor muscles. *Journal of Applied Physiology*, 88, 2131–7.

Hamada, T., Sale, D.G., MacDougall, J.D., *et al.* (2003). Interaction of fibre type, potentiation, and fatigue in human knee extensor muscles. *Acta Physiologica Scandinavica*, 178, 165–73.

Haskell, C.F., Kennedy, D.O., Wesnes, K.A., *et al.* (2005). Cognitive and mood improvements of caffeine in habitual consumers and habitual non-consumers of caffeine. *Psychopharmacology (Berlin)*, 179, 813–25.

Hilfiker, R., Hubner, K., Lorenz, T., *et al.* (2007). Effects of drop jumps added to the warm-up of elite sport athletes with a high capacity for explosive force development. *Journal of Strength and Conditioning Research*, 21, 550–5.

Ingham, S.A., Fudge, B.W., Pringle, J.S., *et al.* (2013). Improvement of 800-m running performance with prior high-intensity exercise. *International Journal of Sports Physiology and Performance*, 8, 77–83.

Jean-St-Michel, E., Manlhiot, C., Li, J., *et al.* (2011). Remote preconditioning improves maximal performance in highly trained athletes. *Medicine and Science in Sports and Exercise*, 43, 1280–6.

Jensen, R.L. and Ebben, W.P. (2003). Kinetic analysis of complex training rest interval effect on vertical jump performance. *Journal of Strength and Conditioning Research*, 17, 345–9.

Kalmar, J.M. (2005). The influence of caffeine on voluntary muscle activation. *Medicine and Science in Sports and Exercise*, 37, 2113–9.

Kamimori, G.H., Karyekar, C.S., Otterstetter, R., *et al.* (2002). The rate of absorption and relative bioavailability of caffeine administered in chewing gum versus capsules to normal healthy volunteers. *International Journal of Pharmaceutics*, 234, 159–67.

Kilduff, L.P., Finn, C.V., Baker, J.S., *et al.* (2013a). Preconditioning strategies to enhance physical performance on the day of competition. *International Journal of Sports Physiology and Performance*, 8, 677–81.

Kilduff, L.P., Owen, N., Bevan, H., *et al.* (2008). Influence of recovery time on post-activation potentiation in professional rugby players. *Journal of Sports Sciences*, 26, 795–802.

Kilduff, L.P., West, D.J., Williams, N., *et al.* (2013b). The influence of passive heat maintenance on lower body power output and repeated sprint performance in professional rugby league players. *Journal of Science and Medicine in Sport*, 16, 482–6.

Lovell, R., Midgley, A., Barrett, S., Carter, D., *et al.* (2013). Effects of different half-time strategies on second half soccer-specific speed, power, and dynamic strength. *Scandinavian Journal of Medicine and Science in Sports*, 23, 105–13.

Masamoto, N., Larson, R., Gates, T., *et al.* (2003). Acute effects of plyometric exercise on maximum squat performance in male athletes. *Journal of Strength and Conditioning Research*, 17, 68–71.

McBride, J.M., Nimphius, S., and Erickson, T.M. (2005). The acute effects of heavy-load squats and loaded countermovement jumps on sprint performance. *Journal of Strength and Conditioning Research*, 19, 893–7.

McMorris, T., Harris, R.C., Swain, J., *et al.* (2006). Effect of creatine supplementation and sleep deprivation, with mild exercise, on cognitive and psychomotor performance, mood state, and plasma concentrations of catecholamines and cortisol. *Psychopharmacology (Berlin)*, 185, 93–103.

Mohr, M., Krustrup, P., Nybo, L., *et al.* (2004). Muscle temperature and sprint performance during soccer matches – beneficial effect of re-warm-up at half-time. *Scandinavian Journal of Medicine and Science in Sports*, 14, 156–62.

Pang, C.Y, Yang, R.Z. Zhong, A., *et al.* (1995). Acute ischaemic preconditioning protects against skeletal muscle infarction in the pig. *Cardiovascular Research*, 29, 782–8.

Rollo, I. and Williams, C. (2011). Effect of mouth-rinsing carbohydrate solutions on endurance performance. *Sports Medicine*, 41, 449–61.

Russell, M., Benton, D., and Kingsley, M. (2012). Influence of carbohydrate supplementation on skill performance during a soccer match simulation. *Journal of Science and Medicine in Sport*, 15, 348–54.

Russell, M. and Kingsley, M. (2011). Influence of exercise on skill proficiency in soccer. *Sports Medicine*, 41, 523–39.

Ryan, E.J., Kim, C.H., Fickes, E.J., *et al.* (2013). Caffeine gum and cycling performance: a timing study. *Journal of Strength and Conditioning Research*, 27, 259–64.

Sargeant, A.J. (1987). Effect of muscle temperature on leg extension force and short-term power output in humans. *European Journal of Applied Physiology and Occupational Physiology*, 56, 693–8.

Seitz, L., Saez de Villarreal, E., and Haff, G.G. (2014). The temporal profile of postactivation potentiation is related to strength level. *Journal of Strength and Conditioning Research*, 28, 706–15.

Skinner, T.L., Jenkins, D.G., Folling, J., *et al.* (2013). Influence of carbohydrate on serum caffeine concentrations following caffeine ingestion. *Journal of Science and Medicine in Sport*, 16, 343–7.

Stuart, G.R., Hopkins, W.G., Cook, C., *et al.* (2005). Multiple effects of caffeine on simulated high-intensity team-sport performance. *Medicine and Science in Sports and Exercise*, 37, 1998–2005.

Tillin, N.A. and Bishop, D. (2009). Factors modulating post-activation potentiation and its effect on performance of subsequent explosive activities. *Sports Medicine*, 39, 147–66.

Van Duinen, H., Lorist, M.M., and Zijdewind, I. (2005). The effect of caffeine on cognitive task performance and motor fatigue. *Psychopharmacology (Berlin)*, 180, 539–47.

West, D.J., Cunningham, D.J., Crewther, B.T., *et al.* (2013a). Influence of ballistic bench press on upper body power output in professional rugby players. *Journal of Strength and Conditioning Research*, 27, 2282–7.

West, D.J., Dietzig, B.M., Bracken, R.M., *et al.* (2013b). Influence of post-warm-up recovery time on swim performance in international swimmers. *Journal of Science and Medicine in Sport*, 16, 172–6.

Zois, J., Bishop, D., Fairweather, I., *et al.* (2013). High-intensity re-warm-ups enhance soccer performance. *International Journal of Sports Medicine*, 34, 800–5.

7

RECOVERY STRATEGIES FOR RUGBY

Jamie Highton and Craig Twist

7.1 Introduction

Encouraging rapid and complete recovery after exercise is important, given the often congested competitive playing and training schedules for modern rugby players. Excluding nutritional intervention (see Chapter 8), this chapter will provide an overview of recovery strategies available to rugby players and will focus predominantly on recovery from exercise-induced muscle damage (EIMD).

7.2 Cryotherapy

Cryotherapy is one of the most common post-exercise recovery strategies used by athletes (Nédélec *et al.* 2013), with rugby players reporting the use of cryotherapy more than hockey, netball, and soccer players (Venter *et al.* 2010). Players also rate ice baths amongst the top five most important recovery strategies available to them, with international players considering their use to be more important than national or club standard players (Venter 2012). However, despite its prevalence and the sound theoretical basis, the evidence that cryotherapy improves post-exercise recovery is inconclusive.

7.2.1 Cryotherapy and functional recovery

The effects of cold-water immersion on recovery from eccentric and high-intensity exercise show moderate reductions in muscle soreness and CK efflux for up to 96 h post-exercise (Bleakley *et al.* 2012; Leeder *et al.* 2012a). However, cold-water immersion provides no further benefit for perceived muscle soreness compared to warm water or contrast water immersion. Bleakely *et al.* (2012) reported no effect of cryotherapy on muscle strength, power, or functional performance. However,

Leeder *et al.* (2012a) stated cold-water immersion improved recovery of muscle power up to 72 h post-exercise. The authors speculated that this could be due to an enhanced recovery of type II muscle fibres with cryotherapy, which are often preferentially damaged during eccentric-biased exercise (Brockett *et al.* 2002).

Cryotherapy can reduce perceived muscle soreness and, biochemical and functional markers of EIMD after intermittent exercise designed to simulate team sports activity. Against control conditions, cold-water immersion (~10–12°C for 10–12 min) applied immediately after prolonged (~60–90 min) exercise promotes recovery of biochemical markers (creatine kinase, myoglobin, and C-reactive protein), perceived soreness, muscle function, and repeated sprint performance in well-trained individuals (Bailey *et al.* 2007; Ascensao *et al.* 2011; Elias *et al.* 2012). Cold-water immersion also alleviates perceived soreness, fatigue, and systemic markers of EIMD and inflammation when conducted daily during tournaments in soccer (Rowsell *et al.* 2009) and basketball (Montgomery *et al.* 2008).

The effectiveness of cryotherapy after exercise that more closely resembles rugby match-play is difficult to determine because studies have used participants of varied training status, different cryotherapy modalities (including type, timing, and duration of exposure), varied control conditions (active vs. passive recovery, compression, stretching), different markers of muscle damage, and differing exercise protocols to elicit EIMD. Italian national rugby union players using five consecutive days of whole-body cryotherapy (30s at -60°C followed by 2 min at -110°C) after training reported lower CK and inflammatory cytokine (IL-2 and IL-8) responses than a control (Banfi *et al.* 2009). Similarly, Gill *et al.* (2006) examined recovery in elite male rugby union players who completed passive or active recovery, compression, or cold-water immersion immediately after a competitive rugby match. Increases in CK after the match were observed in all conditions. However, at 84 hours post-match, creatine kinase had recovered by 85-88% in the active recovery, compression, and contrast water immersion conditions and only by 39% in the passive recovery condition. Unfortunately neither of these studies reported functional markers of recovery.

Very few studies have examined the efficacy of cryotherapy after exercise involving collisions, the number of which are strongly correlated with the degree of EIMD observed after a rugby match (Twist *et al.* 2012). Pointon and Duffield (2012) examined recovery from a simulated match with 60 contacts in sub-elite rugby players exposed immediately to 2 x 9 min of cold-water immersion at 9°C or passive recovery. Voluntary activation of the quadriceps (~5%) and isometric peak torque (~12%) were enhanced immediately after the recovery intervention in the cold-water immersion condition, whilst muscle soreness was reduced (~20%) for up to two hours post-exercise. However, there were no differences between cold-water immersion and passive recovery observed for any markers of EIMD and inflammation at 24 h post-exercise, suggesting that the observed benefits were transient.

7.2.2 Mechanisms of tissue cooling

When cold is applied to the superficial tissue, a temperature gradient is created which results in heat being transferred from body tissues to the surrounding environment. Accordingly, the application of cold temperatures means there is an immediate decrease in skin temperature of approximately 0.35°C per second (Bleakley and Davison 2010). Associated changes in skin temperature with typical immersion protocols can therefore be between 10–20°C (White and Wells 2013).

Of greater clinical importance is the extent to which cryotherapy changes temperature of muscle tissue. Enwekema *et al.* (2002) examined thermodynamics of subcutaneous and muscle tissue before, during, and after a 20-minute application of a cold pack (stored at -15°C) on the quadriceps muscle. In the first five minutes of application, skin and cutaneous tissue 1 cm below the skin temperature lowered by ~2°C, whilst cooling at 2 and 3 cm (~1°C) only occurred one hour after removal of the cold pack. This delay in muscle cooling is caused by heat transfer from deep to superficial tissues and fluid exchange upon the removal of cold temperatures. Other studies have reported that muscle tissue can be cooled by 5–7°C when cold is applied superficially for ~20 min (Jutte *et al.* 2001). Interestingly, Myrer *et al.* (2001) observed that the rate of muscle tissue cooling in participants with <8 mm of subcutaneous adipose tissue was three times that of those with >20 mm (0.72°C per min cf. 0.25°C per min). Therefore, players with a higher body fat percentage (i.e. forwards) might require longer exposure to cryotherapy (~20 min) than backs (~10 min).

A lowered nerve conduction velocity of sensory neurons might explain reduced soreness with cryotherapy. Algafly and George (2007) reported a decrease in nerve conduction velocity of 33% associated with skin cooling to 10°C, equating to a 0.4 m·s⁻¹ decrease for every 1°C drop in skin temperature. This was associated with an increased pain threshold (~89%) and pain tolerance (~76%). Interestingly, one study has reported that cold-water immersion caused lowered nerve conduction velocity of sensory neurons more than application of a cold pack or ice massage (Herrera *et al.* 2011), which persisted for 30 minutes after cold application. The greater area of superficial cooling (where sensory neurons are located) associated with cold-water immersion might explain these observations.

Sensory nerve conduction velocity is slowed more than motor nerve conduction velocity with cryotherapy (Herrera *et al.* 2010), meaning that any ensuing change in muscle function and proprioception (position sense) might increase risk of injury in the period after cold application. Impairments in muscle strength and functional performance with cold application have been reported (Stanley *et al.* 2014), although evidence that joint position sense is altered is currently equivocal (Costello and Donnelly 2010). Nonetheless, athletes should not exercise in the immediate hours after cryotherapy to avoid any potential injury or impaired performance.

Reduced arterial blood flow to the muscle from cold-induced vasoconstriction might improve recovery with cryotherapy (Gregson *et al.* 2011). EIMD is associated with inflammation that results in vasodilation and increased capillary permeability at the site of injury (Smith *et al.* 2008). Increases in blood flow and an influx of inflammatory cells (resulting in an increased osmotic pressure in the muscle cell) increase the risk of oedema and haematoma formation. These processes can induce pain (Cleak and Eston 1992) and cause further damage to skeletal muscle proteins (Lieber and Friden 1999). Thus, a reduced blood flow and capillary permeability associated with cold application could theoretically improve markers of recovery.

Lowering muscle blood flow with cryotherapy potentially reduces the delivery of glucose to the muscle, raising concerns over reduced rates of muscle glycogen synthesis post-exercise. This would be particularly ergolytic for rugby performers, given the relationship between muscle glycogen and performance in team sports (Krustrup *et al.* 2006). However, when CHO (~0.6 g·kg^{-1}·h^{-1}) was provided three hours after glycogen depleting exercise, there were no differences in total glycogen synthesis (160 ± 34 vs. 157 ± 59 mmol·kg^{-1} dw) when completing 10 minutes of cold-water immersion or sitting in normal ambient conditions (Gregson *et al.* 2013). Thus, rugby practitioners need not be concerned with cryotherapy interfering with this facet of nutritional recovery.

7.2.4 Does the type of cryotherapy administered matter?

Cryotherapy can be administered via different techniques, each with different practical considerations and supposed advantages (Table 7.1). For example, an added benefit of cold-water immersion is the exertion of hydrostatic pressure on the body that acts to displace fluids from the periphery towards the central cavity, thus enhancing waste product removal and limiting oedema (Wilcock *et al.* 2006). Similarly, contrast water immersion might induce repeated vasodilation and vasoconstriction that would exert a 'pumping' effect to remove damaging metabolic waste products and oedema more than cold-water immersion alone (Vaile *et al.* 2007). Increases in CK and leukocyte responses (Pournot *et al.* 2011) and reductions in muscle function (Ingram *et al.* 2009) after prolonged intermittent exercise appear less dramatic after cold-water immersion when compared against contrast water immersion. Conversely, improved recovery of muscle function, CK and muscle soreness after a rugby league match was reported with contrast water therapy compared to cold-water immersion (Webb *et al.* 2013). The lack of agreement on studies comparing cold-water immersion and contrast water therapy is probably explained by the heterogeneity of damaging exercise, cryotherapy protocols, and recovery markers (White and Wells 2013). However, both methods appear superior for promoting recovery when compared to temperate water immersion and passive recovery (Pournot *et al.* 2011; Webb *et al.* 2013). Such findings reinforce the additive effect of cold temperature to facilitate recovery.

7.2.5 Timing, duration, and temperature

The typical exposure time and temperature for cryotherapy that show improved recovery are 10–20 min and 10–15°C, respectively (Versey *et al.* 2013). This suggests

TABLE 7.1 Types of cryotherapy used to enhance recovery of performance.

Method	Method details	Temp	Typical exposure	Potential advantages (+) and disadvantages (−)
Ice pack	Ice and gel packs or bagged frozen food applied to skin.		5 to 20 min	+ Applied to localized area + Cheap − Risk of tissue/nerve damage and frostbite if too cold (<0°C) and applied directly
Ice massage	Ice, usually frozen in a paper cup, applied to skin in circular and stroking motion.		5 to 20 min	+ Localized + Added benefits of massage to recovery − Tissue/nerve damage as above
Cold-water immersion/ Ice bath	Immersion in water containing ice/ice bags up to the legs or neck. Water often agitated to prevent thermal boundary layer.	10 to 15°C	10 to 20 min	+ Water might exert beneficial hydrostatic pressure − Logistically difficult to use with a team
Contrast water therapy	Alternating 1 or 2 min cold to hot (can use a hot shower).	Cold − 10°C Hot − 40°C	10 to 15 min	+ Beneficial hydrostatic pressure as above − Logistically difficult − Not as effective as cold–water immersion
Whole-body cryotherapy	Exposure to dry air in a specialised chamber.	−80 to −110°C	1 to 3 min	+ Requires little time − Requires specialist equipment − Expensive − Limited research

muscle tissue can be cooled in this amount of time with adequate participant tolerance and without the risk of nerve or tissue damage. Few attempts have been made to establish a dose–response relationship between time/temperature and recovery. Vaile *et al.* (2008c) compared immersion in 10, 15, and 20°C water for five minutes after 30 minutes of cycling, reporting no difference in recovery of cycling performance 40 minutes after recovery in any condition. Versey *et al.* (2011) further observed that contrast water therapy for six and twelve minutes accelerated recovery of sprint and time-trial cycling performance two hours after 75 minutes of intermittent cycling compared to eighteen-minute exposures. It is interesting that immediate post-exercise cold-water immersion (15°C for 15 min) resulted in enhanced intermittent running capacity 24 hours post-exercise compared to the same immersion protocol completed three hours post-exercise (Brophy-Williams *et al.* 2011). Accordingly, immersion for approximately ~10 min at 10°C immediately after exercise would appear to be the most appropriate method to enhance recovery.

7.3 Compression

The use of compression garments to enhance recovery in team sports is less prevalent than cryotherapy and is deemed less important (Venter 2012). However, the availability, anecdotal evidence, and marketing of these whole and partial body garments mean their popularity is growing. Garments can exert constant pressure or be 'graduated', such that higher pressure is exerted distally (e.g. at the ankle) and a lower pressure is exerted proximally (e.g. at the knee). Commercially available compression garments exert a pressure of ~ 18mmHg (compared to 40–50 mmHg used in clinical settings), whilst graduated compression garments typically exert ~18 mmHg distally and 8–10 mmHg proximally. However, pressures are often not reported in studies, making it difficult to determine the optimal compression garment for recovery.

7.3.1 Mechanisms and practical considerations with compression garments

Mechanisms for enhanced recovery with compression garments have generally been extrapolated from observations in clinical populations, where these items are used to exert a pressure gradient that reduces the available space for swelling to occur (MacRae *et al.* 2011). Reduced oedema and heametoma formation associated with EIMD and subsequent inflammation with compression could theoretically enhance recovery for rugby players. Compression might also reduce muscle oscillation and provide muscle stability to reduce initial EIMD, reduced venous pooling, and enhance venous return, and thus enhance the removal of metabolic waste products and noxious stimuli (Kraemer *et al.* 2004).

Insufficient evidence exists to propose the best compression garment to wear, the duration of compression, the pressure exerted by the garment, or whether graduated compression garments are more effective than constant pressure garments. Higher pressures exerted whilst supine (20–30 mmHg cf. 10 mmHg) result in a higher vein blood flow velocity (Lawrence and Kakkar 1980). However, after standing (Liu et al. 2008) or post-exercise (Mayberry et al. 1991), vein blood flow was not affected by compression pressure. Miyamoto et al. (2011) reported lower post-exercise neuromuscular fatigue when comparing graduated compression stockings of different pressures (ankle = 30 mmHg, calf = 25 mmHg, knee = 10 mmHg c.f. 18, 12, and 17 mmHg at the corresponding sites). Future studies following different forms of exercise, with participants of different training status, are required to support this finding. Studies that have reported positive effects of compression have typically used exposures of 12 to 72 h; therefore, if rugby players do choose to employ compression, this time frame is recommended. However, there is currently no clear association between the duration of compression and rate of recovery. One consideration should be an increase in skin temperature whilst wearing compression garments (Duffield et al. 2010), which could potentially interfere with sleep quality if worn overnight.

7.3.2 Compression, performance, and recovery

Worn during exercise, compression garments are reported to improve proprioception (Kraemer et al. 1998), lower perceived muscle soreness (Ali et al. 2007), increase skin temperature (Duffield et al. 2010), and reduce oxygen cost of running (Bringard et al. 2006). Conversely, wearing compression garments has shown no effect on single and repeated 20-m sprint time, power produced on a single man scrum machine, and jump performance during simulated team sport in rugby players (Duffield et al. 2008; Duffield et al. 2010).

Lower perceived muscle soreness is also reported when compression garments are worn after exercise (Jakeman et al. 2010; Kraemer et al. 2001; Kraemer et al. 2010). However, improved recovery of muscle function (strength and power) and performance after damaging exercise was only reported in two of these studies (Jakeman et al. 2010; Kraemer et al. 2001). Wearing a full-length lower limb compression garment (~18 mmHg) in the post-game and overnight period (~18 h) during a three-day basketball tournament was also no more effective than passive recovery for reducing muscle soreness, CK, myoglobin, and inflammatory markers (Montgomery et al. 2008).

Despite their popularity, the effects of compression garments on functional recovery after rugby-type exercise appears limited. Gill et al. (2006) reported an 84.4% recovery of plasma CK 72 h after elite rugby union players wore a lower body compression garment for 12 h after a rugby union match. This was in contrast to passive recovery that only resulted in a 39% recovery of CK. Hamlin et al. (2012) reported improvements in mean sprint time during 10 x 40 m sprints (~1%) and 3 km run time (~2%) after an 84 min rugby-specific circuit in well-trained male rugby union players. This was accompanied by a ~42% reduction in muscle soreness and no difference in CK 24 hours after. Conversely, Duffield et al. (2008)

reported that wearing a lower body compression garment after a rugby simulation and training activities, compared to normal training attire, did not improve recovery of muscle function, power production during scrummaging, or inflammatory markers. However, perceived muscle soreness was significantly lower 24 h after exercise in the compression condition compared to the control.

7.4 Massage

Whilst elite rugby players often report using massage to help recovery (Venter *et al.* 2010), they do not rank it amongst the top five recovery strategies available to them (Venter 2012). Massage might enhance recovery via an increased muscle blood flow, decreased neuromuscular excitability, reduced passive and active stiffness, prevention of muscle spasm, stimulated parasympathetic activity with associated reduction in resting cortisol concentration, analgesia associated with neurological stimulation of nerve fibres, realignment of muscle fibres, and improved mood (for a review, see Weerapong *et al.* 2005). However, little evidence exists to support many of these mechanisms. For example, the application of massage does not increase muscle blood flow measured using the Doppler ultrasound method (Shoemaker *et al.* 1997). In turn, massage has failed to reduce postexercise lactate (Hinds *et al.* 2004), H^+ accumulation (Wiltshere *et al.* 2010), or neutrophil count (Hilbert *et al.* 2003). Similarly, massage does not offset losses of muscle strength or performance in the days after damaging exercise (Hemmings *et al.* 2000; Hilbert *et al.* 2003). Effects on perceived muscle soreness have been more favourable (Hemmings *et al.* 2000; Hilbert *et al.* 2003), although they are not conclusive. Accordingly, massage is likely to confer little benefit with regard to functional recovery for rugby players.

7.5 Stretching and low-intensity exercise

Stretching (i.e. static, dynamic/ballistic, or proprioceptive neuromuscular facilitation) is commonly incorporated into team sports players' training and pre-exercise warm-ups (Dadebo *et al.* 2004). This is often in an attempt to enhance flexibility, reduce injury risk, and enhance post-exercise recovery. Each of these types of stretching improves range of motion and flexibility (Thacker *et al.* 2004). However, a meta-analysis reported that stretching before and/or after exercise resulted in negligible changes in perceived muscle soreness 24 hours after exercise and that injury risk was not reduced by stretching pre-exercise (Herbert and Gabriel 2002). Dawson *et al.* (2005) reported that 15 minutes of static stretching performed immediately after an Australian Rules football game was no more effective than passive recovery for improving muscle soreness, vertical jump height, and 6 s cycle power output 48 h after exercise. Montgomery *et al.* (2008) also reported that static stretching for 10 min was ineffective in reducing biochemical markers of muscle damage and inflammation in the days after basketball match-play. Thus, there appears to be little beneficial effect of pre- or post-exercise stretching with regard to recovery for rugby players.

Indeed, static stretching can impair immediate repeated-sprint and agility performance in team-sport players (Beckett *et al.* 2009), such that rugby players might wish to avoid stretching inbetween exercise bouts when match-play is imminent, e.g. interchanges.

Low-intensity exercise increases blood flow to damaged muscle, and also improves metabolite clearance post-exercise (Mondero and Donne 2000). Low-intensity exercise (cycling at 60% VO_{2max} and resistance training at <50% 1RM) performed 22 h and 46 h after a soccer match provided no effect on recovery of neuromuscular function, muscle soreness, or biochemical markers of inflammation (Andersson *et al.* 2008; Andersson *et al.* 2010). This is in contrast to studies employing low intensity cycling (Gill *et al.* 2006) or one hour of water-based exercise (Suzuki *et al.* 2004) immediately after a rugby match; such studies have reported lower creatine kinase and an improved mood state in the days after. However, neither of these studies examined recovery of muscle function, and so there is currently insufficient evidence that low-intensity exercise improves post-exercise recovery in rugby players.

7.6 Sleep

Whilst sleep is not a recovery strategy *per se*, adequate quality of sleep is an integral component of successful restoration of athletic performance (Halson 2008). This is particularly important given the positive association between sleep and anabolic processes that promote healing after damaging exercise (Adams and Oswald 1984). Extended periods of sleep deprivation (i.e. >24–30 h) in athletes cause decrements in physiological (Skein *et al.* 2011) and psychological function (Blumert *et al.* 2007). However, rugby players are more likely to experience partial sleep deprivation because of evening matches, travel, social issues, caffeine and alcohol consumption, hyper-hydration, or a combination of these. Such sleep deprivation after a rugby match leads to poorer recovery of jump performance and cognitive function in the days after (Skein *et al.* 2013). Whilst such changes might be an artefact of a nocebo effect, they reinforce that appropriate sleep hygiene (behaviours associated with the quality and quantity of sleep) is important in the recovery process.

Sleep habits of elite athletes compared to age and sex-matched controls over a four-day period indicate longer time in bed (8:36 ± 0:53 h:min) but longer time to fall to sleep (18.2 ± 16.5 min vs. 5.0 ± 2.5 min) and lower sleep efficiency (80.6 ± 6.4 vs. 88.7 ± 3.6%), respectively (Leeder *et al.* 2012b). These data indicate that athletes experience comparable quantity but poorer quality of sleep when compared to the general population. Sleep might also be disturbed before important matches, with two-thirds of athletes reporting poor sleep on at least one occasion in the nights before an important competition (Juliff *et al.* 2014). The main sleep problem specified by athletes was difficulty falling asleep (82.1%) attributed to thoughts about the competition (84%) and nervousness (44%). Interestingly, ~60% of team sport athletes reported having no strategy to overcome poor sleep compared with individual athletes (~33%), who employed relaxation and reading to overcome sleeping problems

(Juliff *et al*. 2014). Rugby players should therefore be encouraged to improve their sleep hygiene by incorporating simple measures such as avoiding caffeine, alcohol, and large volumes of fluid before bedtime; skin warming and cooling in cool and warm environments, respectively; reducing sensory input through eye masks and ear plugs; and adopting a regular bedtime when possible (Halson 2008).

7.7 The repeated-bout effect

Prior exposure to similar exercise affords a protective effect for subsequent exercise bouts termed the 'repeated-bout effect' (RBE). Indeed, prior exposure to damaging exercise attenuates strength loss, muscle soreness, and biochemical disturbances (Nosaka *et al*. 2001b). The mechanism for this protection is poorly understood, but is hypothesised to involve neural, mechanical, and cellular adaptations (McHugh 2003), with the effects reported to last for up to six months (Nosaka *et al*. 2001a).

Whilst RBE could be useful to rugby players to enhance recovery in subsequent bouts of exercise, the majority of studies examining the phenomenon are in untrained populations who have had little or no prior exposure to resistance training. Falvo *et al*. (2007) examined the protective effect of 100 eccentric actions on the bench press two weeks before doing the same exercise in a group of resistance-trained males. Whilst muscle soreness was reduced in the days after the second bout of exercise, there was no attenuated decrement in maximal isometric force production or bench throw power output associated with prior eccentric exercise. In agreement, Falvo *et al*. (2008) reported that the same protocol resulted in no attenuated strength loss or altered electromyographical activity in resistance-trained participants, thus indicating that no neurological adaptation takes place with repeated bouts of damaging exercise in trained individuals. As such, it would appear that adaptation to bouts of damaging exercise is more likely to be observed in individuals who have experienced little adaptation to EIMD associated with training. This has implications for rugby players given their highly trained nature and exposure to previous damaging exercise on a regular basis.

Interestingly, the RBE is not evident when performing repeated bouts of intermittent running. Using well-trained team sport athletes, Leeder *et al*. (2014) examined recovery after completing 90 minutes of intermittent shuttle running on two occasions, 14 days apart. Maximal isometric force production, counter-movement jump height, creatine kinase activity, C-reactive protein, and IL-6 were all equally affected by both bouts of shuttle running, with only muscle soreness being lower after the second trial. Accordingly, exposing rugby players to specific muscle-damaging exercise in an attempt to enhance subsequent post-match recovery is likely to be of little value.

7.8 Athlete perceptions of recovery and the placebo effect

The subjectivity of perceptual measures, coupled with the increased popularity of cryotherapy or compression garments, means an athlete's belief that an intervention will work might be fundamental to the recovery achieved. Indeed, when athletes were falsely instructed (i.e., placebo) that a thermo-neural water immersion condition contained a new recovery oil, recovery of muscle function was superior to a thermo-neural water immersion condition, but similar to cold-water immersion (Broatch *et al.* 2014). Similarly, Cook and Beaven (2013) reported a strong association between an individual's perception of the recovery strategy and its actual effectiveness. Well-trained rugby players used cold-water immersion after an intense training session, with those reporting a more favourable view of the intervention showing better recovery of repeated sprint performance in the days after (Cook and Beaven 2013). Such findings imply that the beneficial effects of the recovery interventions employed by rugby players are, in part, the result of a placebo effect. In employing appropriate recovery strategies, practitioners should base choices on sound underpinning evidence but not be afraid to embrace the potential benefits of a placebo.

7.9 Recovery strategies and training adaptation

Whilst some strategies are likely to exert beneficial effects on post-exercise recovery for rugby players on an acute basis, little is known about the long-term effects of chronic exposure to most recovery strategies. For example, concerns have been raised that chronic exposure to cryotherapy could blunt adaptations to training by interfering with post-exercise inflammation (White and Wells 2013). Inflammation can act as a signal for subsequent regenerative/adaptive processes, including proliferation and incorporation of satellite cells to form new muscle sarcomeres and capillary growth associated with tissue hypoxia (Yamane *et al.* 2006; Toth *et al.* 2011). Further research in this area is warranted to determine if such effects are present in elite athletes. Until clearer insight is provided, it might be considered prudent to limit aggressive recovery treatments in rugby players to periods of the season when training adaptation is not a target or there is a short turnaround time between matches.

7.10 Conclusions

Cryotherapy appears as the most widely used therapeutic recovery modality in elite sport. Whilst more research is required to determine the optimal type, timing, and duration of cryotherapy, immediate post-exercise cold-water immersion for 10 to 15 minutes at 10°C seems likely to elicit the most favourable effects on recovery in rugby players. The efficacy of compression garments with regard to enhancing recovery is currently unclear. Whether it is in recovery from resistance, endurance training or rugby match-play, worthwhile benefits are likely to be confined to improvements in perceived soreness and not functional recovery. Other modes of recovery, such as massage, stretching, and active recovery, seem less appealing to the rugby player. That the benefits associated with several recovery modalities are influenced by the individual's perception of recovery means a potential placebo effect cannot be ruled out. Without increasing the risk of injury or where adaptation is not the focus (i.e. pre-season), practitioners might wish to harness such benefits in an attempt to optimize recovery.

References

Adam, K. and Oswald, I. (1984). Sleep helps healing. *British Medical Journal*, 289, 56–64.

Algafly, A.A. and George, K.P. (2007). The effect of cryotherapy on nerve conduction velocity, pain threshold, and pain tolerance. *British Journal of Sports Medicine*, 41, 365–9.

Ali, A., Caine, M.P., and Snow, B.G. (2007). Graduated compression stockings: physiological and perceptual responses during and after exercise. *Journal of Sports Sciences*, 25, 413–9.

Andersson, H., Behn, S.K., Raastad, T., *et al.* (2010). Differences in the inflammatory plasma cytokine response following two elite female soccer games separated by a 72h recovery. *Scandinavian Journal of Medicine and Science in Sports*, 20, 740–7.

Andersson, H., Raastad, T., Nilsson, J., *et al.* (2008). Neuromuscular fatigue and recovery in elite female soccer: effects of active recovery. *Medicine and Science in Sports and Exercise*, 40, 372–80.

Ascensao, A., Leite, M., Rebelo, A.N., *et al.* (2011). Effects of cold-water immersion on the recovery of physical performance and muscle damage following a one-off soccer match. *Journal of Sports Sciences*, 29, 217–25.

Bailey, D.M., Erith, S.J., Griffin, P.J., *et al.* (2007). Influence of cold-water immersion on indices of muscle damage following prolonged intermittent shuttle running. *Journal of Sports Sciences*, 25, 1163–70.

Banfi, G., Melegati, G., Barassi, A., *et al.* (2009). Effects of whole-body cryotherapy on serum mediators of inflammation and serum muscle enzymes in athletes. *Journal of Thermal Biology*, 34, 55–9.

Beckett, J.R.J., Schneiker, K.T., Wallman, K.E., *et al.* (2009). Effects of static stretching on repeated sprint and change of direction performance. *Medicine and Science in Sports and Exercise*, 41, 444–50.

Bleakley, C. and Davison, G.W. (2010). What is the biochemical and physiological rationale for using cold-water immersion in sports recovery? A systematic review. *British Journal of Sports Medicine*, 44, 179–87.

Bleakley, C., McDonough, S., Gardner, E., *et al.* (2012). Cold-water immersion (cryotherapy) for preventing and treating muscle soreness after exercise. *Cochrane Database of Systematic Reviews*, 2, 1–127.

Blumert, P.A., Crum, A.J., Ernsting, M., *et al.* (2007). The acute effects of twenty-four hours of sleep loss on the performance of national-calibre male collegiate weightlifters. *Journal of Strength and Conditioning Research*, 21, 1146–54.

Bringard, A., Perrey, S., and Belluye, N. (2006). Aerobic energy cost and sensation responses during submaximal running exercise: positive effects of wearing compression tights. *International Journal of Sports Medicine*, 27, 373–8.

Broatch, J.R., Petersen, A., and Bishop, D.J. (2014). Post-exercise cold-water immersion benefits are not greater than the placebo effect. *Medicine and Science in Sports and Exercise*, doi: 10.1249/MSS.0000000000000348

Brockett, C.L., Morgan, D.L., Gregory, J.E., *et al.* (2002). Damage to different motor units from active lengthening of the medial gastrocnemius muscle of the cat. *Journal of Applied Physiology*, 92, 1104–10.

Brophy-Williams, N., Landers, G., and Wallman, K. (2011). Effect of immediate and delayed cold water immersion after a high-intensity exercise session on subsequent run performance. *Journal of Sports Science and Medicine*, 10, 665–70.

Cook, C.J. and Beaven, C.M. (2013). Individual perception of recovery is related to subsequent sprint performance. *British Journal of Sports Medicine*, 47, 705–9.

Costello, J.T. and Donnelly, A.E. (2010). Cryotherapy and joint position sense in healthy participants: A systematic review. *Journal of Athletic Training*, 45, 306–16.

Chesterton, L.S., Foster, N.E., and Ross, L. (2002). Skin temperature response to cryotherapy. *Archives of Physical Medicine and Rehabilitation*, 83, 543–9.

Cleak, M.J. and Eston, R.G. (1992). Delayed onset muscle soreness: mechanisms and management. *Journal of Sports Sciences*, 10, 325–41.

Dadebo, B., White, J., and George, K.P. (2004). A survey of flexibility training protocols and hamstring strains in professional football clubs in England. *British Journal of Sports Medicine*, 38, 388–94.

Dawson, B., Gow, S., Modra, S., *et al.* (2005). Effects of immediate post-game recovery procedures on muscle soreness, power, and flexibility levels over the next 48 hours. *Journal of Science and Medicine in Sport*, 8, 210–21.

Duffield, R., Edge, J., Merrells, R., *et al.* (2008). The effects of compression garments on intermittent exercise performance and recovery on consecutive days. *International Journal of Sports Physiology and Performance*, 3, 454–68.

Duffield, R., Cannon, J. and King, M. (2010). The effects of compression garments on recovery of muscle performance following high-intensity sprint and plyometric exercise. *Journal of Science and Medicine in Sport*, 13, 136–40.

Elias, G.P., Varley, M.C., Wyckelsma, V.L., *et al.* Effects of water immersion on post-training recovery in Australian footballers. *International Journal of Sports Physiology and Performance*, 7, 357–66.

Enwemeka, C.S., Allen, C., Avilla, P., *et al.* (2002). Soft tissue thermodynics before, during, and after cold pack therapy. *Medicine and Science in Sports and Exercise*, 34, 45–50.

Falvo, M.J., Schilling, B.K., Bloomer, R., *et al.* (2009). Repeated bout effect is absent in resistance trained men: an electromyographic analysis. *Journal of Electromyography and Kinesiology*, 19, 529–35.

Falvo, M.J., Schilling, B.K., Bloomer, R.J., *et al.* (2007). Efficacy of prior eccentric exercise in attenuating impaired exercise performance after muscle injury in resistance trained men. *Journal of Strength and Conditioning Research*, 21, 1053–60.

Gill, N.D., Beavan, C.M., and Cook, C. (2006). Effectiveness of post-match recovery strategies in rugby players. *British Journal of Sports Medicine*, 40, 260–3.

Gregson, W., Allen, R., Holden, S., *et al.* (2013). Post-exercise cold-water immersion does not attenuate muscle glycogen resynthesis. *Medicine and Science in Sports and Exercise*, 45, 1174–81.

Gregson, W., Black, M.A., Jones, H., *et al.* (2011). Influence of cold-water immersion on limb and cutaneous blood flow at rest. *American Journal of Sports Medicine*, 39, 1316–23.

Halson, S.L. (2008). Nutrition, sleep, and recovery. *European Journal of Sport Science*, 8, 119–26.

Hamlin, M.J., Mitchell, C.J., Ward, F.D., *et al.* (2012). Effect of compression garments on short-term recovery of repeated sprint and 3km running performance in rugby union players. *Journal of Strength and Conditioning Research*, 26, 2975–82.

Hemmings, B., Smith, M., Graydon, J., *et al.* (2000). Effects of massage on physiological restoration, perceived recovery, and repeated sports performance. *British Journal of Sports Medicine*, 34, 109–15.

Herbert, R.D. and Gabriel, M. (2002). Effects of stretching before and after exercising on muscle soreness and risk of injury: systematic review. *British Medical Journal*, 325, 1–5.

Herrera, E., Sandoval, M.C., Camargo, D.M., et al. (2010). Motor and sensory nerve conduction are affected differently by ice pack, ice massage, and cold water immersion. *Physical Therapy*, 90, 581–91.

Herrera, E., Sandoval, M.C., Camargo, D.M., *et al.* (2011). Effect of walking and resting after three cryotherapy modalities on the recovery of sensory and motor nerve conduction velocity in healthy subjects. *Revista Brasileira de Fisioterapia*, 15, 233–40.

Hilbert, J.E., Sforzo, G.A., and Swensen, T. (2003). The effects of massage on delayed onset muscle soreness. *British Journal of Sports Medicine*, 37, 72–5.

Hinds, T., McEwan, I., Perkes, J., *et al.* (2004). Effects of massage on limb and skin blood flow after quadriceps exercise. *Medicine and Science in Sports and Exercise*, 36, 1308–13.

Ingram, J., Dawson, B., Goodman, C., *et al.* (2009). Effect of water immersion methods on post-exercise recovery from simulated team sport exercise. *Journal of Science and Medicine in Sport*, 12, 417–21.

Jakeman, J.R., Byrne, C., and Eston, R.G. (2010). Lower limb compression garment improves recovery from exercise-induced muscle damage in young, active females. *European Journal of Applied Physiology*, 109, 1137–44.

Juliff, L.E., Halson, S.L., and Peiffer, J.J. (2014). Understanding sleep disturbance in athletes prior to important competitions. *Journal of Science and Medicine in Sport*, doi.org/10.1016/j.jsams.2014.02.007 [Epub ahead of print].

Jutte, L.S., Merrick, M.A., Ingersoll, C.D., *et al.* (2001). The relationship between intramuscular temperature, skin temperature, and adipose thickness during cryotherapy and rewarming. *Archives of Physical Medicine and Rehabilitation*, 82, 845–50.

Kraemer, W.J., Bush, J.A., Newton, R.U., *et al.* (1998). Influence of a compression garment on repetitive power output production before and after different types of muscle fatigue. *Sports Medicine Training and Rehabilitation*, 8, 163–84.

Kraemer, W.J., Bush, J.A., Wickham, R.B., *et al.* (2001). Continuous compression as an effective intervention in treating eccentric exercise-induced muscle soreness. *Journal of Sports Rehabilitation*, 10, 11–23.

Kraemer, W.J., Flannigan, S.D., Comstock, B.A., *et al.* (2010). Effects of a whole body compression garment on markers of recovery after a heavy resistance workout in men and women. *Journal of Strength and Conditioning Research*, 24, 804–14.

Kraemer, W.J., French, D.N., and Spiering, B.A. (2004). Compression in the treatment of acute muscle injuries in sport. *International Journal of Sports Medicine*, 5, 200–8.

Krustrup, P., Mohr, M., Steensberg, A., *et al.* (2006). Muscle and blood metabolites during a soccer game: implications for sprint performance. *Medicine and Science in Sports and Exercise*, 38, 1165–74.

Lawrence, D. and Kakkar, V.V. (1980). Graduated, static, external compression of the lower limb: A physiological assessment. *British Journal of Surgery*, 67, 119–21.

Leeder, J.D.C., Gissane C., van Someren K.A., et al. (2012a). Cold water immersion and recovery from strenuous exercise: A meta-analysis. *British Journal of Sports Medicine*, 46, 233–40.

Leeder, J.D.C., Glaister, M., Pizzoferro, K., *et al.* (2012b). Sleep duration and quality in elite athletes measured using wristwatch actigraphy. *Journal of Sports Sciences*, 30, 541–45.

Leeder, J.D.C., van Someren, K.A., Gaze, D., *et al.* (2014). Recovery and adaptation from repeated intermittent sprint exercise. *International Journal of Sports Physiology and Performance*, 9, 489–96.

Lieber, R.L. and Friden, J. (1999). Mechanisms of muscle injury after eccentric contraction. *Journal of Science and Medicine in Sport*, 2, 253–65.

Liu, R., Lao, T.T., Kwok, Y.L., *et al.* (2008). Effects of graduated compression stockings with different pressure profiles on lower-limb venous structures and haemodynamics. *Advances in Therapy*, 25, 465–78.

MacRae, B.A., Cotter, J.D., and Laing, R.M. (2011). Compression garments and exercise: garment considerations, physiology, and performance. *Sports Medicine*, 41, 815–43.

Mayberry, J.C., Moneta, G.L., DeFrang, R.D., *et al.* (1991). The influence of elastic compression stockings on deep venous hemodynamics. *Journal of Vascular Surgery*, 13, 91–100.

McHugh, M. (2003). Recent advances in the understanding of the repeated bout effect: the protective effect against muscle damage from a single bout of eccentric exercise. *Scandinavian Journal of Medicine and Science in Sports*, 13, 88–97.

Miyamoto, N., Hirata, K., Mitsukawa, N., *et al.* (2011). Effect of pressure intensity of graduated elastic compression stocking on muscle fatigue following calf-raise exercise. *Journal of Electromyography and Kinesiology*, 21, 249–54.

Mondero, J. and Donne, B. (2000). Effect of recovery interventions on lactate removal and subsequent performance. *International Journal of Sports Medicine*, 21, 593–7.

Myrer, J.W., Measom, G., Durrant, E., *et al.* (1997). Cold- and hot-pack contrast therapy: subcutaneous and intramuscular temperature change. *Journal of Athletic Training*, 32, 238–41.

Myrer, J.W., Myrer, K.A., Measom, G.J., *et al.* (2001). Muscle temperature is affected by overlying adipose when cryotherapy is administered. *Journal of Athletic Training*, 36, 32–6.

Nosaka, K., Sakamoto, K., Newton, M., *et al.* (2001a). How long does the protective effect on exercise-induced muscle damage last? *Medicine and Science in Sports and Exercise*, 33, 1490–5.

Nosaka, K., Sakamoto, K., Newton, M., *et al.* (2001b). The repeated bout effect of reduced-load eccentric exercise on elbow flexor muscle damage. *European Journal of Applied Physiology*, 85, 34–40.

Pointon, M. and Duffield, R. (2012). Cold-water immersion recovery after simulated collision sport exercise. *Medicine and Science in Sports and Exercise*, 44, 206–16.

Pournot, H., Bieuzen, F., Duffield, R., *et al.* (2011). Short-term effects of various water immersions on recovery from exhaustive intermittent exercise. *European Journal of Applied Physiology*, 111, 1754–6.

Rowsell, G.J., Coutts, A., Reaburn, P., *et al.* (2009). Effects of cold-water immersion on physical performance between successive matches in high-performance junior male soccer players. *Journal of Sports Sciences*, 27, 565–73.

Shoemaker, J., Tiidus, P., and Mader, R. (1997). Failure of manual massage to alter limb blood flow and long-term post-exercise recovery. *Medicine and Science in Sports and Exercise*, 29, 610–4.

Skein, M., Duffield, R., Edge, J., et al. (2011). Intermittent-sprint performance and muscle glycogen after 30 h of sleep deprivation. *Medicine and Science in Sports and Exercise*, 43, 1301–11.

Skein, M., Duffield, R., Minett, G.M., *et al.* (2013). The effect of overnight sleep deprivation following competitive rugby league matches on post-match physiological and perceptual recovery. *International Journal of Sports Physiology of Performance*, 8, 556–64.

Smith, C., Kruger, M.J., Smith, R.M., *et al.* (2008). The inflammatory response to skeletal muscle injury: Illuminating complexities. *Sports Medicine*, 38, 947–69.

Stackhouse, S.K., Reissman, D.S., and Binder-Macleod, S.A. (2001). Challenging the role of pH in skeletal muscle fatigue. *Physical Therapy*, 81, 1897–903.

Stanley, J., Peake, J.M., Coombes, J.S., *et al.* (2014). Central and peripheral adjustments during high-intensity exercise following cold water immersion. *European Journal of Applied Physiology*, 114, 147–63.

Suzuki, M., Umeda, T., Nkaji, S., *et al.* (2004). Effect of incorporating low intensity exercise into the recovery period after a rugby match. *British Journal of Sports Medicine*, 38, 436–40.

Thacker, S.B., Gilchrst, J., Stroup, D.F., *et al.* (2004). The impact of stretching on sports injury risk: a systematic review of the literature. *Medicine and Science in Sports and Exercise*, 36, 371–8.

Toth, K.G., McKay, B.R., De Lisio, M., *et al.* (2011). IL-6 induced STAT3 signalling is associated with the proliferation of human muscle satellite cells following acute muscle damage. *PLoS ONE*, 6, e17392.

Twist, C., Waldron, M., Highton, J., *et al.* (2012). Neuromuscular, biochemical, and perceptual post-match fatigue in professional rugby league forwards and backs. *Journal of Sports Sciences*, 30, 359–367.

Vaile, J., Gill, N., and Blazevich, A.J. (2007). The effect of contrast water therapy on symptoms of delayed onset muscle soreness (DOMS) and explosive athletic performance. *Journal of Strength and Conditioning Research*, 21, 697–702.

Vaile, J., Halson, S., Gill, N., *et al.* (2008a). Effect of hydrotherapy on recovery from fatigue. *International Journal of Sports Medicine*, 29, 539–44.

Vaile, J., Halson, S., Gill, N., *et al.* (2008b). Effect of hydrotherapy on the signs and symptoms of delayed onset muscle soreness. *European Journal of Applied Physiology*, 102, 447–55.

Vaille, J., Halson, S., and Dawson, B. (2008c). Effect of cold water immersion on repeat cycling performance and thermoregulation in the heat. *Journal of Sports Sciences*, 26, 431–40.

Venter, R.E. (2012). Perceptions of team athletes on the importance of recovery modalities. *European Journal of Sport Science*, 14, S69–76.

Venter, R.E., Potgieter, J.R., and Barnard, J.G. (2010). The use of recovery modalities by elite South African team athletes. *South African Journal for Research in Sport, Physical Education and Recreation*, 32, 133–45.

Versey, N., Halson, S., and Dawson, B. (2011). Effect of contrast water therapy duration on recovery of cycling performance: a dose-response study. *European Journal of Applied Physiology*, 111, 37–46.

Versey, N.G., Halson, S.L., and Dawson, B.T. (2013). Water immersion recovery for athletes: effect on exercise performance and practical recommendations. *Sports Medicine*, 43, 1101–30.

Webb, N.P., Harris, N.K., Cronin, J.B., *et al.* (2013). The relative efficacy of three recovery modalities after professional rugby league matches. *Journal of Strength and Conditioning Research*, 27, 2449–55.

Weerapong, P., Hume, P.A., and Kolt, G.S. (2005). The mechanisms of massage and effects on performance, muscle recovery, and injury prevention. *Sports Medicine*, 35, 235–56.

White, G.E. and Wells, G.D. (2013). Cold-water immersion and other forms of cryotherapy: physiological changes potentially affecting recovery from high-intensity exercise. *Physiology and Medicine*, 2, 26.

Wilcock, I.M., Cronin, J.B., and Hing, W.A. (2006). Physiological response to water immersion: a method for sport recovery? *Sports Medicine*, 36, 747–65.

Wiltshere, E.V., Poitras, V., Pak, M., *et al.* (2010). Massage impairs post-exercise muscle blood flow and 'lactic acid' removal. *Medicine and Science in Sports and Exercise*, 42, 1062–71.

Yamane, M., Teruya, H., Nakamo, M., *et al.* (2006). Post-exercise leg and forearm flexor muscle cooling in humans attenuates endurance and resistance training effects on muscle performance and on circulatory adaption. *European Journal of Applied Physiology*, 96, 572–80.

8

NUTRITION FOR RUGBY

Graeme L. Close and James P. Morton

8.1 Introduction to the role of the sports nutritionist

Sports nutrition is becoming increasingly recognized as one of the most important disciplines of Sports Science, so a rugby club's nutritionist is integral to the support of the team. In most elite rugby clubs, sports nutritionists usually work on a consultancy basis, though some clubs employ individuals on a full-time contract. This trend for employment opportunities likely represents the increased recognition from coaching staff that sound nutrition has a key role to play in maximising performance and promoting training adaptations and recovery. Recent research within elite rugby organizations have suggested that despite the importance of sports nutrition, both players (Walsh *et al.* 2011) and coaches (Zinn *et al.* 2006) demonstrate a lack of nutritional knowledge, further emphasising the need for sports nutrition consultants. The basic role of the sports nutritionist working within rugby clubs can largely be divided into five main tasks:

- Help the player achieve the ideal physique for his or her given position.
- Help the player improve his or her general health through the provision of high quality nutrition.
- Help the player improve game day performance.
- Help the player recover from training and competition.
- Periodize nutrition to maximize adaptions to exercise training.

Specific roles of the nutritionist are outlined in Table 8.1.

In the UK there is no formal sports nutrition career pathway, although The Sport and Exercise Nutrition Register (SENr) standardizes competencies for individuals wishing to deliver sports nutrition services. Regardless of the exact pathway to entering the profession, we consider that all sports nutritionists should

TABLE 8.1 Typical responsibilities of the sports nutritionist working in professional rugby

General Responsibilities	• Develop nutritional structures within the club
	• Set up and monitor supplement policies
	• Design training menus
	• Establish local suppliers of high quality food
	• Develop game day (home and away) strategies
	• Monitor body composition (skin fold testing)
	• Set up hydration policy and monitor hydration status
Individual Responsibilities	• One on one player consultations
	• Write individual plans for players, in relation to body composition, injury/illness, and performance/recovery
	• Liaise with players' parents or partners (where appropriate)
	• Prolong player career through targeted nutrition support
	• Enhance general health of the player
Educational Responsibilities	• Give group talks on hot topics
	• Produce educational materials (posters/hand-outs/booklets)
	• Organize cooking lessons for players
	• Educate staff within the club and run internal CPD programme
Personal Responsibilities	• Understand the science of the discipline
	• Understand the culture of the sport
	• Implement and adhere to own ethical code of conduct
	• Gain appropriate academic and professional qualifications
	• Engage in academic research
	• Develop your own skills through ongoing CPD
	• Engage in reflective practice
	• Keep accurate and professional notes

CPD = Continuing professional development

operate within a multidisciplinary team (e.g. coaches, doctors, physiotherapists, strength and conditioning professionals, sport scientists, chefs) and share common aims and objectives. In the authors' opinion, the goal of the sports nutritionist should be to provide scientifically sound and individualized nutritional interventions that maximize performance, promote training adaptations and recovery whilst maintaining well-being and increasing athlete education at all times.

This chapter provides an overview of sports nutrition issues that are the most relevant when working with rugby players. Unlike some sports, such as soccer, research into nutrition in rugby is somewhat limited with the few papers on rugby tending to be reviews (Casiero 2013; Dziedic et al. 2014) focused on supplements rather than actual food (Cameron et al. 2010; Green 2010; Haywood et al. 2014). Nevertheless, we review the most suitable literature and discuss the macronutrient (carbohydrates, proteins, and fats), micronutrient (vitamins and minerals), and hydration (fluid) requirements for training and competition as well as outlining ergogenic aids (sports supplements) that might aid performance and training adaptation. Personal reflections are offered throughout the chapter as well as unpublished data and observations from the authors' own experiences.

8.2 Carbohydrates

Given that that the body's storage capacity for carbohydrates (CHO) is limited (~500 g) but that muscle glycogen (the body's main store of CHO) is the main fuel source for moderate to high-intensity exercise (typical of a rugby game), an adequate dietary intake of CHO has traditionally been the focus for a rugby player's daily energy requirements. Given the recent debate regarding the role of CHO in an athlete's diet, it is important to consider the CHO requirements for training and for competition separately. Traditionally, CHO have been classified as simple or complex; however the glycemic index classification system might be of much more relevance to the rugby player.

8.2.1 Glycemic index

The classification of CHO purely as simple or complex is too simplistic given, that both CHO types can induce similar post-prandial responses. For this reason, sports nutritionists now pay more attention to the glycemic index (GI). The GI is a numerical scale that classifies CHO foods on their ability to raise blood glucose concentrations. Glucose or white bread is used as the reference food and is given a reference value of 100. Foods that are classified as high-glycemic (HGI), moderate-glycemic (MGI), and low-glycemic (LGI) are typically those with glycemic index scores of >70, 55–70, and <55, respectively. Examples of common CHO foods categorized according to their GI are shown in Table 8.2. For a more complete food list, please see Atkinson *et al.* (2008).

An understanding of the GI is of paramount importance for sports nutritionists, since the GI has the capacity to alter post-prandial responses to feeding as well as influencing substrate oxidation and exercise performance (Donaldson *et al.* 2010). The review suggests that LGI CHO feeding in the hours before exercise confers a metabolic advantage over HGI by inducing a smaller insulin response in the post-prandial period. In this way, there is increased lipid oxidation during exercise coupled with a more stable plasma glucose concentration during exercise, the result of which could be a sparing of muscle glycogen utilization during exercise. LGI foods might therefore prove advantageous not only for competitive situations but also for training, especially when maximizing lipid oxidation is important, such as when athletes need to reduce body fat (Morton *et al.* 2010). Alternatively, because of the capacity of HGI CHO to increase plasma glucose concentrations (and thus promote muscle glucose uptake), HGI foods would be particularly beneficial to consume in the post-exercise period to maximise rates of muscle glycogen re-synthesis and thus promote recovery (Burke *et al.* 1993).

8.2.2 CHO and rugby performance

Although direct evidence for carbohydrate and rugby performance is somewhat limited, there is a wealth of literature on the effects of CHO on soccer performance

TABLE 8.2 Overview of common CHO foods ranked according to their GI rating (adapted from MacLaren and Close (2009)
▨ Indicates LGI (<55) ▨ Indicates MGI (55-70) ▨ Indicates HGI (>70)

		Typical portion size (g)	GI	kcals	CHO (g)
Breakfast	All bran	40	30	108	19
	Crumpets	40	69	71	15
	Porridge (made with water)	250 (ml)	58	216	22
	Croissants	60	67	224	26
	Muesli	40	57	160	25
	Weetabix	40	69	140	30
	Cornflakes	40	72	113	27
	Wholemeal bread	40	74	87	17
	White bread	40	75	94	20
	Bagels	70	72	191	40
Lunch and dinner	Sprouts	80	1	28	3
	Green beans	80	1	20	2
	Kidney beans	80	28	80	14
	Quinoa	40	53	55	10
	Chapatti	38	52	120	20
	Baked beans	135	48	113	20
	Sweet potatoes (boiled)	120	46	101	25
	Egg noodles	200	46	124	26
	White Spaghetti	150	49	156	33
	Wholemeal Spaghetti	150	48	170	35
	Basmati rice	100	58	138	33
	Pita Bread	60	57	153	33
	Brown rice	95	68	106	22
	Udon noodles	95	55	150	31
	Couscous	150	65	168	35
	Potatoes (boiled)	100	78	72	17
	Potatoes (mashed)	100	86	57	14
	White rice	100	73	138	31
	Baguettes	85	95	207	43

	Typical portion size (g)	GI	kcals	CHO (g)
Apricots (fresh)	40	1	76	1
Apricots (dried)	10	30	19	4
Peanuts	25	14	141	3
Cashew nuts	25	22	153	5
Strawberries	100	40	27	6
Oranges	120	43	44	10
Apples	100	36	47	12
Yoghurt (fat free)	200	24	105	14
Apple juice	100	41	38	10
Orange juice	100	50	36	9
Bananas	100	51	91	14
Custard (with skimmed milk)	120	35	125	19
Crisps	35	56	133	12
Popcorn (salted)	50	65	185	23
Malted fruit loaf	35	47	103	23
Honey	25	61	75	18
Milk chocolate	55	41	286	31
Scones	50	92	182	27
Pretzels	10	83	38	8
Doughnuts	75	76	252	37
Waffles	150	76	501	59

(Left margin label spanning rows: *Snacks*)

showing its importance. For example, Krustrup *et al.* (2006) showed pre-game glycogen to be ~450 mmol·kg⁻¹dw that reduced to 225 mmol·kg⁻¹dw post-game. Several important facts can be gained from this study:

1. The players started the game with sub-optimal muscle glycogen, probably due to an inadequate diet in the days leading into the game.
2. Significant reductions in muscle glycogen were observed post-game albeit, in theory, adequate by the end of the game.
3. Despite the total amount of glycogen being adequate at the end of the game, 50% of the muscle fibres were almost empty, mainly in the type II fibres which are recruited for sprinting and high-intensity work.

Given the high-intensity activity in rugby, these data clearly show the important role of glycogen for rugby performance.

8.2.3 Daily CHO requirements for rugby players

It is difficult to provide exact recommendations for rugby players without knowing the specifics of their training programme and the individual requirement of the players (weight gain, weight loss, etc.). It is appropriate to note that the traditional approach of prescribing CHO requirements as a *percentage* of energy intake is a nebulous term that is poorly correlated to the actual amount of CHO consumed and the fuel requirements of the athlete's training and competition demands (Burke *et al.* 2011). Rather, it is more appropriate to discuss CHO requirements in terms of the absolute CHO *availability* (i.e. amount of grams per kg body mass of the athlete) required to meet the actual energy demands associated with the training and competition schedule. This approach makes practical sense given that the energy requirements will vary according to the daily, weekly, and monthly training goals and competition schedules. Suggested doses of CHO are presented in Table 8.3 specific to individual training days and/or specific situations.

TABLE 8.3 Likely daily CHO requirements for rugby players during a typical week

Situation	CHO requirements	Comments
Light training day (skill based field session or standard gym session)	<3 g·kg^{-1}	LGI foods should mainly be consumed
Moderate training day (90 minutes on field intermittent exercise)	3–5 g·kg^{-1}	LGI foods should mainly be consumed
Hard training day (double session, both of which high intensity)	4–6 g·kg^{-1}	LGI foods should mainly be consumed
Day before game	>6 g·kg^{-1}	A mixture of LGI and HGI to increase muscle glycogen stores
Breakfast on game day	1–3 g·kg^{-1}	LGI foods and drinks should be consumed
Pre-match meal	1–3 g·kg^{-1}	LGI foods and drinks should be consumed approx. 3 hours pre-game. This can be breakfast items for early kick-offs.
During the game	30–60 g·h^{-1}	HGI sports drinks (6% glucose are preferable) or gels. These can be consumed during the game or half-time break
Post-match meal	1.2 g·kg^{-1}·h^{-1}	HGI foods to replace glycogen. Can be foods or drinks or both.
Day after game	4–6 g·kg^{-1}	A mixture of LGI and HGI to replace muscle glycogen stores

HGI = High Glycemic Index, LGI = Low Glycemic Index.

8.3 Proteins

Proteins are essential for life and are crucial for a variety of key functions in the human body. The body contains structural proteins, contractile proteins, immuno-proteins, and regulatory proteins. This diverse range of functions is achieved due to the extreme variation in the structure of each protein. Proteins are made from amino acids (usually more than 50 amino acids in each protein) that form together in a specific order. Of the 20 amino acids used to make proteins, nine are classed as essential and the rest non-essential. Essential amino acids must be consumed in the diet, whereas the body can make its own non-essential amino acids. It is crucial to recognise that proteins are continually broken down and re-made throughout the day. This constant turnover allows for damaged proteins to be removed and replaced and for new proteins to be formed in response to exercise training.

8.3.1 Protein requirements of rugby players

Despite protein supplements being the most widely used of all sports supplements, the protein requirement of rugby players is still unclear. Some researchers believe that athletes in general do not require additional protein intake (Rodriguez *et al.* 2009) whilst others suggest that the protein needs of athletes are significantly higher than the 0.8 g·kg⁻¹ recommended to sedentary individuals (Phillips 2004). Others have suggested that if higher needs are required, this is easily achieved through the consumption of a standard diet (Millward 2004), whilst others believe the only way to achieve this is through supplements. Perhaps this debate is heavily influenced by the size of the athletes in question. For example, 2 g·kg⁻¹ can easily be achieved through diet for a 70 kg soccer player, but is much harder to achieve through diet in a 120 kg rugby player. For the 120 kg rugby player, this would involve eating 240 g per day of protein, equivalent to approximately ten chicken breasts. Recent studies from our group have found that, on average, elite rugby players consume ~2.5 g·kg¹ of protein with about 0.5–1.2 g·kg¹ coming from supplements (unpublished observation).

Perhaps instead of focusing on the absolute amount of protein, it might be better for athletes to concentrate on consuming a regular supply of protein throughout the day. As opposed to consuming all of the daily protein in three large meals, we advise that protein is consumed especially prior to and after exercise. This does not necessarily require large doses of protein, with approximately 25–30 g of protein being sufficient (Phillips 2011) (about one large chicken fillet or one 130 g tin of tuna, Table 8.4). Larger rugby players might require slightly more, with the most recent suggestions indicating 0.3 g·kg⁻¹ of protein to be consumed post-exercise and then regularly throughout the day (Phillips 2013).

8.3.2 Timing of protein intake

It is well documented that exercise performed in the fasted state results in a net loss of muscle protein (Phillips *et al.* 1999). This is crucial for rugby players, as exercising in the morning without any food intake might result in a loss of lean muscle

TABLE 8.4 Examples of common protein containing foods

Food	Serving size	Protein content
Chicken breast fillet	1 large (170 g)	35 g
Tin of tuna	1 small can (130 g)	34 g
Greek yoghurt (non fat)	1 small pot (170 g)	17 g
Tin of baked beans	1 large tin (440 g)	19 g
Organic peanut butter	3 tablespoons (100 g)	25 g
Cows milk (semi-skimmed)	500 ml	17 g
Soya milk	500 ml	16.6 g
Yazoo chocolate milk	1 small bottle (500 ml)	15 g
Tinned mackerel fillets in oil	1 small can (125 g)	20 g
Cottage cheese	1 small pot (170 g)	19 g
Typical commercial protein shake	1 serving	20–40 g

mass (Morton *et al.* 2010). The only way to prevent this net loss of muscle protein is to provide protein before (Tipton *et al.* 2001) or immediately post-exercise (Phillips 2011). There has been some debate over the timing of the protein intake, with early studies suggesting that pre-exercise was best and recent work reporting post-exercise is equally effective (Phillips 2011). Practically, the consumption of 20–25 g of high-quality protein taken prior to and after exercise might be the best way to ensure maximum rates of muscle protein synthesis.

8.3.3 Source of protein intake

Whey protein results in greater muscle protein synthesis post-exercise compared with both casein or soya based protein (Phillips *et al.* 2009). This is likely to represent the speed in which whey increases blood amino acid concentrations compared with casein and soya. Milk (80% casein, 20% whey) has also been compared with soya protein with data demonstrating that milk is superior to soya in stimulating muscle protein synthesis (Phillips *et al.* 2009). Interestingly, in this study, the soya protein resulted in a more rapid increase in total amino acids in the blood but a slower increase in blood leucine concentration, suggesting that leucine availability is crucial in stimulating muscle protein synthesis. Moreover, it appears that leucine plays a key role in switching on muscle protein synthesis, acting as a metabolic regulator (Phillips 2011). However, because casein results in a slower appearance of amino acids in the circulation, it might be beneficial to consume this protein source prior to sleeping so as to provide a sustained delivery of amino acids during the overnight fast and thus attempt to promote protein synthesis during this time (Res *et al.* 2012).

8.4 Fats

Fat has historically been viewed negatively, and as such, many rugby players believe that they should eliminate all fats from their diets. Over the last decade a number of studies have challenged this belief, even questioning the assumption that all saturated fats are problematic (Hu 2010). Although excessive intake of fat is a problem for general health and weight control (as is over consumption of any macronutrient), too little dietary fat is also a problem for optimal health. The body needs sufficient supply of essential fatty acids (omega-3 and omega-6 fatty acids) as well as the fat-soluble vitamins A, D, E, and K. Finally, fats are also required during exercise as an energy store, especially when carbohydrate stores become depleted such as when the exercise is greater than 90 minutes.

8.4.1 Types of dietary fat

Fats are generally classified as saturated ('bad fats') or unsaturated ('good fats'), based on their chemical structure. Unsaturated can then be further subdivided into mono-unsaturated (MUFA) or poly-unsaturated (PUFA). Despite some foods being described as saturated or unsaturated fats, all fats contain a mixture of fatty acids, and they are simply classified according to the majority fat source they contain.

A major problem with removing saturated fats from the diet is what to replace them with. Studies have demonstrated that reducing saturated fat intake will be of no benefit and can even cause more harm if the saturated fats are replaced with refined carbohydrates such as sugary drinks, mashed potatoes, and white bread (Hu 2010). In contrast, replacing some saturated with unsaturated fats including foods such as salmon, nuts, avocados, and seeds has been shown to improve health. Moreover, individual saturated fatty acids have differing effects on blood lipid concentrations, depending upon their composition. For example, lauric acid (found in high concentrations in coconut oil), despite being a saturated fatty acid, actually decreases the total-to-HDL cholesterol ratio, due to an increase in HDL cholesterol (Mensink *et al.* 2003). Therefore, rather than advising players on the types of fatty acids, better advice might simply be on the types of food to eat (Astrup *et al.* 2011). The simple message to the rugby player is to choose 'natural' fats and avoid processed ones, especially trans fats which should without question be eliminated from a rugby player's diet. Trans fats provide no benefit to human health, increasing LDL cholesterol and lowering HDL and are therefore a major risk factor for cardiovascular disease (Mozaffarian *et al.* 2006). Typically, these fats are found in some margarines and some deep fried foods.

A further class of PUFA are the essential fatty acids, which are classified as omega-3 (n-3) and omega-6 (n-6) fatty acids and must be taken through the diet to achieve optimal health. Western diets typically have an omega 6:3 ratio of about 16:1, whereas the ratio should be somewhere in the region of 4:1 or even lower (Simopoulos 2002). However, few athletes achieve this ratio. The main dietary source of omega-3 is oily fish (mackerel, salmon, tuna, herring, etc.) and therefore athletes should be encouraged to eat these on a regular basis or consider a high-quality fish oil supplement.

8.5 Hydration

During rugby training and games, core (and muscle) temperatures can increase to >39°C. The main biological mechanism for losing heat during exercise is through evaporation of sweat. Potential mechanisms underpinning dehydration-induced decrements in physical and mental performance include increased core temperature, increased cardiovascular strain, increased muscle glycogen utilization, and impaired brain function (See Chapter 9). In addition to fluid loss *per se*, sweat also contains electrolytes such as sodium, chloride, potassium, calcium, and magnesium. Loss of sodium is the most significant for rugby players, with salt losses between 2–13 g observed during training and competition for team sports (Maughan *et al.* 2004; Kurdak *et al.* 2010). The importance of high salt losses are underscored by observations linking them to exercise-related muscle cramps (Bergeron 2003), so it is important to identify rugby players who are 'salty sweaters' and tailor hydration strategies to each individual. Simple monitoring strategies such as examining clothing post-exercise for salt stains might help identify such players, though sweat patch testing (e.g. Maughan *et al.*, 2004) is the preferred objective method.

8.5.1 Assessment of hydration status in the rugby player

In developing individualized hydration strategies, it is important to perform regular estimations of pre-exercise hydration status in order to identify those athletes who may need particular attention. Within the field setting, assessments of pre-exercise urine osmolality and colour provide reasonably inexpensive but informative measures. Osmolality values <700 mOsmol·kg^{-1} are suggestive of a normal state of hydration (i.e. euhydration; Sawka *et al.* 2007), as is a urine colour that is pale yellow (Armstrong 2005). Studies in elite rugby have demonstrated that up to 80% of players can commence training in a hypo-hydrated state and might not hydrate correctly during training (Cosgrove *et al.* 2014).

Urine indices of hydration are sensitive to changes in posture, food intake, and body water content, and for these reasons a urine sample passed upon waking is often advised as the criterion sample (Sawka *et al.* 2007). However, values indicative of dehydration at this time (e.g. 7 AM) might not mean the athlete is dehydrated upon commencing training several hours later, assuming that appropriate fluid intake has been consumed upon waking and with breakfast. The same can be said for competition, in that samples suggestive of dehydration collected prior to the pre-competition meal might not mean athletes are dehydrated at the onset of competition itself. Where practical, athletes should therefore be assessed at both the former and latter time-points, so as to initially identify those athletes who are causes for concern, but to also verify that any subsequent hydration strategies implemented are effective to ensure euhydration prior to competition.

8.5.2 Fluid requirements for rugby players

In an attempt to ensure pre-exercise euhydration, it is recommended that 5–7 ml·kg^{-1} of fluid is consumed at least four hours prior to exercise (Sawka *et al.* 2007).

Additionally, if the individual does not produce urine or the urine remains dark coloured, a further 3–5 ml·kg[-1] could be consumed about two hours before exercise. Drinking within this time schedule should allow for fluid absorption and enable urine output to return to normal (Sawka *et al.* 2007). Consumption of sports drinks at this time, as opposed to water, is also beneficial given that they not only contain electrolytes but also additional carbohydrates. The fluid requirements of rugby players can be divided into pre, during, and post-exercise requirements. In order to offset the negative effects of dehydration on performance, the American College of Sports Medicine advises fluid ingestion at a rate that limits body mass loss to <2% of pre-exercise values (Sawka *et al.* 2007). Under no circumstances, however, should rugby players aim to drink to gain mass during exercise as this can lead to water intoxification, which in extreme cases can be fatal (Almond *et al.* 2005). Cold beverages (10°C) are beneficial to reduce the rise in body temperature during exercise (Lee and Shirreffs 2007). On training days (as opposed to competition), players might wish to consume water or low-calorie sports drinks only, given that carbohydrate ingestion during exercise might attenuate skeletal muscle adaptations to training as well as reduce lipid oxidation (Morton *et al.* 2009).

After training or competition, the goal is to replace any fluid and electrolyte loss incurred by the exercise sessions. The extent of the drinking strategy is dependent on the time-scale with which re-hydration must occur. Current guidelines recommend 1.5 kg of fluid for every 1 kg body mass loss induced by exercise (Sawka *et al.* 2007). Furthermore, fluids should be consumed (with electrolytes) over time as opposed to large boluses (Kovacs *et al.* 2002), so as to maximise fluid retention. Any players identified as salty sweaters may benefit from the addition of extra sodium to promote fluid retention and stimulate thirst (Maughan and Shirreffs 2008).

8.6 Micronutrients

Micronutrients are compounds that are required in small quantities (<1 g) to maintain normal physiological function and are broadly divided into vitamins and minerals. Although micronutrients do not directly supply energy for human performance, they play essential roles in many metabolic pathways. Whilst it is accepted that deficiency in most micronutrients could adversely affect health and performance, it is also known that some micronutrients taken in excess could be equally harmful to health.

8.6.1 Vitamins

Vitamins are organic compounds that are essential for normal physiological functioning of the body. Vitamins are only required in small amounts; however, they must be consumed in the diet (with the exception of vitamin D, which is mainly obtained from sunlight). Vitamins are generally categorized as fat-soluble (A, D, E, and K) or water-soluble (e.g. the B vitamins, C).

8.6.1.1 Fat-soluble vitamins

The fat-soluble vitamins are predominantly stored in the liver and in adipose tissue for later delivery into other tissues. The major advantage of fat-soluble vitamins over water-soluble vitamins is that they can be stored. This means that, if the daily intake is low, then the body can turn to its stores for a supply, and when intake is high, the stores can be replaced. The storage capacity of vitamins is particularly important when trying to establish if a rugby player's diet lacks any fat-soluble vitamin. Food diaries completed for three to five days are typically used to assess a player's diet, although this might not be long enough to detect deficiencies in fat-soluble vita-mins. A second important consideration regarding fat-soluble vitamins is that because the body stores them, excessive intake can be a problem to health. Vitamin D is somewhat unique given that it mainly synthesized from sunlight exposure. During the winter months in the UK, if sunscreen is applied or if players cover their skin, vitamin D cannot be synthesized, and this might render at risk of deficiencies. There is growing evidence that athletes should be tested for Vitamin D deficiencies given its unique route of entry (Close *et al.* 2012).

8.6.1.2 Water-soluble vitamins

Water-soluble vitamins include C and the B vitamins and, unlike fat-soluble vitamins, are not stored in the body. Excessive intake of water-soluble vitamins results in tissue saturation and those vitamins surplus to requirements are excreted in the urine. High doses of water soluble vitamins are unlikely to be toxic if taken in excess, although there are some exceptions to this such as vitamin B_6, which can result in peripheral nerve damage (Cohen and Bendich 1986). The inability to store water-soluble vitamins means that if daily intake is low, tissue concentrations are low, as there are no stores to draw upon. It is therefore important that the daily requirements of these vitamins are met to ensure adequate status. Many rugby players have been advised that high doses of B vitamins (energy) and C (immune function) are beneficial to health and performance. Whilst low B vitamins could be a problem, in reality this is rarely the case. Moreover, if a rugby player does indeed have low B vitamin status it would be more beneficial to treat the cause of this (usu-ally inadequate calorie intake or poor food choices) rather than simply supplement with B vitamins. A commercially available vitamin C supplement can contain 1,000 mg, which is 25 times the recommended nutrient intake (RNI) for this vita-min (the RNI in the UK is 40 mg). The reasons given to increase vitamin C intake are to increase immune function and to boost antioxidants, although the evidence is questionable (Close *et al.* 2006; Gleeson 2007) and probably reflects commercial sales rather than scientific fact.

8.6.2 Minerals

Minerals are essential inorganic compounds that are crucial for normal physio-logical function, as well as being important in many aspects of metabolism.

Minerals, of which there are at least 20 that must be consumed in adequate amounts to allow normal physiological function, are stored in the human body in various tissues. There is evidence some mineral deficiencies can occur in athletes attempting to lose weight or undertaking vigorous training regimes (Clarkson 1991; Manore 2002). The minerals that are most likely to be deficient during low-calorie diets are calcium, iron, and zinc. The bioavailability (ability to absorb it from the diet) is also lower in minerals (Turnlund 1991) than vitamins and, as such, it can sometimes be harder to ensure adequate mineral status. However, most research has suggested that – providing athletes are not eliminating food groups, are eating a well-balanced diet, and are consuming adequate calories in relation to their energy expenditure – there should be no major risk of inadequate mineral intake (e.g. Imamura *et al.* 2013). Unlike vitamins, there is generally a small margin of safety between the RNI and toxicity, so particular care should be taken when using mineral supplements.

8.6.3 Assessing if a rugby player is deficient in micronutrients

Factors that could contribute to micronutrient deficiencies include:

* Eliminating food groups from diets either due to food dislikes, allergies, or moral reasons
* Low-calorie diets often utilized when attempting to reduce body fat
* Very low-fat diets, which could affect the fat-soluble vitamins
* A lack of variety in the diet
* Lack of sunlight exposure (including constant use of sunscreens or protective clothing)

In practice, unless the rugby player fits into one of the scenarios above, it is highly unlikely that he will be deficient in any micronutrients. The first course of action if an athlete (or coach) is concerned about the micronutrient intake is to complete a detailed food diary and get this analyzed by a suitably qualified individual (dietician or sports nutrition consultant). If there is cause for concern after dietary analysis, subsequent blood analysis might be required. Caution should be taken using companies that claim to measure micronutrient deficiencies for athletes and then promote the use of their own mega-dose expensive supplements to correct these 'deficiencies'.

8.7 Sports supplements and ergogenic aids

There is a common misconception with many rugby players that supplements are essential to a successful nutritional plan. However, supplements are supplements, not a substitute, and there is little point supplementing an inadequate diet. Once an athlete's diet is as good as it can be, there are some instances where a targeted supplement plan *might* be of use. However, only qualified individuals who are up-to-date with the current rugby-specific doping regulations should prescribe supplements. If a rugby player does use supplements, he should only use those from companies that have their products independently batch tested. A laboratory that performs such testing is the HFL laboratory (www.HFL.co.uk), which lists companies that routinely test their products on its website. Rugby players should also be aware that although a product has been tested, this does not guarantee the supplement is drug free. In the authors' own practice the following questions help determine if a supplement will be advised:

- Is there a need for the supplement (cannot get in a normal diet)?
- Is there a clear scientific rationale for the use of the supplement?
- Is there no health risk associated with the use of the supplement?
- Is the supplement free of any prohibited substances?
- Is there an independently tested product available?

If the answer to all five of these is *yes*, then there might be grounds to consider the use of such a supplement.

It is not possible within this chapter to cover all those supplements available to rugby players and the reader is therefore referred to the A–Z of sports supplements published in *The British Journal of Sports Medicine*. Table 8.5 presents the main non-prohibited supplements typically used by rugby players, and it summarizes their efficacy with regards to performance. Supplements that are banned but might improve athletic performance are not covered.

8.8 Final thoughts on working in applied practice

The present chapter has attempted to outline the fundamental principles with regards to sports nutrition in a specific context for the rugby coach and player. In reality however, when working with elite athletes, the sports nutritionist needs more than the fundamental scientific literature. At the start of this chapter the five major goals of the nutritionist were outlined. Whilst these are unquestionably the major goals of the sports nutritionist, we also feel that it is imperative the sports nutritionist establishes his or her own ethical code of conduct. From our practice this can be summarized by the three rules below, which we make no apology for listing in order of importance:

1. Do no harm
2. Improve health
3. Improve performance, enhance training adaptions, and promote recovery

Experience has shown us that focusing on points 1 and 2 provides a strong platform to subsequently develop point 3. Whilst some practitioners might focus upon short-term performance gains, it is our belief that the focus should always be on the long-term health of the athlete.

TABLE 8.5 Summary of the major non-prohibited supplements used by athletes

Supplement	Ergogenic claims	Reasons not to take	Common dose	Key reference
Creatine	Improve speed, strength, and power	Increase mass, anecdotal reports of increased cramping, risk of contamination, and failed drug tests	5 g four times per day for 4–5 days followed by 3 g per day or 3 g per day for 30 days	Tarnopolsky (2010)
Caffeine	Prolong endurance performance, increase lipid oxidation, and increase mental alertness	Some players naïve to caffeine might get side effects including nausea, headache, and tremors at high dose	2–4 mg·kg^{-1} body mass Take 45–60 min pre-exercise	Tarnopolsky (2010)
Beta Alanine	Increases muscle carnosine, which is the main intracellular buffer of hydrogen ions, thus improving high-intensity exercise	Some athletes will experience skin tingling that may cause distress. Risk of contamination and failed drug tests.	3–6 g per day Must be taken daily for ~4 weeks before benefits are noticed.	Hobson et al. (2012)
BCAA	Prevent central fatigue, increase lean mass	Little evidence to support central fatigue hypothesis. Little evidence to support increase in lean mass if consuming an appropriate diet.	5 g taken 2–3 times per day	Blomstrand (2001)
Green Tea Extract	High in green tea catechins and epigallocatechin gallate (EGCG), which is claimed to increase fat oxidation during exercise	Contains caffeine that might not be desired by all athletes. Most of the evidence so far is in animal studies. Risk of contamination and failed drug tests.	The amount in a cup of green tea is likely to be too small. 300 mg taken 3 times per day used in research studies.	Venabales et al. (2008)

(continued)

TABLE 8.5 (Continued)

Supplement	Ergogenic claims	Reasons not to take	Common dose	Key reference
HMB	A derivative of leucine that can increase muscle mass and strength through its anti-catabolic properties. Reduce post exercise muscle damage/soreness	Limited evidence of effects in trained individuals. Risk of contamination and failed drug tests.	3 g per day	Zanchi et al. (2011)
Vitamin D	Correction of a deficiency is claimed to improve bone health and muscle function	High dose supplementation could result in problems such as hypercalcaemia and kidney stones	Requires individual consultation with a clinician	Willis et al. (2008)
Bovine Colostrum	Rich in immune and growth factors. Increase lean mass, improve immune function, and promote gut health.	Potential for elevated IGF–1 and thus failed drug test. Evidence is at best equivocal, especially in relation to immune function.	Various doses used usually between 10–20 g per day	Shing et al. (2009)
CLA	Essential fatty acids reported to promote loss of body fat and increase lean muscle mass	Limited studies in athletes. Most positive data is from animal studies. Risk of contamination and failed drug tests.	1.4–6.8 g per day	Schoeller et al. (2009)

BCAA = Branched-Chain Amino Acids; HMB = Beta-Hydroxy Beta-Methylbutyrate; CLA = Conjugated Linoleic Acid

A huge supplement culture exists in elite rubgy, often with athletes taking (at best) useless or (at worse) dangerous or prohibited supplements. It is the role of the nutrition consultant to ensure rugby players understand the importance of food over supplements, and the pitfalls of uncontrolled supplement usage. This requires not only an in-depth knowledge of fundamental nutrition, but the ability to build working relationships with the players based upon mutual trust and respect.

In terms of knowledge, it is often surprising the level of detail that some players want with regards to nutrition. Whilst some rugby players simply ask what to eat and when to eat it, we have had conversations on the fundamental principles of digestion and absorption, and the mechanism by which beta alanine buffers hydrogen ions (players' request). It is imperative that the sports nutritionist not only knows what to advise, but that she also has the scientific knowledge and academic qualifications to understand why she is giving the advice.

A major problem working in rugby is the limited time available with the players. Whilst many teams now have an ever-increasing number of full-time support staff, the nutritionist is still often a consultancy role. In reality, very little can be done in these limited time frames and often the job is more about 'putting out fires' than building solid nutrition programmes. As a consequence, full-time support staff should understand the concepts of nutrition outlined in this chapter so that they might provide appropriate and factual advice. It is the authors' wish that clubs will appreciate the importance of the nutritionist, and more full-time opportunities will arise in professional rugby.

Finally, we are often asked what comes first: the science or the practice? In our opinion, this is as hard to answer as the proverbial chicken and egg debate. Whilst it is fundamental to understand in detail the core scientific literature and be able to implement this research into real world advice, practical knowledge will sometimes take precedence over the science. Ultimately, the very best sports nutritionists have the common sense to understand that both theory and applied experience are essential and have the wisdom to know when one takes priority over the other.

Case study: assessing energy expenditure and intake of an elite rugby player during pre-season

Graeme L. Close and Warren Bradley

Introduction

To allow scientifically valid nutrition plans to be written, it is important to understand the energy requirements and the typical energy intakes of athletes engaged in a given sport. However, to date, these data are not available within a rugby setting (league or union). Moreover, the macronutrient intake and composition of elite players' diets are also unknown. This case study therefore describes the assessment of energy expenditure during a pre-season training day and the corresponding dietary intake of an elite rugby union player competing in the RaboDirect Pro12 League.

TABLE 8.6 Training content for a typical week

	Mon	Tue	Wed	Thur	Fri	Sat	Sun
AM	Gym	Gym	Rest	Gym	Field	Rest	Rest
PM	Field	Field	Rest	Gym (conditioning)	Gym		

Case presentation

The player was a 33-year-old forward, (110 kg body mass) who had played over 100 games for his club as well as being a current international player. Further details on the player are not provided to maintain player confidentiality. The data reported in the present case study are from the pre-season of 2013/2014. At the time of the case study, the player was looking to make small reductions in body fat whilst maintain lean mass. Data for a typical training week during the collection period are shown in Table 8.6.

To assess energy expenditure, the given player was asked to wear a Sensewear Armband every day for a week (Bodymedia, USA). The band was worn at all times (including sleeping), apart from during full-contact sessions or when bathing. At the end of the week, the armband was collected and the data downloaded. Energy expenditure data are presented as the mean for the week. The player was also asked to complete a 24-h dietary recall for a typical training day within the assessment week. During the training week, Global Positioning System (GPS) data were also recorded (Minimax S4 GPS unit, Catapult Innovations, Australia), sampling at 10 Hz with data presented as mean of the week. A summary of the intake, expenditure, and distance covered during the week can be seen in Table 8.7.

Discussion

The aim of this case study was to identify the energy intake and expenditure of an elite rugby union player during the course of a typical pre-season week, whilst at the same time quantifying typical distances covered during a training week. Analysis of the dietary recall suggested that the daily intake was relatively low and

TABLE 8.7 Mean energy expenditure, energy intake, and distances covered during a typical pre-season training week (excluding a rest day)
The expenditure and intake represent the mean daily values, whereas the distances covered represent weekly data.

Expenditure	4,200 Kcal
Intake	3,894 Kcal
CHO	4.1 g·kg^{-1} body mass
Fat	1 g g·kg^{-1} body mass
Protein	2.5 g·kg^{-1} body mass
Distance covered	9,898 m
Distance covered >4.4 m·s^{-1}	1,800 m

not too dissimilar to values reported in professional soccer players (Maughan 1997). This is somewhat surprising, given the large difference in body mass between rugby and soccer. However, most methods of assessing energy intake suffer from reliability issues and the possibility of athletes under-reporting nutrition intake.

Mean daily energy expenditure was only 3,894 Kcal, despite this being measured over the course of a pre-season training week. These data might reflect the growing trend within elite sport to focus training upon quality over quantity. Indeed it was observed that over a training week <10 km was covered by the player, of which only 1.8 km was at high intensities (speeds >4.4 m·s^{-1}).

During a pre-season training week the player was only consuming 4.1 g·kg^{-1} body mass of carbohydrates per day, which is significantly lower than suggested intakes for athletes engaged in rugby (approximately 6 g·kg^{-1} body mass; Burke et al. 2011). One interpretation of these data could be that the player is consuming insufficient carbohydrates, and the nutritionist should advise the player to increase his carbohydrate intake accordingly. However, if the player were to consume 6 g·kg^{-1} of carbohydrates, this would involve an additional 880 Kcal per day (approximately four additional jacket potatoes per day) that might have resulted in the player gaining unwanted mass. It could therefore be argued that the carbohydrate intake of the player is in fact adequate to fuel the training whilst maintaining body mass. Carbohydrate guidelines based upon g·kg^{-1} body mass could result in over-consumption in athletes with extremely large muscle mass, such as rugby players. However, future research collected over a longer period of time and on more players is now required to make definitive conclusions on the carbohydrate requirements of rugby players. Moreover, whether this carbohydrate intake is adequate for optimal match day performance is unclear.

Protein intake of the athlete was within the guidelines recommended for athletes engaged in training designed to reduce fat mass but maintain muscle mass (Mettler et al. 2010). The athlete consumed 2.5 g·kg^{-1} of protein that was predominantly from food with an average of 2 x 30 g consumed in the form of protein shakes. The supplements were taken for convenience and consumed post-training. This timing of protein intake appears logical given that protein consumed post-exercise is beneficial in promoting muscle protein synthesis (Rasmussen et al. 2000).

In conclusion, the present case study provides the first evidence of typical energy intake and expenditure in an elite rugby union player. The data suggest that the intakes of the athlete are perhaps not in keeping with current guidelines, although they may be appropriate for the athlete given their training demands.

References

Almond, C.S., Shin, A.Y., Fortescue, E.B., et al. (2005). Hyponatremia among runners in the Boston Marathon. *New England Journal of Medicine*, 352, 1550–6.

Armstrong, L.E. (2005). Hydration assessment techniques. *Nutrition Reviews*, 63, S40–54.

Astrup, A., Dyerberg, J., Elwood, P., et al. (2011). The role of reducing intakes of saturated fat in the prevention of cardiovascular disease: where does the evidence stand in 2010? *American Journal Clinical Nutrition*, 93, 684–8.

Atkinson, F.S., Foster-Powell, K., and Brand-Miller, J.C. (2008). International tables of glycemic index and glycemic load values. *Diabetes Care*, 31, 2281–3.

Bergeron, M.F. (2003). Heat cramps: fluid and electrolyte challenges during tennis in the heat. *Journal of Science and Medicine in Sport*, 6, 19–27.

Blomstrand, E. (2001). Amino acids and central fatigue. *Amino Acids*, 20, 25–34.

Burke, L.M., Collier, G.R., and Hargreaves, M. (1993). Muscle glycogen storage after prolonged exercise: effect of the glycemic index of carbohydrate feedings. *Journal of Applied Physiology*, 75, 1019–23.

Burke, L.M., Hawley J.A., Wong, S.H., et al. (2011). Carbohydrates for training and competition. *Journal od Sports Science*, 29, S17–27.

Cameron, S.L., McLay-Cooke, R.T., Brown, R.C., et al. (2010). Increased blood pH but not performance with sodium bicarbonate supplementation in elite rugby union players. *International Journal of Sports Nutrition and Exercise Metabolism* 20, 307–21.

Casiero, D. (2013). Fueling the rugby player: maximizing performance on and off the pitch. *Current Sports Medicine Reports*, 12, 228–33.

Clarkson, P.M. (1991). Minerals: exercise performance and supplementation in athletes. *Journal of Sports Science*, 9, 91–116.

Close, G.L., Ashton, T., Cable, T., et al. (2006). Ascorbic acid supplementation does not attenuate post-exercise muscle soreness following muscle-damaging exercise but may delay the recovery process. *British Journal of Nutrition*, 95, 976–81.

Close, G.L., Russell, J., Cobley, J.N., et al. (2012). Assessment of vitamin D concentration in non-supplemented professional athletes and healthy adults during the winter months in the UK: implications for skeletal muscle function. *Journal of Sports Sciences*, 31, 344–53.

Cohen, M. and Bendich, A. (1986). Safety of pyridoxine—a review of human and animal studies. *Toxicology Letters*, 34, 129–39.

Cosgrove, S.D., Love, T.D., Brown, R.C., et al. (2014). Fluid and electrolyte balance during two different preseason training sessions in elite rugby union players. *Journal of Strength and Conditioning Reseach*, 28, 520–27.

Donaldson, C.M., Perry, T.L., and Rose, M.C. (2010). Glycemic index and endurance performance. *International Journal of Sport Nutrition and Exercise Metabolism*, 20, 154–65.

Dziedzic, C.E. and Higham, D.G. (2014). Performance nutrition guidelines for international rugby sevens tournaments. *International Journal of Sport Nutrition and Exercise Metabolism*, 24, 305-14.

Gleeson, M. (2007). Immune function in sport and exercise. *Journal of Applied Physiology*, 103, 693–9.

Green, G. (2010). Creatine supplementation and DHT:T ratio in male rugby players. *Clinical Journal of Sports Medicine*, 20, 220–2.

Haywood, B.A., Black, K.E., Baker, D., et al. (2014). Probiotic supplementation reduces the duration and incidence of infections but not severity in elite rugby union players. *Journal of Science and Medicine in Sport*. 17, 356-60.

Hobson, R.M., Saunders, B., Ball, G., et al. (2012). Effects of beta-alanine supplementation on exercise performance: a meta-analysis. *Amino Acids*, 43, 25–37.

Hu, F.B. (2010). Are refined carbohydrates worse than saturated fat? *American Journal of Clinical Nutrition*, 91, 1541–2.

Imamura H., Iide K., Yoshimura, Y., et al. (2013). Nutrient intake, serum lipids, and iron status of colligiate rugby players. *Journal of the International Society of Sports Nutrition*, 10, 9.

Kovacs, E.M., Schmahl, R.M., Senden, J.M., *et al.* (2002). Effect of high and low rates of fluid intake on post-exercise rehydration. *International Journal of Sports Nutrition and Exercise Metabolism*, 12, 14–23.

Kurdak, S.S., Shirreffs, S.M., Maughan, R.J., *et al.* (2010). Hydration and sweating responses to hot-weather football competition. *Scandinavian Journal of Medicine and Science in Sports*, 20, 133–9.

Krustrup, P., Mohr, M., Steensberg, A., *et al.* (2006). Muscle and blood metabolites during a soccer game: implications for sprint performance. *Medicine and Science in Sports and Exercise*, 38, 1165–74.

Lee, J.K., Shirreffs, S.M. (2007). The influence of drink temperature on thermoregulatory responses during prolonged exercise in a moderate environment. *Journal of Sports Science*, 25, 975–85.

MacLaren, D.P. and Close, G.L. (2009). Glycemic index and glycemic load: relevance for athletes in training. *Professional Strength and Conditioning*, April.

Maughan, R.J. (1997). Energy and macronutrient intakes of professional football (soccer) players. *British Journal of Sports Medicine*, 31, 45–7.

Maughan, R.J. and Shirreffs, S.M. (2008). Development of individual hydration strategies for athletes. *International Journal of Sports Nutrition and Exercise Metabolism*, 18, 457–42.

Maughan, R.J., Merson, S.J., Broad, N.P., *et al.* (2004). Fluid and electrolyte intake and loss in elite soccer players during training. *International Journal of Sports Nutrition and Exercise Metabolism*, 14, 333–46.

Manore, M.M. (2002). Dietary recommendations and athletic menstrual dysfunction. *Sports Medicine*, 32, 887–901.

Mensink, R.P., Zock, P.L., Kester, A.D.M., *et al.* (2003). Effects of dietary fatty acids and carbohydrates on the ratio of serum total to HDL cholesterol and on serum lipids and apolipoproteins: a meta-analysis of 60 controlled trials. *American Journal of Clinical Nutrition*, 77, 1146–55.

Mettler, S., Mitchell, N., and Tipton, K.D. (2010). Increased protein intake reduces lean body mass loss during weight loss in athletes. *Medicine and Science in Sports and Exercise*, 42, 326–37.

Millward, D.J. (2004). Protein and amino acid requirements of athletes. *Journal of Sports Sciences*, 22, 143–4.

Morton, J.P., Robertson, C., Sutton, L., *et al.* (2010). Making the weight: a case study from professional boxing. *International Journal of Sports Nutrition and Exercise Metabolism*, 20, 80–5.

Morton, J.P., Croft, L., Bartlett, J.D., *et al.* (2009). Reduced carbohydrate availability does not modulate training-induced heat shock protein adaptations but does upregulate oxidative enzyme activity in human skeletal muscle. *Journal of Applied Physiology*, 106, 1513–21.

Mozaffarian, D., Katan, M.B., Ascherio, A., *et al.* (2006). Trans fatty acids and cardiovascular disease. *New England Journal of Medicine*, 354, 1601–13.

Phillips, S.M. (2004). Protein requirements and supplementation in strength sports. *Nutrition*, 20, 689–95.

Phillips, S.M. (2011). The science of muscle hypertrophy: making dietary protein count. *Proceedings of Nutrition Society*, 70, 100–3.

Phillips, S.M. (2013). Protein consumption and resistance exercise: maximizing anabolic potentialsports. *Science Exchange*, 26, 1–5.

Phillips, S.M., Tipton, K.D., Ferrando, A.A., *et al.* (1999). Resistance training reduces the acute exercise-induced increase in muscle protein turnover. *American Journal of Physiology*, 276, E118–24.

Phillips, S.M., Tang, J.E., and Moore, D.R. (2009). The role of milk- and soy-based protein in support of muscle protein synthesis and muscle protein accretion in young and elderly persons. *Journal of the American College of Nutrition*, 28, 343–54.

Rasmussen, B.B., Tipton, K.D., Miller, S.L., *et al.* (2000). An oral essential amino acid-carbohydrate supplement enhances muscle protein anabolism after resistance exercise. *Journal of Applied Physiology*, 88, 386–92.

Res, P.T., Groen, B., Pennings, B., *et al.* (2012). Protein ingestion before sleep improves post-exercise overnight recovery. *Medicine in Science in Sports and Exercise*, 44, 1560–9.

Rodriguez, N.R., DiMarco, N.M., and Langley, S. (2009). Position of the American Dietetic Association, Dietitians of Canada, and the American College of Sports Medicine: Nutrition and athletic performance. *Journal of the American Dietetic Association*, 109, 509–27.

Sawka, M.N., Burke, L.M., Eichner, E.R., *et al.* (2007). American College of Sports Medicine position stand: Exercise and fluid replacement. *Medicine in Science in Sports and Exercise*, 39, 377–90.

Schoeller, D.A., Watras, A.C., and Whigham, L.D. (2009). A meta-analysis of the effects of conjugated linoleic acid on fat-free mass in humans. *Applied Physiology Nutrition and Metabolism*, 34, 975–8.

Shing, C.M., Hunter D.C., Stevenson, L.M. (2009). Bovine colostrum supplementation and exercise performance: potential mechanisms. *Sports Medicine*, 39, 1033–54.

Simopoulos, A.P. (2002). The importance of the ratio of omega-6/omega-3 essential fatty acids. *Biomedicine & Pharmacotherapy*, 56, 365–79.

Tarnopolsky, M.A. (2010). Caffeine and creatine use in sport. *Annals of Nutrition and Metabolism*, 57, 1–8.

Tipton, K.D., Rasmussen, B.B., Miller, S.L., *et al.* (2001). Timing of amino acid-carbohydrate ingestion alters anabolic response of muscle to resistance exercise. *American Journal of Physiology, Endocrinology and Metabolism*, 281, E197–206.

Turnlund, J.R. (1991). Bioavailability of dietary minerals to humans: the stable isotope approach. *Critical Reviews in Food Science and Nutrition*, 30, 387–96.

Venables, M.C., Hulston, C.J., Cox, H.R., *et al.* (2008). Green tea extract ingestion, fat oxidation, and glucose tolerance in healthy humans. *American Journal of Clinical Nutrition*, 87, 778–84.

Walsh, M., Cartwright, L., Corish, C., *et al.* (2011). The body composition, nutritional knowledge, attitudes, behaviors, and future education needs of senior schoolboy rugby players in Ireland. *International Journal of Sports Nutrition and Exercise Metabolism*, 21, 365–76.

Willis, K.S., Peterson, N.J., and Larson-Meyer, D.E. (2008). Should we be concerned about the vitamin D status of athletes? *International Journal of Sports Nutrition and Exercise Metabolism*, 18, 204–24.

Zanchi, N.E., Gerlinger-Romero, F., Guimaraes-Ferreira, L., *et al.* (2011). HMB supplementation: clinical and athletic performance-related effects and mechanisms of action. *Amino Acids*, 40, 1015–25.

Zinn, C., Schofield, G., and Wall, C. (2006). Evaluation of sports nutrition knowledge of New Zealand premier club rugby coaches. *International Journal of Sports Nutrition and Exercise Metabolism*, 16, 214–25.

9

RUGBY AND THE ENVIRONMENT

Rudi Meir

9.1 Introduction

Rugby is played in a wide range of environmental settings, ranging from the cool to cold conditions of winter in the north of England to the very warm humid conditions of Far North Queensland in Australia. This variability means that players can experience a range of environmental conditions across the entire playing season.

Professional and representative players of both rugby codes are required to cope with rapid changes in the environmental conditions brought about by extended national and international travel. It is commonplace for teams to train in one climatic zone and then travel to and play in a different one (in terms of the ambient conditions). For example, athletes based in Melbourne, Australia, will play their home games in very different ambient conditions in June to those they will experience when required to play regular competition games in completely different climate zones. Melbourne is classified as being in Australia's temperate zone and has a mean maximum temperature at 15:00 h in June (winter) of 13.7°C with mean relative humidity (RH%) of 63%. If the team plays a scheduled match away in North Queensland, which is located in a tropical climate zone, the mean maximum temperature at 15:00 h in June will be 24.4°C (RH% = 52%). Such variation in ambient conditions could place additional stress on players resulting in a negative impact on their performance.

9.1.1 Body temperature regulation: a brief overview

Humans are warm-blooded (i.e. homeothermic) and, independent of environmental temperature, can maintain a remarkably constant internal body temperature between 35.5 and 37.7°C. Body temperature is subject to change across the day (diurnal), being higher in the late afternoon/early evening and lower in the early hours of the morning. It has been established for some time (e.g. Iampietro *et al.* 1957) that whilst exercise influences diurnal body temperature, such changes are associated with the ingestion of food. This notwithstanding, rises in an athlete's body temperature are typically associated with an increase in exercise intensity, exercise duration, and warm humid environmental conditions. If allowed to progress unchecked, body temperature can rise to a level that can be fatal (Hargreaves 2008). In fact, exercising body temperature can rise to dangerous levels even in relatively mild or even cool conditions (Maughan and Shirreffs 2010).

Humans regulate temperature either behaviourally or physiologically (Sawka *et al.* 2012). Behavioural control is a product of conscious decisions to influence heat storage, e.g. changing the type of clothes worn or altering physical activity. For example, Aughey *et al.* (2013) reported that team sport athletes, when playing in hot (27 ± 2°C; RH% 58 ± 15%) compared to cool conditions (17 ± 4°C; RH% 51 ± 11%), reduce the amount of low-intensity activity to maintain high-intensity running in the second half of matches. Such observations are an example of a feed-forward mechanism that initiates a conscious decision to down-regulate exercise intensity (Tucker *et al.* 2006). Physiological control includes redistribution of body heat by either vasodilation or vasoconstriction and sweating (Sawka *et al.* 2012). For temperature to remain constant, the amount of heat lost must equal the amount gained. On this basis, if heat gain is greater than that lost there will be a net gain in heat, resulting in increased body temperature (Marino *et al.* 2000).

Temperature regulation is controlled almost entirely by nervous feedback mechanisms, virtually all of which operate through the hypothalamus (Wendt *et al.* 2007; Silverthorn 2010). The primary function of the hypothalamus is to make the appropriate adjustments necessary to maintain core temperature by setting into motion heat-regulating mechanisms which protect the body from heat loss or gain (Boulant 2000; Wendt *et al.* 2007). It is responsive to increased local temperature in the form of blood perfusing the anterior hypothalamus, which is primarily responsible for dealing with increases in body heat (Powers and Howley 2012). It will respond initially to increased temperature by increasing effector nervous impulses to the skin, resulting in vasodilation of blood vessels in the periphery, bringing blood closer to the surface, and thereby facilitating heat dissipation from the body. These nervous impulses decrease once temperature decreases. If this response is insufficient to reduce temperature, the anterior hypothalamus will stimulate the sweat glands to 'off-load' heat by the mechanism of evaporation (Boulant 2000).

The system of temperature regulation operates around an apparent set-point, sometimes referred to as resetting the hypothalmic thermostat (Gisolfi and Wenger 1984). Sensor signals located within the skin and core have opposite temperature response characteristics, i.e. cold signals from skin receptors and warm signals from the core. An exponential rise in core temperature signals (resulting from increased core temperature) is balanced by skin temperature signals (which increase with falling skin temperature). The system is at set-point when these signals match each other. Should core temperature deviate from the set-point, a load error initiates a proportional response of heat dissipation or heat production by effector mechanisms (e.g. shivering, sweating, increased or decreased blood flow, and dilation or constriction of superficial veins) (Powers and Howley 2012).

Should temperature continue to rise once the heat dissipating mechanism is operating at maximum capacity, further increases in core temperature will result, possibly reaching dangerous levels (i.e. hyperthermia). Effector mechanism activation thresholds are raised in the case of fever, or lowered in the case of heat acclimation and endurance training (Gisolfi and Wenger 1984; Boulant 2000). As long as the conditions causing the hypothalmic thermostat to be reset at the new value continue their effect, temperature will be regulated in more or less the same way, but at the new set-point value.

9.1.2 Mechanisms of heat exchange

Heat tends to pass from locations of high temperature (e.g. core) to locations of lower temperature (e.g. skin). The body has four mechanisms of heat transfer: conduction, convection, radiation, and evaporation. Combined, all four mechanisms allow the body to maintain thermal balance by losing body heat to the environment (Cheuvront and Haymes 2001; Wendt *et al.* 2007).

Heat is gained from the environment and an individual's metabolism (Figure 9.1). Increased body temperature represents the storage of metabolic heat, which is a by-product of skeletal muscle contraction (Armstrong 2003). At the onset of exercise there is an immediate increase in metabolic rate; thereafter, core temperature

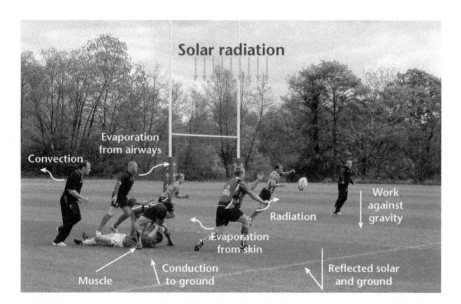

FIGURE 9.1 Mechanisms of heat exchange for the rugby player

increases at a reduced rate until heat loss equals production and steady-state values are achieved (Wendt *et al.* 2007). The process of converting fuel energy to mechanical work results in the production of large quantities of heat; only approximately 20–25% of the total energy production is utilized for mechanical work. The remaining 75–80% of metabolism is in the form of heat energy, and can cause a potentially dangerous rise in core temperature (Åstrand *et al.* 2003; Silverthorn 2010). In addition, the greater the intensity of exercise, the greater the total heat production will be (Dennis and Noakes 1999).

9.1.3 Measurement of body temperature in rugby

Despite inter-site variations, core temperature during exercise can be measured primarily at one of five sites: the rectum, mouth, oesophagus, tympanum (eardrum), or auditory meatus (ear canal) (Sawka *et al.* 2012). Measurement of internal temperature is achieved by use of mercury or infrared thermometers, with skin temperature measured by thermocouples or thermistors placed at various locations on the body. Temperatures at the ear canal, eardrum, or mouth are easy to measure but are influenced by movement of air over the skin, ambient temperature, and breathing. The values recorded at the oesophagus or rectum are more accurate, with oesophageal temperature responding rapidly to the onset of exercise whilst rectal temperature tends to have a lag time (thermal inertia) of five to ten minutes (Sawka *et al.* 2012). However, such methods are typically confined to the clinical or sport science laboratory setting and are not generally considered practical in a field setting. Infrared tympanic thermometers have been used in the field with professional rugby league players for some time (Meir *et al.* 1990; Meir *et al.* 2003). This device estimates core body temperature via the amount of infrared radiation emitted by the tympanic membrane. Ingestible wireless telemetric temperature pills (e.g. CorTEmp®) have also become increasingly popular during athletic events (e.g. Aughey *et al.* 2013), and provide a practical alternative that seems more favourable than oesophageal and rectal temperatures for measuring core temperature during exercise (Byrne and Lim 2007). Users should conduct appropriate calibration of the device beforehand and ensure ingestion takes place eight to twelve hours before measurements. Despite their practicality, users should be mindful of issues with reliability, data loss through apparatus malfunction, electromagnetic interference, and the potential for sensors to be expelled before data collection (Byrne and Lim 2007).

9.2 Possible effects of rising core temperature on the rugby player

Meir *et al.* (2003) recorded mean tympanic temperatures during elite rugby league matches played in England. Matches were played mostly in the evening in relatively mild conditions (April to May, 12.3 ± 6.0°C, RH% 83.3 ± 11.4%), meaning the moisture content in the air (i.e. dew point) was low compared with that associated with higher ambient temperatures. This relatively low thermal load is reflected, to some extent, by the range in absolute changes of tympanic temperature over the course of the matches of -1.8 to +3.4°C. Indeed, some players recorded post-match tympanic temperatures that were lower than their pre-match values. There was also no difference in body temperature between playing positions, and none of the players recorded tympanic temperatures above 38.3°C. These observations contrast to Australian professional rugby league players playing in the warmer humid conditions of the Southern hemisphere's autumn (23–24°C, RH% 67–73%), recording mean peak tympanic temperatures of 38.8 ± 0.4°C for forwards and 38.5 ± 0.7°C for backs. Indeed, a number of players in this environment produced readings above 39°C with the highest temperature recorded as 39.9°C. (Meir *et al.* 1990). Again, there was no difference in tympanic temperature between playing positions.

The external load imposed on the rugby player during training or matches is likely to result in an increase in body temperature and will also become more difficult if heat loss is restricted (e.g. wearing non-permeable clothing). Combined with oppressive environmental conditions, these factors might cause increases in core temperature of ~2–3°C above resting values with continuing exercise (Maughan and Shirreffs 2010). This rise in exercising body temperature will result in alterations to energy metabolism, cardiovascular function, fluid balance, central nervous system function, motor drive, and perceptions of fatigue (Hargreaves 2008).

Core body temperatures greater than 38.5°C are considered hyperthermic (Mora-Rodriguez 2012) yet, as shown above, do not appear to place players at increased risk of heat injury. However, there is clear evidence that hyperthermia can impact on a range of physiological parameters, causing alterations in moderate to high-intensity exercise performance (González-Alonso *et al.* 2008; Nybo and Nielsen 2001; Maughan *et al.* 2010). The competing blood flow demands associated with active muscle (to meet the energy demands of the activity) and blood flow to the skin (to help maintain core temperature within tolerable limits) combine to compromise cardiac output. This ultimately compromises the ability to sustain high-intensity exercise and the process of temperature regulation (González-Alonso *et al.* 2008). Increases in core temperature above 38°C are also associated with impaired muscle function (Nybo and Neilsen 2001; Drust *et al.* 2005). As core and skin temperature approximate 38°C, a concomitant levelling off of cutaneous blood flow, and the ability to dissipate heat occurs. Furthermore, such temperature increases (~38°C) can be achieved even in mild conditions. For example, Drust *et al.* (2000) reported increases in core temperature >39°C during the later stages of an intermittent exercise protocol lasting ~46 minutes in 18.0 ± 3.3°C and RH% 54 ± 12%.

Changes to prolonged intermittent exercise in hot environmental conditions provide the most appropriate insight into how increased core temperature would affect rugby performance. Whilst increasing body temperature via pre-warming can enhance sprint performance (Lacerda *et al.* 2007; Linanne *et al.* 2004), the ability to produce high-intensity efforts in hot conditions is reduced towards the end of prolonged intermittent exercise (Morris *et al.* 2005; Drust *et al.* 2005). In addition, a strong negative relationship exists between rate of increase in rectal temperature and distance covered during intermittent shuttle running, i.e. participants reach exhaustion sooner in the hot versus thermoneutral conditions (Morris *et al.* 2005). Muscle function is also impaired in hot conditions, with reductions in maximal voluntary contractions of knee extensors (Nybo and Nielsen 2001) and greater decrements in vertical jump performance after competitive soccer matches (Mohr and Krustrup 2013). Sunderland and Nevill (2005) have also reported deteriorations in skill performance, but not decision making, during intermittent exercise in hot conditions.

Elevated body temperature is perhaps the key factor limiting performance of prolonged, intermittent, high-intensity exercise when the ambient temperature is high. Metabolic disturbances (e.g. increased glycogen utilization) do not entirely explain reductions in high-intensity exercise performance. Elevations in muscle and core temperature during intermittent exercise are also associated with alterations in the central drive to the active musculature that leads to reductions in motor output (Drust *et al.* 2005) and an increased sense of effort (Sunderland and Nevill 2005). Alterations to central drive are manifest in players consciously modifying their exercise intensity when exercising in the heat in an attempt to maintain performance. For example, players adopting pacing strategies that reduces the amount of low and moderate intensity activity to ensure that high-intensity running could be preserved throughout a match (Duffield *et al.* 2009; Aughey *et al.* 2013).

Several studies have reported heavier individuals experience greater heat stress when exercising in warm and humid conditions (Dennis and Noakes 1999; Marino *et al.* 2000; Buresh *et al.* 2005). Compared to their lighter contemporaries, heavier athletes produce and store more heat that results in a shorter time to exhaustion caused by a faster time to limiting core temperature of ~39.5°C (Buresh *et al.* 2005). Accordingly, heavier rugby players, such as forwards, might be disadvantaged when training and playing in warm environmental conditions. Forwards playing in warm conditions would require a different interchange strategy to that used in cooler conditions to avoid an earlier onset of fatigue resulting in impaired performance.

9.3 Strategies to counter heat-induced reductions in rugby performance

Playing rugby in mild to hot conditions may require strategies to control body temperature within tolerable limits and minimize any negative impact on player performance. Discussed below are some of the approaches that might be adopted by coaches.

9.3.1 Pre-cooling strategies

Pre-cooling has potential benefits for the rugby player competing and training in warm to hot humid environments. The proposed mechanisms of action is a reduction in core temperature prior to exercise, slowing the rate at which core body temperature rises during exercise and lowering the increased sense of effort normally associated with exercise in the heat (Wegmann et al. 2012). Increased heat storage capacity (Marino 2002) would also enable team sport players to better regulate their work during prolonged intermittent exercise in hot conditions (Duffield and Marino 2007; Duffield et al. 2009). Strategies include cold-water immersion, the wearing of ice garments (e.g. vests, chilled towels draped over the head, shoulders, and upper back, or ice-packs), ice slurry ingestion, fans dispersing chilled water vapour over the body, or a mix of these methods.

The effect of pre-cooling on repeat-sprint performance in the heat is unclear, with studies reporting either no (Drust et al. 2000; Brade et al. 2013), small, (Duffield et al. 2003; Castle et al. 2006; Duffield and Marino 2007; Duffield et al. 2011) or large (Minnet et al. 2011) beneficial ergogenic effects. Given the dose-dependent response to cooling (Castle et al. 2006), the use of combined methods (e.g. internal and external, or head, body, and limb cooling) seems logical. However, the performance benefits are again equivocal, with studies reporting both positive (Duffield and Marino 2007; Minnet et al. 2011; Brade et al. 2012) and negative responses (Duffield et al. 2012; Brade et al. 2013). Studies that found no effect of combined pre-cooling methods adopted a field-based approach, high-lighting the potentially poor transfer of laboratory-based findings to a real–world environment. Pre-cooling also appeared to have little practical importance on those athletes that were acclimatised to heat (Brade et al. 2013). This notwith-standing, there was no negative effect of mixed-method pre-cooling; such strate-gies could therefore still prove marginally beneficial for unacclimatised players competing in warm, humid environments.

The application of some pre-cooling strategies in an applied rugby setting are prohibited by the logistical constraints involved in cooling large numbers of play-ers at one time and the equipment required. A more practical approach might simply be the use of chilled towels (soaked in 5°C water; Figure 9.2) or ice vests worn during the warm-up period prior to play and at interchange and half-time breaks. The use of an ice slurry (-1°C) sports drink consumed before play might also be useful in lowering core temperature (Siegel et al. 2010; Dugas 2011). The mechanism here being that a greater heat energy is required to change its state from a solid to a liquid; therefore more internal heat is used compared to ingest-ing liquid alone (Siegel et al. 2010). A combination of external and internal body cooling techniques seem to provide most ergogenic benefit to repeated sprint performance in the heat compared to individual cooling methods alone (Brade et al. 2014).

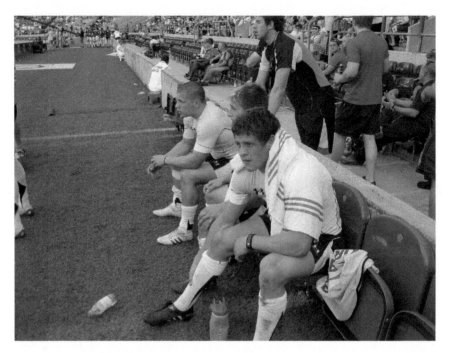

FIGURE 9.2 Welsh IRB rugby sevens players cooling off on the touchline by using chilled towels immersed in cold water.

9.3.2 Fluid loss and replacement during exercise in hot environments

Increases in body temperature during team sport training and matches results in disruption to the body's fluid and electrolyte balance (Kurdak *et al.* 2010; Duffield *et al.* 2012). This means players in the heat experience significant increases in sweat rate ($\geq$1-1.5 $l \cdot h^{-1}$) and fluid loss (Kurdak *et al.* 2010; Duffield *et al.* 2013; Mohr and Krustrup, 2013), a response that seems highly variable between individuals (Kurdak *et al.* 2010) and can occur despite water being freely available for consumption throughout the event (Kurdak *et al.* 2010; Duffield *et al.* 2012). The rate of change in core temperature during intermittent training is strongly related to the mean running speed, the individual's overall perceived exertion, loss of potassium, rate of sweating, and total sweat loss (Duffield *et al.* 2012). Sodium and potassium losses are also positively related to the total distance covered during exercise in the heat (Duffield *et al.* 2012). Any reduction in body water will result in increased cardiovascular and thermoregulatory stress during exercise (Maughan and Shirreffs 2010; Duffield *et al.* 2013). Therefore it is vital to monitor changes in hydration status in an effort to minimise any detrimental effect to exercise performance and health caused by inadequate hydration (Sawka *et al.* 2007; Maughan and Shirreffs 2010). This is particularly important given that many rugby players actually present for competition with some degree of hypohydration (O'Hara *et al.* 2010). Individuals who are dehydrated by as little as 1–22% of body mass before commencing exercise will not only experience an amplification of the effects of fluid deficit incurred during exercise, but also a reduction in overall performance compared with a euhydrated state prior to commencing exercise (Sawka *et al.* 2007; Maughan and Shirreffs 2010).

Notwithstanding the pre-exercise state of hydration, individuals exercising in warm–hot environments will experience varying degrees of fluid loss dependent upon the intensity and duration of activity (Maughan *et al.* 2010; Duffield *et al.* 2013). Exercise sweat loss equating to >2% of body mass could result in greater reductions in high-intensity running performance in the final 15 minutes of matches (Mohr *et al.* 2010) and the ability to perform repeated explosive muscle actions after prolonged intermittent exercise in the heat (Mohr and Krustrup 2013). In contrast, Australian Football players with ~2.5% reduction in body mass during a match have shown no change in sprint performance or jump performance towards the end of a game (Duffield *et al.* 2009). These differences might be explained by players adopting pacing strategies to preserve high-intensity running in the final stages of a game (Duffield *et al.* 2009; Aughey *et al.* 2013).

Impaired skill performance occurs during exercise in the heat (Sunderland and Nevill 2005), which might be attributed to the dehydration's negative influence on cognitive function (Cian *et al.* 2001; Grandjean and Grandjean 2007). Cian *et al.* (2001) concluded that dehydration (body mass loss of ~2.8%) increased reaction time, decreased tracking performance, and reduced short-term memory capacity after exercise in the heat. Conversely, Bandelow *et al.* (2010) investigated the effects of dehydration on cognitive function during football matches (mean temperatures ranging from 33.8-34.4°C) and observed that mild dehydration of up to 2.5% of body mass had no clear effect on cognitive function, but did result in slowing psycho-motor speed and increased accuracy. Bandelow *et al.* (2010) also reported that when a sports drink was taken to increase plasma glucose, performance time on relevant cognitive tests improved but accuracy decreased. Such findings suggest that a 'trade-off' exists between performance and accuracy and might help explain observed changes in skill performance but not decision making (e.g. Sunderland and Nevill 2005). Such findings also highlight the inherent difficulty in translating laboratory-based findings to field-based settings.

9.3.2.1 Monitoring and management of fluid loss

In an effort to monitor the hydration status of players, many professional teams undertake daily monitoring of squad members. This can involve using one or more strategies that include assessing urine osmolality using a hand held refractometer, urine colour (assessed against a urine colour chart), or simply recording daily pre- and post-training body mass (Armstrong 2007; Harvey *et al.* 2008; O'Hara *et al.* 2010). Collection of urine samples is not always practical in the context of a team environment, where players and coaches often require minimal intrusion and disruption before and after games. In addition, it is worth noting that urine colour can be affected by factors unrelated to hydration such as food, medications, illness, and ingestion of large volumes of hypotonic fluid (Shirreffs 2000; Oppliger and Bartok 2002). Therefore, recording pre- and post-match body mass changes and correcting for fluid intake and urine output is often all that is required to monitor fluid loss from sweating (Armstrong 2007; Maughan and Shirreffs 2010; Sawka et al. 2007), with a 1 g change in body mass representing approximately a 1 ml change in water status (Shirreffs 2000). Indeed, research by Harvey et al. (2008), which also utilized urine specific gravity, urine colour, and body mass changes before and after football matches, found that recording body mass alone is an effective method of monitoring dehydration.

Reported changes in body mass in the Australian professional rugby league have been suggested to reflect an inability to adequately replace body water when training and competing on consecutive days (Meir and Murphy 1998), possibly leading to chronic dehydration. Indeed, Maughan and Shirreffs (1997) acknowledge the importance of recovery and rehydration for athletes competing in multiple events or competitions in the space of a few days. Research involving English Premiership rugby union players showed that forwards typically record significantly greater fluid losses from play compared with backs (Meir et al. 2011). Whilst not surprising given the increased workloads often experienced by forwards compared with backs in a game of rugby, the issue for coaches and players is that individuals experiencing greater fluid losses will typically take longer to restore their body mass to pre-exercise values (Meir and Murphy 1998). Indeed, forwards more than backs struggled to restore their body mass back to pre-match values when provided with a three-day recovery period before their next scheduled training session (Meir et al. 2011). Interestingly, forwards found it easier to achieve target body mass values when the recovery period was only one or two days. It was speculated that when players only had a short turnaround time before their next training session they were more conscious of the need to replace their lost fluids. With longer recover periods (i.e. three days), some players might have felt they had more time to restore their fluid levels and so were less compliant with their rehydration regime (Meir et al. 2011).

It must be stressed that body mass changes alone are a conservative estimate of actual fluid loss, and in order to increase the accuracy of this measure, total fluid intake and excretion should also be recorded (Harvey et al. 2008; Shirreffs 2010). Recording body mass changes alone allows players to be readily kept informed of their hydration status and the effectiveness of their re-hydration regime, particularly when faced with exercising in hot and humid conditions. To further increase the effectiveness of such a strategy, all players should be regularly counselled about the need to monitor and be aware of their fluid requirements and to use changes in body mass as a useful guide to the amount of fluid loss they need to restore from one occasion to the next. Further, players also need to be made aware that voluntary fluid intake may not be adequate to counteract body fluid lost from sweating

(Carey 2001). A more aggressive regime of fluid intake, which combines sodium and electrolytes with water for the restoration and maintenance of hydration, is recommended (Meir *et al.* 2011; Shirreffs 2010). Sodium is the electrolyte that is lost in the largest quantities in sweat, whilst other electrolytes, such as chloride, potassium, calcium, and magnesium, are lost in smaller quantities (Shirreffs 2010; Shirreffs and Maughan 1997). Research shows that there is considerable variation between individuals with respect to sodium loss, and Shirreffs (2010) suggests that there may be some benefit in identifying those players who are heavy 'salty sweaters', so their fluid replacement strategy can reflect this consideration.

Players should have their body mass recorded each day, prior to the start of training. If their body mass is below the individual's established playing mass by more than 500 g, they should be advised to increase their fluid intake (Meir 2012). It should be the goal of each player to be hyperhydrated prior to each match. Accordingly, each players' hyperhydrated mass should be the reference that all measures are assessed against. Replacement fluid should be consumed immediately after training/play at a rate equal to or greater than that lost (e.g. 1 kg reduction in body mass = 1.5 litres of fluid to be ingested), to compensate for on-going loss due to urination and sweating (Sawka *et al.* 2007; Shi and Gisolfi 1998). However, some individuals will find ingesting large quantities of fluid difficult, even over several hours between multiple training sessions on the same day. As a result, it is easier in many cases to ensure that adequate fluid breaks are provided during training sessions (e.g. consume fluid at a rate of ~100 ml every 15-20 minutes), particularly in warmer, more humid environments. Such a strategy will help replace lost fluid from sweat and reduce the net effect of fluid loss. Sawka *et al.* (2007) also recommends consuming beverages and snacks that contain sodium, thus stimulating the thirst mechanism and encouraging the player to drink more fluid. It is worth noting that there is debate within the literature as to whether or not the goal should be to replace all lost fluid from sweating (Noakes 2007). Such a strategy may not even be desirable, since there are examples of successful elite standard endurance athletes experiencing dehydration equal to 8–10% of body mass with no negative impact on their performance (Noakes 2007; Sharwood *et al.* 2004).

9.4 Conclusion

Rugby league and rugby union are high-intensity, intermittent collision sports that are often played in mild to warm environmental conditions. Combined, these demands can produce significant increases in a player's core body temperature, which has the potential to lead to heat stress and a reduction in performance. The body has an amazing capacity to control body temperature with changes reflecting the physiological stress being placed on the body during exercise. The primary concern for the rugby player is overheating resulting from elevated core temperature, which can lead to impaired performance. Temperatures above 38.5°C are considered hyperthermic, yet rugby players can record temperatures during play significantly higher than this without any apparent risk to their health. However, rising body temperature should not be allowed to go unchecked, and players and support staff need to understand how to limit its consequences. The primary mechanism for removing excess heat from the body during exercise is through the process of sweating and evaporative heat loss. However, profuse sweating can lead to a significant loss of body fluid that will increase both thermal and cardiovascular strain. As a result, much attention needs to be placed on replacing the fluid lost due to sweating. A simple strategy that can provide useful information about a player's hydration status is to record body mass changes pre- and post-match and again upon return to training. Generally speaking, the negative effects of fluid loss (e.g. cardiovascular and thermoregulatory stress) will be negligible if fluid losses are kept to within less than 2% of optimal body mass. To this end, the need to be fully hydrated, or even slightly hyperhydrated, prior to a match should be clear. Players should return to each training session with knowledge of the fluid lost from sweating in the previous session and attempt to replace this amount.

Case study: pre- and post-game body mass changes during an international rugby tournament: a practical perspective

Meir and Halliday (2005) examined the changes in pre- and post-match body mass during an international age-grade (England Under-21) rugby union tournament played in Australia. This competition was conducted over a ten day period, in mild conditions during the Southern hemisphere winter (average temp. across all games = 18.5 ± 1.6°C; RH% 39.5 ± 17.7% and required members of the team (n=28; 15 forwards and 13 backs) under investigation to play four games during this period. The method of monitoring fluid status during this tournament was the use of changes in body mass, which was recorded pre- and post-match across all four games (three pool games and a final game). These changes were compared with a reference mass recorded prior to departure from England. Prior to departing for the competition, players were provided with material and a presentation on the need for fluid replacement throughout the tour.

The issue for coaches during a competition like this is ensuring that players are adequately hydrated prior to their next training session or game. Consequently, all players had their body mass recorded daily using digital scales (Seca, Hamburg, Germany) measured to the closest 0.1 kg. Post-game body mass was recorded with the players in their underwear only and towelled dry to remove surface sweat. Upon entering the changing room after each game, players were asked to abstain from ingesting any more fluid until they had been weighed. This process typically took 5–10 minutes to complete from the completion of the game.

The average body mass loss, expressed by changes in pre- to post-match body mass, for the group was 0.94 ± 0.94 kg, which is lower than that reported previously (e.g. Meir et al. 2003; Meir et al. 2011). This possibly reflects the mild conditions experienced by players throughout the tournament and the possibility that the total work performed, and therefore the total thermal stress for international age-grade rugby, is less than experienced at higher standards.

Players were constantly reminded in regular tour meetings about ensuring good drinking habits. In addition, squad members were required to record their individual body mass twice daily (i.e. before breakfast and dinner) in a tournament diary. This provided them with a very simple yet effective reminder of the need to constantly replenish lost fluid from training and games. Players also recorded their estimated daily fluid intake in their diary, which was checked every two to three days by the coaching staff. As can be observed in Figure 9.3, participants had a 'reference' body mass recorded prior to departure from England, which players had difficulty maintaining prior to games one and two. This is likely due to a combination of the travel, environmental conditions and multiple daily training on consecutive days leading up to games one and two. However, this reference body mass was marginally exceeded prior to games three and four (reference = 94.7 ± 10.7 kg; pre-game 3 = 95.3 ± 9.9 kg; pre-game 4 = 94.9 ± 10.1 kg), suggesting that the behavioural practices of players in terms of fluid intake was sufficient to replace the fluid lost from the earlier games and training.

This case study illustrates that training and playing in an international rugby tournament that requires international travel can have an impact on the hydration status of players even when played in relatively mild environmental conditions. However, if effective strategies and education of participants about the importance of appropriate fluid intake prior, during, and after training and play are implemented, then body mass can be maintained at reference values when playing multiple games over a short period of time. Such strategies are therefore able to maximize performance and minimize heat and dehydration related health risks. On this basis, recording body mass daily and pre- and post-game is a worthwhile and simple measure of fluid status that can be readily undertaken at little cost and without inconvenience to the player.

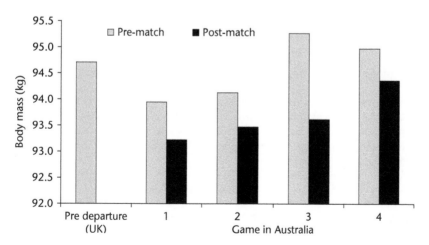

FIGURE 9.3 Mean body mass (kg) changes prior to and during competition in international age group rugby union tournament (n=28).

References

Aughey, R.J., Goodman, C.A., and McKenna, M.J. (2013). Greater chance of high core temperatures with modified pacing strategy during team sport in the heat. *Journal of Science and Medicine in Sport*, 17, 113–8.

Armstrong, L.E. (2003) *Exertional heat illness*. Champaign, IL: Human Kinetics.

Armstong, L.E. (2007). Assessing hydration status: The elusive gold standard. *Journal of the American College of Nutrition*, 26, 575S–584S.

Åstrand, P.O., Rodahl, K., Dahl, H.A., *et al.* (2003). *Textbook of work physiology: Physiological bases of exercise*, 4th ed. Champaign, IL: Human Kinetics.

Bandelow, S., Maughan, R., Sherriffs, S., *et al.* (2010). The effects of exercise, heat, cooling and rehydration strategies on cognitive function in football players. *Scandinavian Journal of Medicine and Science in Sports*, 20, 148–60.

Boulant, J.A. (2000). Role of the preoptic-anterior hypothalamus in thermoregulation and fever. *Clinical Infectious Diseases*, 31, S157–61.

Buresh, R., Berg, K., and Noble, J. (2005). Heat production and storage are positively correlated with measures of body size/composition and heart rate drift during vigorous running. *Research Quarterly for Exercise and Sport*, 76, 267–74.

Brade, C.J., Dawson, B.T., and Wallman, K.E. (2013). Effect of pre-cooling on repeat-sprint performance in seasonally acclimatised males during an outdoor simulated team-sport protocol in warm conditions. *Journal of Sports Science and Medicine*, 12, 565–70.

Brade, C.J., Dawson, B.T., and Wallman, K.E. (2014). Effects of different precooling techniques on repeat sprint ability in team sport athletes. *European Journal of Sports Science*, 14, S84–91.

Byrne, C. and Lim, C.L. (2007). The ingestible telemetric body core temperature sensor: a review of validity and exercise applications. *British Journal of Sports Medicine*, 41, 126–33.

Carey, B. (2001). Hard to swallow. *Strength and Conditioning Journal*, 2, 55–6.

Castle, P.C., MacDonald, A.L., Philp, A., *et al.* (2006). Precooling leg muscle improves intermittent sprint exercise performance in hot, humid conditions. *Journal of Applied Physiology*, 100, 1377–84.

Cheuvront, S.N. and Haymes, E.M. (2001). Thermoregulation and marathon running. *Sports Medicine*, 31, 743–62.

Cian, C., Barraud, P.A., Melin, B., *et al.* (2001). Effects of fluid ingestion on cognitive function after heat stress or exercise induced dehydration. *International Journal of Psychophysiology*, 42, 243–51.

Dennis, S.C. and Noakes, T.D. (1999). Advantages of a smaller body mass in humans when distance-running in warm, humid conditions. *European Journal of Applied Physiology*, 79, 280–4.

Drust, B., Rasmussen, P., Mohr, M., *et al.*, (2005). Elevations in core and muscle temperature impairs repeated sprint performance. *Acta Physiologica Scandinavica*, 183, 181–90.

Drust, B., Reilly, T., and Cable, N.T. (2000). Physiological responses to laboratory-based soccer-specific intermittent and continuous exercise. *Journal of Sports Sciences*, 18, 885–92.

Duffield, R., Dawson, B., Bishop, D., *et al.* (2003). Effect of wearing an ice cooling jacket on repeat sprint performance in warm/humid conditions. *British Journal of Sports Medicine*, 37, 164–9.

Duffield, R., Bird, S.P., and Ballard, R.J. (2011). Field-based pre-cooling for on-court tennis conditioning training in the heat. *Journal of Sports Science and Medicine*, 10, 376–84.

Duffield, R., Coutts, A., McCall, A., *et al.* (2013). Pre-cooling for football training and competition in hot and humid conditions. *European Journal of Sport Science*, 13, 58–67.

Duffield, R., Coutts, A., and Quinn, J. (2009). Core temperature responses and match running performance during intermittent-sprint exercise competition in warm conditions. *Journal of Strength and Conditioning Research*, 23, 1238–44.

Duffield, R. Green, R., Castle, P., *et al.* (2012). Precooling can prevent the reduction of self-paced exercise intensity in the heat. *Medicine and Science in Sports and Exercise*, 42, 577–84.

Duffield, R. and Marino, F.E. (2007). Effects of pre-cooling procedures on intermittent-sprint exercise performance in warm conditions. *European Journal of Applied Physiology*, 100, 727–35.

Duffield, R., Steinbacher, G., and Fairchild, T.J. (2009). The use of mixed-method, part-body pre-cooling procedures for teamsport athletes training in the heat. *Journal of Strength and Conditioning Research*, 23, 2524–32.

Duffield, R., McCall, A., Coutts, A.J., *et al.* (2012). Hydration, sweat, and thermoregulatory responses to professional football training in the heat. *Journal of Sports Sciences*, 30, 957–65.

Dugas, J. (2011). Ice slurry ingestion increases running time in the heat. *Clinical Journal of Sports Medicine*, 21, 541–2.

Gisolfi, C.V. and Wenger, C.B. (1984). Temperature regulation during exercise: Old concepts new ideas. *Exercise and Sport Science Reviews*, 12, 339–72.

González-Alonso, J., Grandall, G.G., and Johnson, J.M. (2008). The cardiovascular challenge of exercising in the heat. *Journal of Physiology*, 586, 45–53.

Grandjean, A.C. and Grandjean, N.R. (2007). Dehydration and cognitive performance. *Journal of the American College of Nutrition*, 26, 549S–554S.

Hargreaves, M. (2008). Physiological limits to exercise performance in the heat. *Journal of Science and Medicine in Sport*, 11, 66–71.

Harvey, G. Meir, R. Brooks, L., *et al.* (2008). The use of body mass changes as a practical measure of dehydration in team sports. *Journal of Science and Medicine in Sport*, 1, 600–3.

Iampietro, P.F., Buskirk, E.R., Bass, D.E., *et al.* (1957). Effect of food, climate, and exercise on rectal temperature during the day. *Journal of Applied Physiology*, 11, 349–52.

Kurdak, S.S., Shirreffs, S.M., Maughan, R.J., *et al.* (2010). Hydration and sweating responses to hot-weather football competition. *Scandinavian Journal of Medicine and Science in Sports*, 20, 133–9.

Lacerda, A.C., Gripp, F., Rodrigues, L.O., *et al.* (2007). Acute heat exposure increases high-intensity performance during sprint cycle exercise. *European Journal of Applied Physiology*, 99, 87–93.

Linnane, D.M., Bracken, R.M., Brooks, S., et al. (2004). Effects of hyperthermia on the metabolic responses to repeated high-intensity exercise. *European Journal of Applied Physiology*, 93, 159–66.

Marino, F.E. (2002). Methods, advantages, and limitations of body cooling for exercise performance. *British Journal of Sports Medicine*, 36, 89–94.

Marino, F.E., Mbambo, Z., Kortekass, E., *et al.* (2000). Advantages of smaller body mass during distance running in warm, humid environments. *European Journal of Physiology*, 441, 359–67.

Maughan, R.J. and Shirreffs, S.M. (2010). Dehydration and rehydration in competitive sport. *Scandinavian Journal of Medicine and Science in Sports*, 20, 40–7.

Maughan, R.J. and Shirreffs, S.M. (1997). Preparing athletes for competition in the heat: Developing an effective acclimatization strategy. *Sports Science Exchange*, 65.

Maughan, R.J., Shirreffs, S.M., Ozgünen, K.T., *et al.* (2010). Living, training, and playing in the heat: Challenges to the football player and strategies for coping with environmental extremes. *Scandinavian Journal of Medicine and Science in Sports*, 20, 117–24.

Meir, R. (2012). Training for and competing in Sevens rugby: Practical considerations from experience in the International Rugby Board World Series. *Strength and Conditioning Journal*, 34, 76–86.

Meir, R., Brooks, L., and Rogerson, S. (2011). What do changes in pre-match vs. post-match, 1, 2, and 3 days post-match body weight tell us about fluid status in English Premiership rugby union players? *Journal of Strength and Conditioning Research*, 25, 2337–43.

Meir, R., Brooks, L., and Shield, T. (2003). Body weight and tympanic temperature change in professional rugby league players during day and night games: A study in the field. *Journal of Strength and Conditioning Research*, 17, 566–72.

Meir, R.A., Davie, A.J., and Ohmsen, P. (1990). Thermoregulatory responses of rugby league footballers playing in warm humid conditions. *Sport Health*, 8, 11–4.

Meir, R. and Halliday, A. (2005). Pre- and post-game body mass changes during an international rugby tournament: A practical perspective. *Journal of Strength and Conditioning Research*, 19, 713–6.

Meir, R. and Murphy, A. (1998). Fluid loss and rehydration during training and competition in professional rugby league. *Coaching and Sport Science Journal*, 3, 9–13.

Minett, G., Duffield, R., Marino F., *et al.* (2011). Volume-dependent response of precooling for intermittent-sprint exercise in the heat. *Medicine and Science in Sports and Exercise*, 43, 1760–9.

Mohr, M., Mujika, I., Santisteban, J., *et al.* (2010). Examination of fatigue development in elite soccer in a hot environment: A multi-experimental approach. *Scandinavian Journal of Science and Medicine in Sports*, 20, 125–32.

Mohr, M. and Krustrup, P. (2013). Heat stress impairs repeated jump ability after competitive elite soccer games. *Journal of Strength and Conditioning Research*, 27, 683–9.

Mora-Rodriguez, R. (2012). Influence of aerobic fitness on thermoregulation during exercise in the heat. *Exercise and Sport Sciences Reviews*, 40, 79–87.

Morris, J.G., Nevill, M.E., Boobis, L.H., *et al.* (2005). Muscle metabolism, temperature, and fatigue during prolonged, intermittent, high-intensity running in air temperatures of 33°C and 17°C. *International Journal of Sports Medicine*, 26, 805–14.

Noakes, T.D. (2007). Drinking guidelines for exercise: What evidence is there that athletes should drink 'as much as tolerable', 'to replace the weight lost during exercise', or '*ad libitum*'. *Journal of Sports Sciences*, 25, 781–96.

Nybo, L. and Nielsen, B. (2001). Hyperthermia and central fatigue during prolonged exercise in humans. *Journal of Applied Physiology*, 91, 1055–60.

O'Hara, J.P., Jones, B.L., Tsakirides, C., *et al.* (2010). Hydration status of rugby league players during home match play throughout the 2008 Super League season. *Applied Physiology, Nutrition and Metabolism*, 35, 790–6.

Oppliger, R.A. and Bartok, C. (2002). Hydration testing of athletes. *Sports Medicine*, 32, 959–71.

Powers, S.K. and Howley, E.T. (2012). *Exercise physiology: Theory and application to fitness and performance*, 8th ed. New York: McGraw Hill. pp. 260–80.

Sawka, M.N., Burke, L.M., Eichner, E.R., *et al.* (2007). Exercise and fluid replacement: Position stand of the American College of Sports Medicine. *Medicine and Science in Sports and Exercise*, 39, 377–90.

Sawka, M.N., Young, A.J., Castellani, S.M., *et al.* (2012). Physiological systems and their responses to conditions of heat and cold. In P.A. Farrell, M.J. Joyner, and V.J Caiozzo, (Eds.), *ACSM's Advanced Exercise Physiology*, 2nd ed. Philladelphia: Lippincott Williams and Wilkins, pp. 567–02.

Sharwood, K.A., Collins, M., Goedecke, J.H., *et al.* (2004). Weight changes, medical complications, and performance during an Ironman triathlon. *British Journal of Sports Medicine*, 38, 718–24.

Shi, X. and Gisolfi, C. (1998). Fluid and carbohydrate replacement during intermittent exercise. *Sports Medicine*, 25, 157–72.

Siegel, J., Maté, M., Brearley, G., *et al.* (2010). Ice slurry ingestion increases core temperature capacity and running time in the heat. *Medicine and Science in Sports and Exercise*, 42, 717–25.

Shirreffs, S.M. (2000). Markers of hydration status. *Journal of Sports Medicine and Physical Fitness*, 40, 80–4.

Shirreffs, S.M. (2010). Hydration: Special issues for playing football in warm and hot environments. *Scandinavian Journal of Medicine and Science in Sports*, 20, 90–4.

Shirreffs, S.M. and Maughan, R.J. (1997). Whole body sweat collection in man: An improved method with preliminary data on electrolyte content. *Journal of Applied Physiology*, 82, 336–41.

Silverthorn, D.U. (2010). *Human physiology: An integrated approach*, 5th ed. San Francisco: Pearson Benjamin Cummings.

Sunderland, C. and Nevill, M.E. (2005). High-intensity intermittent running and field hockey skill performance in the heat. *Journal of Sports Sciences*, 23, 531–40.

Tucker, R., Marle, T., Lambert, E.V., *et al.* (2006). The rate of heat storage mediates an anticipatory reduction in exercise intensity during cycling at a fixed rating of perceived exertion. *Journal of Physiology*, 574, 905–15.

Wegmann, M., Faude, O., Poppendieck, W., *et al.* (2012). Pre-cooling and sports performance: a meta-analytical review. *Sports Medicine,* 42, 545–64.

Wendt, D., van Loon, L.J.C., and van Marken Lichtenbelt, W.D. (2007). Thermoregulation during exercise in the heat. *Sports Medicine*, 37, 669–82.

10

PRACTICAL CONSIDERATIONS FOR TEAM TRAVEL, THE LIFESTYLE OF ELITE ATHLETES, TRAVEL FATIGUE, AND COPING WITH JET LAG

Ben J. Edwards, Colin M. Robertson, and Jim M. Waterhouse

10.1 Introduction

International rugby players and their support staff compete or undertake specialized training all over the world; hence, there is a need to travel. For example, the Rugby World Cup has been hosted in New Zealand and Australia (1987), Australia (2003), and New Zealand (2011), and will be held in Japan in 2020.

Any travel, regardless of the transport used, can lead to 'travel fatigue' that persists for up to ~24 h after arrival at the destination. This can be minimized by detailed planning of the trip, including before, during, and after arrival at the destination. Flights that rapidly cross time zones also result in jet lag, which takes several days to address. Both travel fatigue and jet lag can be debilitating and may distract the athlete from the final preparations such as training, and from optimal performance at the competition itself. Further, the management and support team who are generally older and less fit are also susceptible to jet lag and this may affect their decisions, actions, and mentoring of athletes as they adjust to the new time zone. Accordingly, key staff might arrive at destination a number of days or weeks before the athletes. Many Olympic and international squads are given formal advice, normally in the form of a booklet as a complement to personal counselling. In the case of the Great Britain Olympic team (Team GB), this advice was the culmination of two years of research, in which a 'dry run' was conducted the year before the 2000 Games. Each athlete who participated received a feedback report on his/her adjustment. This targeting and specific educational programme prior to the Games led to a good compliance of staff and athletes at the preparation camp in the Gold Coast (Australia), and identified those individuals who had severe symptoms and a slower rate of adjustment.

This chapter will outline current views on the nature and origin of these problems, and offer advice on how to minimise their adverse effects. Recent reviews of this field include Forbes-Robertson *et al.* (2013), Edwards and Waterhouse (2012), Leatherwood and Dragoo (2013), Samuels (2012), Waterhouse *et al.* (2007)

and position statements by the European College of Sport Science (Reilly *et al.* 2007).

10.2 Travel fatigue vs. jet lag

'Travel fatigue' is associated with any long journeys, irrespective of mode of transport or number of time zones crossed (Reilly *et al.* 2007; Waterhouse *et al.* 2007). Its symptoms include disorientation, general weariness, and increased incidence of headaches. The severity of these symptoms can vary between individuals, and normally disappear substantially by the next day, after a shower, sufficient rehydration, and a good night's sleep. Nocturnal sleep should present no problems, since night at the destination and at the place of departure coincide. A recent study has shown travel fatigue does not appear to negatively impact elite rugby league players' ability to perform strength and power tasks (McGuckin *et al.* 2014).

By contrast, a flight across three or more time zones gives rise to 'jet lag' in the new time zone (Waterhouse *et al.* 2007). Jet lag is caused by the sluggish readjustment of the circadian timing mechanism to the new environment and lasts until full adjustment has occurred; hence, it is essentially different from travel fatigue. Other explanations for jet lag include the following:

- The hassle of the flight
- The new lifestyle, food, and culture at the destination
- The excitement of attending important events
- The length of the flight

However, jet lag can be induced in an isolation chamber (where no travel has been undertaken). Jet lag is also found after returning home to a normal routine, and its severity is related to the number of time zones crossed, not the flight length. The symptoms of jet lag, which are likely to result in decreased ability to train and perform well, include:

- Fatigue
- Sleep disturbance (either the inability to get to sleep or an earlier waking time)
- Inappropriately-timed hunger or loss of appetite
- Losses of concentration and drive
- Headaches

10.2.1 How long does it take to get over jet lag?

Generally, symptoms are more severe and readjustment takes longer the greater the number of time zones involved. Flights to the west (requiring a delay of the body clock) are generally better tolerated and associated with less jet lag for the following reasons:

- It is easier to get to sleep following increased time awake.
- The first day in the new time zone is lengthened, enabling the body's biological rhythms to extend in line with the person's free-running period of about 25 h and thus catch up. (see section 10.3)

- Exposure to the natural light–dark cycle at the destination promotes appropriate adjustment of the body clock.

Further, after an eastward journey across ten time zones (an advance of local timing), current guidelines suggest that, for the purposes of the use of light as a readjustment strategy, it should be treated as a transition of 14 hours to the west (requiring a delay of the body clock). This tendency for the body clock to adjust by a delay rather than an advance after crossing ten to twelve time zones in an easterly direction (where destination time is advanced by ten to twelve hours with regard to departure time) is termed an antidromic effect (as opposed to an orthodromic effect, where the adjustment is in the expected direction of travel).

In studies where the symptoms and rating of jet lag are taken routinely (and at multiple times) at the destination during the solar day, although fatigue is present until adjustment occurs, the importance of other symptoms depends upon the time of day these are assessed. Hence, jet lag in the morning is associated with poorer sleep the previous night, whilst jet lag during the day is associated with decreased abilities to concentrate and maintain motivation. In the evening, jet lag is associated with not feeling ready for the next sleep (Waterhouse et al. 2005). The amount of jet lag experienced differs between individuals, but there has been little success in predicting those who will be most affected (for summary, see Waterhouse et al. 2007). For example, it has been argued that jet lag will be less marked in subjects who are younger, more physically fit, and have flexible sleeping habits, but supporting evidence is poor, especially in the case of well-motivated and experienced travellers (Waterhouse et al. 2000).

10.3 Where is the body clock located, and what is its purpose?

The internal timing mechanism that mediates these rhythms (the body clock) is located at the base of the hypothalamus in paired suprachiasmatic nuclei (SCN). Through cyclic interactions between 'clock genes', 'clock proteins', and their products, a biochemical cycle arises in the activity of SCN cells (Reppert and Weaver 2001). The cells have receptors for melatonin (the hormone released by the pineal gland), receive information directly from the eyes (the retinohypothalamic tract), and obtain information about physical activity and general 'excitement' via the intergeniculate leaflet. There may also be some input due to 'feeding' (Raphe-hypothalamic tract) via the Raphe nuclei – although the effect of this is thought to be weak in humans. The body clock's influence pervades the whole body since it is near brain areas that regulate temperature, hormone secretion, the autonomic nervous system, sleep–wake cycles, and feeding cycles. Although there are peripheral clocks throughout the body, the SCN-based body clock has been likened to the conductor in an orchestra, keeping the other clocks in rhythm and in harmony.

The purpose of body clock is to prepare the body for waking and mental activity in the light and for sleeping and nocturnal inactivity (consolidated sleep and restitution) when it is naturally dark. Both changes require ordered sequences of biochemical and physiological events. These effects of the body clock are altered after timezone transitions and are responsible for jet lag. Temporal isolation studies, in which subjects have been kept in caves or isolation chambers with constant environments, have shown that one of the inherent characteristics of the body clock is that it free-runs with a period of ~24.5 hours, so it tends to become phase delayed. This inexact timing mechanism is set to an exact 24 hour day by so-called zeitgebers (German: time givers), rhythms resulting from the environment. These rhythms include the light–dark cycle, the sleep–wake cycle, rhythms in socialising, eating, and, possibly, based on some recent evidence, rhythms of activity and exercise (See reviews by Atkinson *et al.* 2007 and Edwards *et al.* 2009).

In humans, the most important zeitgebers are the light–dark cycle and the rhythm of melatonin secretion. The activity of the body clock cannot be measured directly in humans, so there is need to rely on 'marker rhythms'. The most widely used marker rhythms are the pineal secretory product, melatonin, and core body temperature. In the case of the 24 hour rhythm of core temperature found in the majority of the population (intermediate types), when subjects are living normally, values peak in the evening (17:00 h) and are at their lowest at night (05:00 h), when cosinor analysis has been performed upon 24 hour data. When morning–evening (chronotype) preference is assessed by a simple questionnaire (Smith *et al.* 1989), Morning types (larks) show rhythms of temperature that occur earlier by ~1 h, and evening types (owls) later by ~1 h. This difference in phase of the core body temperature due to chronotype complicates the timing of an adaption strategy, giving rise to the idea that, prior to travel, athletes should have their phase assessed.

A 'constant routine' allows us to separate the internal (or endogenous clock driven) and external (environmental driven) components of any rhythms by minimising environment and lifestyle input. In such a protocol which lasts for >24 h, subjects remain awake and inactive in a constant environment (temperature, humidity, and light), whilst maintaining the same posture and engaging in quiet activities. In this protocol, the subjects also eat identical isocaloric meals at regular intervals. Results indicate that in the case of core temperature, although the rhythm is reduced, the rhythm of body temperature persists (Figure 10.1).

Circadian rhythmicity in human physiology has been reported extensively – that is, rhythms that manifest themselves over a 24 hour solar day (see Drust *et al.* 2005). In regard to sporting performance and in relation to jet lag, it is worth noting that, before travel:

*   Circadian rhythms in gross muscular tasks such as strength (regardless of site of measurement), power, and time-trial performance show peaks and minima in parallel to those of core body temperature (Table 10.1).

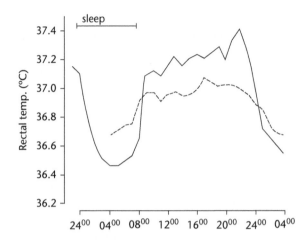

FIGURE 10.1 Mean circadian changes in core (rectal) temperature measured hourly in 8
subjects: Living normally and sleeping from 24:00 to 08:00h (solid line);
then awoken at 04:00h and spending the next 24h on a 'constant routine'
(dashed line). (based on Reilly *et al.* 1997).

- Those tasks that have a high cognitive component and require greater central processing (such as accuracy of tennis or badminton serves) peak around 13:00–15:00 h due to homeostatic and circadian components.
- Those tasks that require fine motor coordination, relate to learning, or require game tactics are suggested to be better in the morning (see Drust *et al.* 2005).

Evidence that jet lag affects the sporting performance of athletes is sparse due to an uncertainty about how to measure performance in a way that replicates performance but does not cause serial fatigue, how frequently measurements should be made each day, and how many days the study should last having reached the destination. The rationale for the adjustment strategies recommended for athletes crossing multiple time zones can be found elsewhere (see Waterhouse *et al.* 2007 and Reilly and Waterhouse 2009).

10.4 Behavioural advice on dealing with jet lag before and during a flight

The body clock will not have time to adjust if the stay in the new time zone lasts only a few days. Therefore, if the event involves only a brief visit at a destination to compete, then the athlete should arrange activities to coincide with daytime in the time zone just left (coincident with 'body time') and avoid times coincident with night on body time (Lowden and Åkerstedt 1998). Accordingly, after eastward flights, local afternoons or evenings are preferable to morning; after westward

TABLE 10.1 Circadian variation in a range of performance measures for males

Performance	Peak time (decimal time, h)	Amplitude (% of 24-h mean)	Reference
Rectal temperature	17.29	0.8	Giacomoni et al. (2005)
Isometric			
Grip strength	20.00	6.0	Atkinson et al. (1994)
Leg strength: **Knee** **extensors**	16.17	4.5	Giacomoni et al. (2005)
Back strength	16.53	10.6	Coldwells et al. (1994)
Dynamic strength			
Knee extensors			
1.05 rad.s^{-1}	16.58	2.8	Giacomoni et al. (2005)
3.14 rad.s^{-1}	17.06	2.6	Giacomoni et al. (2005)
Anaerobic Power			
Broad jump	17.45	3.4	Reilly and Down (1986)
Stair run	17.26	2.1	Reilly and Down (1992)
Time-trial			
Swimming 100 m	18.03	3.4	Kline et al. (2007)
Running 10 km	17.41	6.3	Edwards et al. (2008)
Intermediately complex **hand–eye coordination skill**	15.20	9.8	Edwards and Waterhouse (2009)

flights, mornings and early afternoons are preferable to late afternoons and evenings (see Table 10.2 for examples for +3 eastward and –3 westward time zone transition). For complete adaptation, current advice suggests that athletes should schedule their arrival well in advance of competition, allowing one day for each time zone travelled to the west and 1.5 days for each time zone travelled in an easterly direction (Klein and Wegmann 1974). This allowance may be an overestimation and would be impractical, as it would require an athlete travelling from the UK to arrive 15 days prior to any competition on the east coast of Australia (10 time zones to the east). It has prompted a more realistic suggestion of leaving one day for each time zone crossed in either a westward or eastward journey (Waterhouse et al. 2007).

TABLE 10.2 Is there an optimal timing of performance after three time zones travel eastward or westward?

Body clock time	23:00	05:00	11:00	17:00	23:00
Local time Easterly **travel (+3 time zones)**	02:00	08:00 Disadvantage Morning	14:00	20:00 Advantage Evening	02:00
Local time Westerly **travel (–3 time zones)**	20:00	02:00 Disadvantage Early Morning	08:00	14:00 Advantage Early Afternoon	20:00

10.4.1 Pre-adjustment strategy

Theoretically, adjustment of sleep–wake habits before the flight could begin to alter the normal circadian rhythm in the desired direction prior to departure. This strategy involves sending the athletes to bed earlier and getting them up earlier for an eastward journey, and retiring and rising later for a westward journey. The strategy for a westward flight is tolerated more easily than that for a flight to the east as, when sent to bed earlier (eastward flight), athletes find it hard to get to sleep until the normal time (biological time) – and then are expected to wake earlier than usual. As a result, some sleep deprivation results (see Reilly and Edwards 2007). In order to avoid disrupting the individual's ability to integrate with the rest of society whilst still in the home time zone, and to allow the athlete to continue to train normally, an adjustment of the sleep–wake cycle by no more than one to two hours and for no more than one to two days is recommended.

10.4.2 Travel times

Some of the factors that can be changed relatively easily are the time of flight departure, and hence time of arrival, along with the decision whether or not to incorporate a stop-over. Arriving as close to night-time in the new time zone as schedules allow is advantageous due to the smaller accumulation of fatigue during the flight; this tactic means that the new sleep–wake cycle (and its zeitgeber effects) are experienced as soon as possible (Waterhouse *et al.* 2002). If the journey (such as one from the UK to the East coast of Australia) is broken up, with a stop-over in Singapore for a few days, this aids adjustment at the final destination, as it gives the body clock a chance to adjust partially when exposed to the environment at the place of stop-over. In practice, this break in the journey involves additional disruption for the athlete in terms of maintaining quality of training. Also, it could add complications such as heat and humidity in the stop-over environment, and these present their own problems for the athlete (see Chapter 9).

10.4.3 During the flight

Generally, when on-board the idea is to change the timing of the behaviour of the athlete as much as possible to that which is appropriate to destination time in terms of activity, sleep and wakefulness, and eating meals. Travellers should set watches to destination time, and use this to decide whether or not to take a nap, the best time for a nap being when it is night in the destination time zone. Sleepiness will be greatest when it is night in the time zone just left, but napping at this time will hinder adjustment to destination time. These strategies should be conveyed to the cabin crew, to avoid confusion and inappropriate times of waking the athlete – for example, for meals. Further, there is a need to replenish the fluid loss (about 15 to 20 ml extra fluid per hour), preferably fruit juice or water, to compensate for the loss of water from the upper respiratory tract attributable to inhaling dry cabin air

(Reilly *et al.* 2007). Drinks containing caffeine or alcohol should be avoided during the flight, as they are diuretics and would accentuate dehydration, which could persist into the early days in the new time zone. Following reports of the increase in incidence of deep vein thrombosis associated with inactivity in a cramped environment, performing isometric exercises and leaving the seat to walk around the plane are advised (Philbrick *et al.* 2007), with some senior staff advised to wear compression stockings (Sajid *et al.* 2006).

10.5 Pharmacological advice on dealing with jet lag

10.5.1 Melatonin

The use of chronobiotics such as melatonin and its synthetic analogues, which directly shift the body clock or indirectly aid adjustment due to their soporific properties that aid getting to sleep at the new nighttime, has received some attention in the research literature (Waterhouse *et al.* 2007; Altun and Ugur-Altun 2007). When given approximately two hours before the desired bedtime, the soporific effects of melatonin are being invoked. However, if melatonin is to adjust the body clock appropriately, ingestion time depends upon the flight direction and number of time zones crossed. There has been some concern with the appropriate timing of melatonin to aid in readjustment of the body clock after an easterly transition across ten time zones. Further, when strict control of light-avoidance and exposure is not adhered to (this exerting a powerful zeitgeber effect upon the body clock), the effectiveness of melatonin is reduced (Edwards *et al.* 2000). The current position statement of the British Olympic Association advises athletes against using melatonin. Furthermore, in the UK, pure melatonin is available only when prescribed by a physician (Reilly *et al.* 1998). Evidence failing to support the value of melatonin in dealing with a variety of sleep problems, including sleep restriction after time zone transitions, was presented in a meta-analysis by Buscemi *et al.* (2006). Interestingly, this meta-analysis also provided evidence that melatonin was safe with use up to a period of three months.

10.5.2 Sleeping pills

Sleeping pills have been used by some travelling athletes to induce sleep during flights. Drugs such as benzodiazepines (particularly the short-acting benzodiazepines) are effective in inducing sleep, but they do not guarantee a prolonged period asleep. For example, they were ineffective in accelerating adjustment of the body clock in a group of British Olympic athletes travelling to the United States (Reilly *et al.* 2001). In additon, these drugs have not all been satisfactorily tested for subsequent residual effects on motor performances such as sport skills and may, in fact, be counterproductive if administered at the incorrect time. Sedatives such as zopiclone and zolpidem have fewer side effects and minimal interference with normal sleep architecture (Lemmer 2007). Also, there is a current trend for athletes, specifically rugby players, to use hypnotics habitually; to this end, over the last ten years, the main advice requested by medics has been how much of these drugs can be prescribed before performance is adversely affected. The caveat regarding the use of such drugs is that, if athletes are going to use hypnotics or melatonin, they should do so only with the support of the team doctor and should also inform the sport scientist, who can check an individual's response to such medications.

10.5.3 Caffeine and promoting alertness

Caffeine (equivalent to two cups of coffee) temporarily improves alertness during a night without sleep (Wright *et al.* 1997). It also increases nocturnal sleep latency and decreases the amount of slow wave sleep (recuperative sleep). Its effects upon daytime sleep (following one night of total sleep deprivation) seem more marked (Carrier *et al.* 2007), a result that might be particularly relevant since sleep in the new time zone might coincide with 'daytime' by body time. The best advice is to drink coffee at the new breakfast time to promote wakefulness and to avoid it in the evening.

10.6 Behavioural advice on dealing with jet lag

The behavioural strategy involves the appropriate use of the zeitgebers (time-givers) that aid entrainment: the light–dark and the sleep–wakefulness cycles, diet and meal-times, activity and exercise, and melatonin ingestion. A combined approach of light exposure and avoidance and melatonin ingestion (incorporating exercise regimens, mealtimes and social factors – all of which might act to emphasise rhythms in the new time zone) would seem an attractive proposition (Cardinali *et al.* 2006; Barion and Zee 2007; Lack and Wright 2007). Further work is required to establish the value of such 'package deals'. There is also little scientific evidence in favour of promoting clock adjustment by consuming protein in the morning to promote arousal and carbohydrates at nighttime to promote sleep (Leathwood 1989). Rather, it seems that meals can be used to emphasize the timing of rhythms in the new time zone.

In implementing adjustment strategies aimed at shifting the human circadian rhythm, an indirect marker for the body clock is used. In this and the following examples, the reference point will be the body temperature minimum of ~05:00 ± 1 h (though this is chronotype-dependent), this profile having been previously established by cosine analysis of 24 hours of temperature data (see Figure 10.2). Light is the strongest zeitgeber, and the effect of light depends upon the time of exposure, as described by a phase–response curve (Czeisler *et al.* 1989; Honma and Honma 1988; Minors *et al.* 1991). Exposure to light during the six hours before the temperature minimum results in a delay in the body clock, and in the six hours after the temperature minimum, a phase advance. Exposure to bright light at other times results in no phase shift and this is referred to as a 'dead–zone' (Khalsa *et al.* 2003). The size of phase shifts depends upon light intensity, domestic lighting (~200 lux) exerting

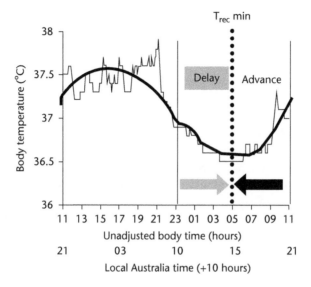

FIGURE 10.2 Circadian rhythm of rectal temperature with a cosine curve superimposed on 24 hours of raw data. Body temperature minimum and direction of resultant phase-shift produced by light given six hours before and six hours after this minimum are indicated. Local time is superimposed with an example of the strategy for light exposure and avoidance after an eastward transition across 10 time zones.

smaller effects than natural light (>10000 lux). Natural light passing through windows and domestic lighting normally combine to adjust the body clock to a 24 hour rhythm (Waterhouse *et al.* 1998).

If we now use an example of a phase-delaying strategy, in the case of a ten time zone transition to the east (UK to the east coast of Australia) for intermediate type athletes (05:00 h body temperature minimum), we can superimpose local time on body clock time (see Figure 10.2). The unadjusted body clock produces a temperature minimum at 15:00 h by new local time. This would require exposure to light between 10:00 h and 15:00 h (local time) on Day 1 (to produce a phase delay), and avoiding light between 15:00 h and 21:00 h (which would cause a phase advance). On Day 2 (as the body temperature minimum would have been delayed by about two hours to 17:00 h by local time), the next day's light exposure would be recommended to be between 11:00 h and 17:00 h, and avoidance between 17:00 h and 23:00 h, and so on for subsequent days. If a phase-advance strategy were used for the same journey, then the times of light avoidance and exposure would be the opposite. This would produce an advance rather than delay of the body clock on the first day, and then would continue to be advanced by two hours per day on subsequent days. It is generally observed that readjustment tends to follow an exponential function, with greater adjustment occurring in the first few days (Wegmann *et al.* 1983), and those rhythms with a greater internal (body clock) component taking longer to adjust, hence requiring an order to adjustment.

Figure 10.3 shows the advantage of adjustment by a phase delay (14 hours) rather than advance after a time zone transition of 10 hours. When adjusted to the local time zone, peak performance generally occurs in the early evening (17:00 h) and the temperature minimum, associated with greatest sleepiness and lowest performance, is found towards the end of sleep. The cosine curve fitted to such results has been transposed onto the local time in the new time zone, showing the timing of the performance rhythm with complete lack of adjustment, partial adjustment, and complete adjustment shown. Immediately after arrival, peak temperature and performance will be at about 03:00 h local time, and the minimum temperature value and worst performance at 15:00 h hours. If a phase delay occurs, peak performance progressively delays and soon coincides with times awake, and sleepiness moves later through the evening and soon coincides with the time when sleep is wanted. This adaptation means that there is some time of the day (mornings, when body temperature is high) when high-quality training can take place during the process of adjustment. By contrast, an advance of the body clock by ten hours advances the peaks of temperature and performance through the night in the new time zone, so hindering

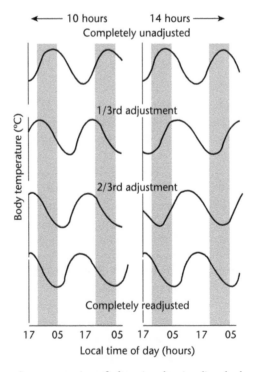

FIGURE 10.3 Schematic representation of advancing the circadian rhythm of rectal temperature by 10 hours or delaying it by 14 hours after an eastward flight across 10 time zones. Shading indicates night time.

sleep. Also, the temperature minimum and maximum sleepiness advance through the afternoon and morning. Therefore, impaired sleep and performance will be inconvenient for a greater number of days. These results suggest a practical advantage if adjustment after an eastward journey across ten time zones is by a delay rather than an advance of the body clock. It also is more convenient with regard to light exposure for individuals arriving in the early morning in the new time zone (which is what, in practice, happens with most long-haul flights to the east).

There are, however, difficulties in translating theory into practice. In the field study upon 85 individuals before the Sydney Olympics (summer 2000), adjustment was consistent with a delay for 35 individuals, with an advance of the body clock for 23. For 27 individuals, it was unclear whether adjustment was by an advance or delay (Reilly *et al.* 2003; Waterhouse *et al.* 2002). Such differences in adjustment would have made it difficult to manage daily preparations in Australia after arrival. Nevertheless, taking into consideration also the departure and arrival times, and attempting to promote adjustment in one direction for the team as a whole, a 'phase-advance' strategy was chosen. This most appropriate strategy involved light-avoidance in the morning, no morning training for three to four days, and a lie-in for the first three days after arrival.

Another method to readjust the body clock to the new time zone is exercise. This is intuitively attractive as this is the medium that athletes already use, and so warrants further investigation. Like light, a partial phase response curve to exercise has been recently reported (Atkinson *et al.* 2007; Edwards *et al.* 2009), but the practicalities of using this are still unclear. This notwithstanding, one study has successfully used a practical amount of exercise as pre-adaptation strategy to improve performance the day before a competition (Edwards *et al.* 2005).

In most cases, the individual phase position of an athlete is not known, and taking these measures is not practical. Therefore, if we take a window of $\pm 1\,h$ from 05:00 h to take into account chronotype (morning–eveningness), we can provide a table of recommended use of bright light to adjust the body clock after time zone transitions. These 'body times' must be converted to the new local times. Table 10.3 shows this conversion applied to the first day in the new time zone (when body time coincides with local time in the time zone just left). It should also be remembered that eastward flights across more than ten time zones should be treated as ones to the west (requiring a delay of the body clock), because large delays of the body clock are easier to accomplish than large advances.

10.7 Advice on training schedules

Athletes will want to continue training and preparing for competition before adjustment of the body clock is complete. There is no single 'correct' approach; it must be individually tailored. The advice acted upon should be determined by personal preference, following discussions between interested parties (athlete, coach, trainer, etc.). This advice is formalized in Table 10.4.

TABLE 10.3 Recommendation for the use of bright light to adjust the body clock after time zone transitions.

	Good local times (h) for exposure to light	Bad local times (h) for exposure to light
Time Zones to the West (h)		
3	19:00–01:00†	03:00–09:00★
4	18:00–24:00†	02:00–08:00★
5	17:00–23:00†	01:00–07:00★
6	16:00–22:00†	24:00–06:00★
7	15:00–21:00†	23:00–05:00★
8	14:00–20:00†	22:00–04:00★
9	13:00–19:00†	21:00–03:00★
10	12:00–18:00†	20:00–02:00★
11	11:00–17:00†	19:00–01:00★
12	10:00–16:00†	18:00–24:00★
13	09:00–15:00†	17:00–23:00★
14	08:00–14:00†	16:00–22:00★
Time Zones to the East (h)		
3	09:00–15:00★	01:00–07:00†
4	10:00–16:00★	02:00–08:00†
5	11:00–17:00★	03:00–09:00†
6	12:00–18:00★	04:00–10:00†
7	13:00–19:00★	05:00–11:00†
8	14:00–20:00★	06:00–12:00†
9	15:00–21:00★	07:00–13:00†
10	Treat as 14h to the west‡	Treat as 14h to the west‡
11	Treat as 13h to the west‡	Treat as 13h to the west‡
12	Treat as 12h to the west‡	Treat as 12h to the west‡

† Promotes a phase delay of the body clock
★ Promotes a phase advance of the body clock
‡ Body clock adjusts to large delays easier than to large advances
This table is based on T_{min} of 05:00 h

10.8 Summary

Travel fatigue and jet lag are inevitable consequences of travel. Though symptoms present themselves in a similar manner, they are caused by different aspects of travel. Travel fatigue typically subsides after one day, but jet lag takes longer (about one day per time zone crossed). Advice in regard to preparation prior to, during, and after arrival at the destination can help reduce the symptoms of jet lag. Behavioural strategies such as light avoidance and exposure should be preferentially adopted rather than pharmacological methods. An educational programme providing feedback to athletes by oral presentations and in written form works well and provides informed advice as what to expect when suffering from jet lag. Once the decision of the appropriate strategy has been made, all athletes in the team should

TABLE 10.4 Comments and considerations related to performance, timing of training, and roles of naps and habit in time of training.

Considerations	Comments
Poorer performance	In the build-up to a competition, performance (especially that requiring cognitive skills) will be reduced and motivation will fall. This is normal and, as adjustment to the new time zone progresses, performance, sleep, and motivation will improve.
Times of training	There are 'best' and 'worst' times to train for competition, where worst times coincide with night in the time zone just left and the best (least bad!) to late afternoon by this time. Individuals can choose: *either* to adjust immediately their training schedules to accord with new local time, accepting that results will initially be poorer: *or* to adjust training schedules to accord with *home* time for the first days in the new time zone, gradually adjusting the time to the new local time (about 2 h per day, in step with adjustment of the body clock).
Role of naps	Taking naps to compensate for sleep loss is useful; naps lasting only a few minutes provide some benefit, but naps should not be long enough to hinder nocturnal sleep. Lastly, although individuals will feel most tired during night-time in the time zone just departed, napping then is not advised, since it will hinder adjustment of the body clock.
Role of habit in time of training	We have shown that training at a particular time of day may produce a more marked improvement when tested at the same time (Edwards *et al.* 2005). One explanation is that there might be an effect of habituation. Again, therefore, a choice arises: *either* to train at the accustomed time of day (so adjusting habits to the new time zone), which might help 'settling down' in the new time zone: *or* to train at the same time as when the competition will be held. Importantly, an individual should understand that options exist, the rationale for adoption of one strategy, and then (after consultation) act accordingly *but stick with one strategy*.

be informed with the expectation that all follow this programme. Some individuals take longer to adjust and report heightened symptoms, and should be monitored until complete adjustment has occurred. It is good practice to send key athlete support staff to the destination before the athletes' arrival, to ensure the support staff are prepared for the athletes – when they have to be fully alert for work and for their monitoring role – rather than recovering from jet lag themselves.

Case study: preparation and performance of a representative team for the Rugby League World Cup in Australia 2008

Introduction

The case study integrates the scientific theory behind jet lag strategies with applied real world rugby practice and application, and shows how the 'gold standard' recommendations sometimes have to be modified for practical reasons.

Case presentation

The flight departed from Manchester, United Kingdom, at 21:00 h on the 13th of October 2008, bound for the Rugby League World Cup in Australia (ten time zones eastwards). The first decision was whether to advance (11 hours; taking into account daylight savings time) or delay the clock. A 13 hour delay strategy, for the reasons given previously, was adopted. The moment the team boarded the flight, the adaption strategy was reinforced by the managers, staff, and players, as a result of which the flight time became Day 1 of the adjustment strategy. This view was strengthened since the confines of the aeroplane provided an artificial environment which could be controlled with regard to exposure to light and ingestion of meals. The athletes had a thorough hydration strategy on the plane and promoted activity and stretching on board. The activity for the five days after arrival and light/dark predetermined map of adjustment, as well as comments on the day, are given in Table 10.5.

Discussion: issues relating to athletes and jet lag coping strategies

In previous implementation of jet lag re-adjustment strategies, we found those athletes who were the more compliant to the advice given tended to adjust faster than those who were resistant to this advice. The 'poor adjusters' tended to be led by coaches and managers who were resistant, but rather stuck to 'what they always did', irrespective of the multiple time zone transition involved. To this end, reinforcing a 'team' approach, with all staff and athletes agreeing what was being done and why it worked well, improved compliance and reduced any barriers to uptake. This strategy entailed educating the athlete as to what jet lag is, explaining what strategies should be adopted to minimize it, and encouraging perseverance, compliance, and a positive attitude – all of which helped to promote and manage adjustment to the new time zone. Training at a lower intensities and durations than normal for the first couple of days after arrival was advocated, to help reduce possible problems with injury. Even so, the good dialogue between athletes and staff that existed enabled the athletes to input their views on how they were feeling (e.g. tiredness) and performing, and this led to a change in structure of one of the training days. Timing exercise to be undertaken outdoors at times advocated for light exposure (in the morning), and discussing tactics indoors when light should be avoided, worked well for the team and was well tolerated. Further, maximizing the use of the location and environment (beach and sea in Australia) enabled a progressive increase in training, even with fatigue present and without any complaints from the athletes.

One of the problems at the destination was 'anchor sleep', which refers to a short sleep period at the time the individual would normally have been asleep if living on home time. Such sleep contrives to 'anchor' circadian rhythms to home time and this opposes adaptation to the new local time. For this reason, we instructed the athletes not to nap for the first few days after arrival at the destination. However, sleep deprivation, due to cumulative sleep loss from the time of arrival to Day 4 after arrival, was apparent in the squad, and this was taken into account by changing the

TABLE 10.5 Day(s) from arrival, light/dark strategy, activity undertaken and comments

All times are expressed in local time. The strategy is based on a progressive 1-hour (black) or 2-hour (*italics*) delay in the rhythm each day after arrival.

Day	Light seeking	Avoidance	Activity
Day 0 arrival **15th October**. Sydney airport at 08:00 h	08:00–14:00 h	16:00–22:00 h	Further travel to the training ground in Narrabeen, and generally settling into camp – room and kit allocations, team meetings.
Comment: All of this made for an easy first full day's adjustment – as the players and staff had no training demands placed on them, and we could arrange these activities to coincide easily with the predetermined 'activity light seeking' and 'light avoidance' times.			
Day 1 after arrival **16th of October** Session 1 (06:30 h) Session 2 (14:00–15:40 h)	09:00–15:00 h *10:00–16:00 h*	17:00–23:00 h *18:00–24:00 h*	1) 2-mile run at 60–70% heart rate max. Then forwards and backs were split into 2 groups 1) gym and 2) grappling sessions (65% of typical workloads) – these sessions were rotated. 2) Skill-based, focusing on local muscular endurance, specifically around the shoulders and upper limbs at moderate intensity.
Comment: The session worked well and served its purposes; drawing the squad closer to the level of intensity they would need to be training fully. It was quite apparent that all of the players felt as though they'd had more than enough.			
Day 2 after arrival **17th October** Session 1 (09:00 h)	11:00–16:00 h *14:00–20:00 h*	18:00–24:00 h *20:00–02:00 h*	Plan was to take the team into Manly and make use of the training ground situated two minutes from the beach. The skills session at the training ground then run the squad over to the beach and take them through some real grunt work on the sand and in the water.
Comment: This was a very physically demanding session, set at an intensity reaching very close to 100%. Had such an intense session been conducted in a gym or on a wet and windy field in the UK, it would be very likely that after one effort you would have a squad of disgruntled and complaining athletes on your hands. The session worked much better than planned, and that only ever happens once in a very long whilst. Importantly though, we were obviously approaching full acclimation and the full squad was starting to look like it might be ready and able to cope with high-intensity training loads and demands.			
Day 3 after arrival **18th October** Session 1 (09:00 h) Session 2 (14:00–15:40 h)	12:00–17:00 h *16:00–22:00 h*	19:00–01:00 h *22:00–04:00 h*	1) Squad broken down into forwards and backs the second real weights session 2) Skill work – primarily focusing on grip and passing drills.
Comment: I was starting to have some concerns. The squad was all training well, ahead of schedule from a physical point of view, but there were still problems with sleep patterns, and some of the players weren't getting off to sleep until the very early hours. With a schedule like ours that could only ever last for a limited period of time. There were more than just a few complaints made during this session, the squad was visibly tired and, as such, it was affecting their motivation to train. The players had a senior's meeting with the head coach and requested that they be given some respite and an easier day (the strong man event, which would involve tyre-flips, tug-o-war and Atlas stones). That night we all – players, coaches and management alike – slept a lot better.			
Day 4 after arrival **19th October** Session 1 (**09:00 h**)	13:00–18:00 h *18:00–24:00 h*	20:00–02:00 h *24:00–06:00 h*	Athletes self-selected their activity
Comment: So the strong man event was off. Some of the squad were disappointed and only too pleased to air their objection. The athletes were given free-rein over what they decided to do in the gym. The first match (against Tonga) wasn't until the 27th of the month, so we still had eight days to go, and two days before we started our game-specific preparations. Also, allowing any athletes to self-select their activity has always proven – in my experience – to do them more good than harm. It was like being stood in the middle of 'Globo Gym'; there was a good energy in the gym'.			

nature and structure of a training day. On restarting normal training practices, we monitored the athletes whilst they were still adjusting, and everybody's (both coaches' and athletes') expectations of performance reflected this lack of full adjustment.

In conclusion, this case study of a representative Rugby League squad competing in the 2008 World Cup in Australia, highlights the benefits of inclusion of coaches and managers as well as athletes in team strategies that had been learnt from successful international and Olympic preparation camps, as well as from an understanding of the importance of monitoring the progress of training and symptoms in all individuals in the team.

References

Altun, A. and Ugur-Altun, B. (2007). Melatonin: therapeutic and clinical utilization. *International Journal of Clinical Practice*, 61, 835–45.

Atkinson, G. (1994). Effects of age on human circadian rhythms in physiological and performance measures. PhD thesis. Liverpool: John Moores University.

Atkinson, G., Edwards, B., Reilly, T., *et al.* (2007). Exercise as a synchroniser of human circadian rhythms: an update and discussion of the methodological problems. *European Journal of Applied Physiology*, 99, 331–41.

Barion, A. and Zee, P. (2007). A clinical approach to circadian rhythm sleep disorders. *Sleep Medicine*, 8, 566–77.

Buscemi, N., Vandermeer, B., and Hooton, N. (2006). Efficacy and safety of exogenous melatonin for secondary sleep disorders and sleep disorders accompanying sleep restriction: meta-analysis. *British Medical Journal*, 332, 385–8.

Cardinali, D., Furio, A., and Reyes, M. (2006). The use of chronobiotics in the resynchronization of the sleep–wake cycle. *Cancer Causes and Control*, 17, 601–9.

Carrier, J., Fernandez-Bolanos, M., and Robillard, R. (2007). Effects of caffeine are more marked on daytime recovery sleep than on nocturnal sleep. *Neuropsychopharmacology*, 32, 964–72.

Coldwells, A., Atkinson, G., and Reilly, T. (1994). Sources of variation in back and leg dynamometry. *Ergonomics*, 37, 79–86.

Czeisler, C., Kronauer, R., Allan, J., *et al.* (1989). Bright light induction of strong (type 0) resetting of the human circadian pacemaker. *Science*, 244, 1328–33.

Drust, B., Waterhouse, J., Atkinson, G., *et al.* (2005). Circadian rhythms in sports performance: an update. *Chronobiology International*, 22, 21–44.

Edwards, B.J., Atkinson, G., Reilly, T., *et al.* (2000). Use of melatonin on recovery from jet-lag following an easterly flight across 10 time-zones. *Ergonomics*, 43, 1501–13.

Edwards, B.J., Boyle, B., Doran, D., *et al.* (2008). Effect of time of day on 10km time-trial running performance. Abstract for the E.C.S.S. 13th annual congress. Estoril, Portugal. 9–12 July.

Edwards, B.J., Edwards, W., Atkinson, G., *et al.* (2005). Can performance in a morning time-trial be improved by morning exercise the day before? *International Journal of Sports Medicine*, 26, 651–6.

Edwards, B.J., Reilly, T., and Waterhouse, J. (2009). Zeitgeber-effects of exercise on human circadian rhythms: what are alternative approaches to investigating the existence of a phase-response curve to exercise? *Biological Rhythm Research*, 40, 53–69.

Edwards, B.J. and Waterhouse, J. (2009). Effects of one night of partial sleep deprivation upon diurnal rhythms of accuracy and consistency in throwing darts. *Chronobiology International*, 26, 756–68.

Edwards, B.J. and Waterhouse, J. (2012). Effects of long-distance journeys upon endurance training: travel fatigue and jet lag. In I. Mujika (ed), *Endurance Training – Science and Practice* Basque Country: S.L.U. pp. 293–03.

Forbes-Robertson, S., Dudley, E., Vadgama, P., *et al.* (2012). Circadian disruption and remedial interventions: effects and interventions for jet lag for athletic peak performance. *Sports Medicine*, 42, 185–208.

Giacomconi, M., Edwards, B., and Bambaeichi, E. (2005). Gender-related differences in the circadian variations in muscle strength. *Ergonomics*, 48, 1473–87.

Honma, K. and Honma, S. (1988). A human phase response curve for bright light pulses. *Japanese Journal of Psychiatry Neurology*, 42, 167–8.

Khalsa, S., Jewett, M., Cajochen, C., *et al.* (2003). A phase response curve to single bright light pulses in human subjects. *Journal of Physiology*, 549, 945–52.

Klein, K.E. and Wegmann, H.M. (1974). The resynchronisation of human circadian rhythms after transmeridian flights as a result of flight direction and mode of activity. In L.E. Scheving, F. Halberg, and J.E. Pauly (Eds.), *Chronobiology* Tokyo: Igku Shoin, pp. 564–70.

Kline, C.E., Durstine, J.L., Davis, J.M., Moore, T.A., Devlin, T.M., Zielinski, M.R., and Youngstedt, S.D. (2007). Circadian variation in swim performance. *Journal of Applied Physiology*, 102, 641–9.

Lemmer B. (2007). The sleep–wake cycle and sleeping pills. *Physiology and Behaviour*, 90, 285–93.

Lack, L. and Wright, H. (2007). Chronobiology of sleep in humans. *Cellular and Molecular Life Sciences*, 64, 1205–15.

Leathwood, P. (1989). Circadian rhythms of plasma amino acids, brain neurotransmitters, and behaviour. In J. Arendt, D. Minors, and J. Waterhouse (Eds.). *Biological Rhythms in Clinical Practice* Guildford: Butterworths, pp. 136–59.

Leatherwood, W.E., and Dragoo, J.L. (2013). Effect of airline travel on performance: A review of the literature. *British Journal of Sports Medicine*, 47, 561–7.

Lowden, A. and Åkerstedt, T. (1998). Retaining home-base sleep hours to prevent jet lag in connection with a westward flight across nine time zones. *Chronobiology International*, 15, 365–76.

McGuckin, T.A., Sinclair, W.H., Sealey, R.M., *et al.* (2014). The effects of air travel on performance measures of elite Australian rugby league players. *European Journal of Sport Science*, 14, S116–22.

Minors, D., Waterhouse, J.M., and Wirz-Justice, A. (1991). A human phase-response curve to light. *Neuroscience Letters*, 133, 36–40.

Philbrick, J., Shumate, R., and Siadaty, M. (2007). Air travel and venous thromboembolism: A systematic review. *Journal of General Internal Medicine*, 22, 107–14.

Reilly, T., Atkinson, G., and Budgett, R. (2001). Effect of low-dose temazepam on physiological variables and performance tests following a westerly flight across five time zones. *International Journal of Sports Medicine*, 22, 166–74.

Reilly, T., Atkinson, G., Edwards, B., *et al.*, (2007). Coping with jet lag: a position statement for the European College of Sport Science. *European Journal of Sport Science*, 7, 1–7.

Reilly, T., Atkinson, G., and Waterhouse, J. (1997). *Biological Rhythms and Exercise*. Oxford: Oxford University Press.

Reilly, T. and Down, A. (1986). Circadian variation in the standing broad jump. *Perceptual and Motor Skills*, 62, 830.

Reilly, T. and Down, A. (1992). Investigation of circadian rhythms in anaerobic power and capacity of the legs. *Journal of Sports Medicine and Physical Fitness*, 32, 343–7.

Reilly, T. and Edwards, B. (2007). Altered sleep-wake cycles and physical performance. *Physiology and Behavior*, 90, 274–284.

Reilly, T. and Waterhouse, J. (2009). Sports performance; is there evidence that the body clock plays a role? *European Journal of Applied Physiology*, 106, 321–32.

Reilly, T., Edwards, B.J., and Waterhouse, J. (2003). Lang-haul travel and jet-lag: Behavioural and pharmacological approaches. *Medicina Sportiva*, 7, E115–22.

Reilly, T., Maughan, R., and Budgett, R. (1998). Melatonin: A position statement of the British Olympic Association. *British Journal of Sports Medicine*, 32, 99–100.

Reppert, S. and Weaver, D. (2001). Molecular analysis of mammalian circadian rhythms. *Annual Review of Physiology*, 63, 647–78.

Sajid, M., Tai, N., and Goli, G. (2006). Knee versus thigh length graduated compression stockings for prevention of deep venous thrombosis: A systematic review. *European Journal of Vascular and Endovascular Surgery*, 32, 730–6.

Samuels, C.H. (2012). Jet lag and travel fatigue: A comprehensive management plan for sport medicine physicians and high-performance support teams. *Clinical Journal of Sports Medicine*, 22, 268–73.

Smith, C.S., Reilly, C., and Midkiff, K. (1989). Evaluation of three circadian rhythm questionnaires with suggestions for an improved measure of morningness. *Journal of Applied Psychology*, 74, 728–38.

Waterhouse, J., Nevill, A., Finnegan, J., *et al.* (2005). Further assessments of the relationship between jet lag and some of its symptoms. *Chronobiology International*, 22, 107–22.

Waterhouse, J., Reilly, T., Atkinson, G., *et al.* (2007). Jet lag: trends and coping strategies. *Lancet*, 369, 1117–29.

Waterhouse, J., Edwards, B., Nevill, A., *et al.* (2000). Do subjective symptoms predict our perception of jet-lag? *Ergonomics*, 43, 1514–27.

Waterhouse, J., Edwards, B., Nevill, A., *et al.* (2002). Identifying some determinants of 'jet lag' and its symptoms: a study of athletes and other travelers. *British Journal of Sports Medicine*, 36, 54–60.

Waterhouse, J., Minors, D., Folkard, S., *et al.* (1998). Light of domestic intensity produces phase shifts of the circadian oscillator in humans. *Neuroscience Letters*, 245, 97–100.

Wegmann, H., Klein, K., Conrad, B., *et al.* (1983). A model for prediction of resynchronization after time zoneflights. *Aviation, Space and Environmental Medicine*, 54, 524–7.

Wright, K., Badia, P., and Myers, B. (1997). Combination of bright light and caffeine as a countermeasure for impaired alertness and performance during extended sleep deprivation. *Journal of Sleep Research*, 6, 26–35.

11

PSYCHOLOGICAL PREPARATION FOR THE RUGBY PLAYER

Adam R. Nicholls

> 'A slight crosswind was blowing from left to right, but it was not enough to affect the flight of the ball and the kick at goal. My mental state, however, was not correct. I approached the ball off a shortened run up and stabbed the ball wide. I had actually strangled myself in the lead up to the kick by not giving it the respect it deserved. The team entrusted me with these duties, and I did not duly oblige'.
> *– Jon Callard (Nicholls and Callard 2012, p.101).*

11.1 The importance of psychology in rugby

Participating in rugby has the potential to be very stressful, as the quotation from Jon Callard, a former English rugby union international player, reveals. It is clear that players need to prepare psychologically as well as physically, to be able to perform at their best. The ex-England head coach, Brian Ashton MBE, stated that the mental side of the game – the 'glue that holds together the technical, physical, and tactical sides of the game under the most hostile pressure – is the least understood and practiced' (Nicholls and Calla.rd 2012, p. vii). In order to prepare players psychologically, it is important that coaches, psychologists, and players are aware of some of the stressors and demands associated with rugby.

11.1.1 The psychological demands of rugby

There have been a number of studies published that have explored the demands (i.e. stressors) that cause players to worry. One of the first studies to explore stressors among rugby players was carried out by Nicholls *et al.* (2006), who examined eight players from a leading Irish club. These players kept a stressor and coping diary over a period of 28 days, which included two Heineken Cup matches and two Celtic league matches. Overall, the players reported 24 different stressors, with nine of these accounting for 79% of all stressors. Further, the top four most reported stressors (i.e. injury, which was cited 35 times, mental error [28], physical error [22], and performance/outcome worries [19]) accounted for 44% of all stressors reported, suggesting that a small number of stressors reoccur on a frequent basis. Interestingly, the players reported the most stressors during the Heineken Cup matches, which are deemed to be more high profile than Celtic league matches. From a coaching perspective, this suggests that players need more psychological skills training in preparation for the most important matches.

It also appears that age is another factor to consider when examining the stressors that rugby players will experience. Nicholls and Polman (2007) studied a group of England Under-18 rugby union players and found that there were many similarities with the findings of Nicholls et al. (2006). Mental errors, physical errors, and injuries were common stressors among these younger players. However, there were also some subtle differences. Receiving parental and coach criticism and observing an opponent play well were the second and fifth most cited stressors, respectively. As such, coaches should recognize that younger players might report coach criticism as a stressor more frequently than older players. A limitation of the aforementioned papers by Nicholls and colleagues (2006, 2007) is that they have focussed exclusively on stressors that occur during training and matches. As such, these papers have failed to explore the overall stressors that players might encounter, such as non-sport stressors (e.g. education and relationships). There is, however, one study that has explored sport and non-sport stressors among a sample of professional rugby union players (e.g. Nicholls et al. 2009). In their study, Nicholls et al. found that non-sport stressors included the players' diet, home life, and sleep. Sleep is very important in helping players recover more effectively and experience less stress, according to Polman et al. (2007), who found that professional rugby league players reported poor sleep correlated with tension and misery. In order to prevent stressors having a negative effect on an individual's psychological well-being and rugby performance, players should be introduced to a variety of psychological strategies by either their coach or sport psychologist, which they can practice and utilize in matches. What follows are some examples of appropriate strategies that might be used with rugby players.

11.2 Psychological preparation

Empirical research regarding how to prepare rugby players for matches is somewhat limited. Nicholls and Callard (2012) provided some guidelines that players could use to mentally prepare themselves, which involved segmenting preparation into the day before a match, mental preparation before the match starts on match day, preparation during the breaks in play of the first-half, half-time, and during breaks in play in the second-half.

In terms of the day before a match, Nicholls and Callard (2012) suggested that players engage in mental imagery (see 11.3.3) and imagine what they want to achieve in the following day's match, playing to strengths, attacking/defensive formations, and team roles. Players could spend 10 to 15 minutes engaging in this mental preparation. It is also important that players spend time preparing for the match by establishing routines (e.g. listening to music on the coach to a match, establishing a standard physical warm-up, and performing with the appropriate intensity during the physical warm-up). During breaks in play in the first and second half, players can focus on their own role and what they want to happen during set plays, such as scrums, line outs, or kicks to touch. Half-time represents a period in which players can prepare for the second-half of the game. They can do this by thinking about things they did well in the first half and focussing on what they want to achieve in the second-half and how they will achieve this.

11.2.1 Goal setting

A goal, according to Locke and Latham (2002), relates to an objective that a rugby player has, a target within rugby, or a desired standard that a player wants to achieve within a set time frame. Having a goal has been associated with enhanced performance (for a review see Locke and Latham 2002), enhanced self-efficacy, confidence, and reduced anxiety (Kingston and Hardy 1997).

Rugby players can be taught to set different goals, with Burton *et al.* (2001) suggesting three goal types: outcome, performance, and process goals. An outcome goal refers to a specific desired result in a particular rugby match (e.g. win next home match) or competition (e.g. finish first in the league). Although it is important that rugby players are taught to set outcome goals, it is equally important that coaches and sport psychologists realise that these types of goals are only partially controllable. This is because outcomes in rugby are dependent on other teams, other players, and even officials. Performance goals involve rugby players wanting to achieve certain standards of performance. A goal kicker, for example, might want to improve his or her kick success rate from 65 to 75%. Finally, process goals encourage rugby players to focus on the actions that are associated with successful performance. For example, keeping their head down and following through with the kicking leg. In addition, the setting of outcome, performance, and process goals should be over the short- (i.e. next match), medium- (i.e. over a season), and long-term (i.e. the next four years).

To maximize the potential effectiveness of goal setting, Smith (1994) proposed an acronym: SMARTS – Specific, Measurable, Action-oriented, Realistic, Time, and Self-determined. Goals should be specific in that the rugby player states exactly what it is he or she wants to achieve (i.e. selection for the county team). Goals should be measurable so that a player can determine the extent to which a goal has been accomplished. Goals should be action-oriented, in which they encourage a rugby player to consider what he or she has to do in order to achieve them. Goals should be realistic, so that the rugby player will be able to achieve the goals. And finally, all goals should be self-determined and decided by the athlete within a specific time frame.

11.2.2 Performance profiling

The performance profile, which was developed by Butler (1989) and based upon Kelly's personal construct theory (1991), facilitates self-awareness among athletes regarding the characteristics required to be successful. Performance profiling is known to help players identify their own strengths and weaknesses, enhance motivation, facilitate discussion between a coach and player, and also enhance communication between team mates (Dale and Wrisberg 1996; D'Urso *et al.* 2002; Jones 1993; Weston *et al.* 2011). However, given the individuality of positional requirements, it is likely that the successful characteristics that define one player will differ from another. For example, the characteristics that a hooker needs to be successful are very different than those of a flanker or full-back.

In order to complete the performance profile, players are required to complete three stages. Firstly, the player writes down a list of the most important characteristics required to be successful in his or her position within physical, technical, tactical, and psychological categories. The player then ranks the 12 most important characteristics and writes down the meaning of each characteristic. It is important to note that players will often have their own meaning for the same characteristics. The final process involves the player plotting this information on a performance profile and rating his or her own score out of 10 relative to each of the 12 characteristics they have previously identified and defined. Players can monitor progress on a regular basis. Coaches can also ask their players to complete a team performance profile, in which the players complete the aforementioned processes, but in relation to the characteristics that make a successful team (Nicholls and Jones 2012).

11.2.3 Mental imagery

Mental imagery has the potential to benefit rugby players because it has been associated with skill acquisition (Beauchamp *et al.* 1996), increased confidence (Callow and Walters 2005), and increased recovery from injury (Ievleva and Orlick 1991). Mental imagery is the 'quasi-sensory and quasi-perceptual experiences of which we are self-consciously aware and which exist for us in the absence of those stimulus conditions that are known to produce their genuine sensory perceptual counterparts' (Richardson 1969. p.2-3). It is important to note that mental imagery does not just include images in the mind, it also includes noises, smells, and feeling associated with rugby (Munroe *et al.* 2000).

When rugby players engage in mental imagery, some players might see the images from the view they would see if they were performing the actual rugby skill, and is referred to as an 'internal perspective' (Murphy *et al.* 2008). Alternatively, other rugby players might see themselves as though they are watching their actions through a camera lens, known as an 'external perspective' (Murphy *et al.* 2008).

In terms of teaching rugby players how to use mental imagery techniques, Holmes and Collins (2001) developed a model known as the PETTLEP approach, with the acronym standing for Physical, Environment, Task, Timing,

Learning, Emotion, and Perspective. These are described accordingly (Holmes and Collins 2001):

1. *Physical.* When engaging in mental imagery, rugby players should include a physical element to this skill. For example, wearing the kit they would when whilst holding a rugby ball (Murphy *et al.* 2008). Players could also be taught to incorporate movement within their imagery (e.g. a goal kick).
2. *Environment.* Players should also imagine the setting in which they will be playing. If a pitch or stadium for an upcoming match has unique features, these should be incorporated within the player's images.
3. *Task.* Players should concentrate on what they would normally be thinking about when they perform a specific skill. For example, hookers might stop negative thoughts and engage in positive self-talk when they take lineout throws.
4. *Timing.* The mental imagery of different skills should be carried out at the speed they would occur in real life. If a kicker's routine lasts for 10 seconds, then when the player imagines this routine, it should also last for 10 seconds.
5. *Learning.* Mental imagery should reflect a rugby player's current level of proficiency. If a player is learning a new skill and is not as proficient as he would like to be, this should be represented in the mental images. However, players could also imagine themselves making small improvements.
6. *Emotion.* Rugby players should consider the emotions they felt in their most successful performances and re-create these emotions whilst engaging in mental imagery.
7. *Perspective.* Players should choose the perspective they wish to use, regardless of whether it is an external or internal perspective.

11.2.4 Coping effectiveness training

Coping effectiveness training (Chesney *et al.* 1996) includes 'constantly changing cognitive and behavioural efforts to manage specific external and/or internal demands that are appraised as taxing or exceeding the resources of the person' (Lazarus and Folkman 1984, p. 141).

Coping strategies are often classified within one of three dimensions, namely problem-focussed coping, emotion-focussed coping, and avoidance coping (Kowalski and Crocker 2001). Problem-focussed coping strategies alleviate the problem that causes the person to experience stress. These include problem solving, such as working out why a particular stressor is occurring (Holt and Hogg 2002), time management (Gould *et al.* 1993), and increasing physical effort during times of stress as opposed to disengaging and reducing effort (Reeves *et al.* 2009). Conversely, emotion-focussed coping strategies regulate a rugby player's emotional responses to stress, and include praying (Gould *et al.* 1993) and seeking support from others (Poczwardowski and Conroy 2002). Avoidance coping includes blocking negative thoughts (Reeves *et al.* 2009).

Coping effectiveness training (Chesney *et al.* 1996) is based upon the goodness-of-fit approach (Folkman 1984), which states that problem-focussed coping strategies will be the most effective when rugby players can control the stressors they are encountering (e.g. poor performance). Alternatively, emotion-focussed and avoidance coping strategies will be more effective when players are unable to control the stressors they are encountering (e.g. performance of opposition). As such, coping effectiveness training involves several inter-linked sessions in which rugby players are taught about the principles of learning to cope more effectively. To date, coping effectiveness training has not been tested in rugby players. However, applying this strategy with a sample of adolescent soccer players from a Football Association Premier League Academy (Reeves *et al.* 2011) revealed that it reduced stress and enhanced performance.

11.2.5 Mental toughness training

Mental toughness is one of the most important psychological characteristics that determines success in sport (Gould *et al.* 1987). Clough and Strycharczyk (2011) defined mental toughness as 'the quality which determines how people deal effectively with challenge, stressors and pressure… irrespective of prevailing circumstances' (p. 1). As such, individuals who are mentally tough are able to maintain and even thrive in highly pressurised situations.

Given that improved mental toughness is thought to enhance the ability of an athlete to perform well under pressure (e.g. Clough and Strycharczyk 2011; Gucciardi *et al.* 2009a, 2009b), it would seem advantageous for coaches and sport psychologists to focus on its development. Interventions to improve mental toughness have been used with cricketers and swimmers (Gucciardi *et al.* 2009b; Sheard and Golby 2006). These studies provided the framework for some guidelines developed by Nicholls and Jones (2012), and included coach behaviour, sport intelligence, coping effectiveness training, optimism training, concentration training, and confidence training.

To develop mental toughness in rugby players, it is important that coaches do not let their own desires for success override the requirements of the players. Coaches should create an environment in which players can develop (Gucciardi *et al.* 2009a) and focus their endeavours on helping rugby players improve. Coaches should also reward improvement and effort. A sporting environment in which coaches reward improvement is referred to as a mastery motivational climate, whereas an environment that rewards players who do the best is a performance mastery environment (Amorose 2007). Nicholls and Jones (2012) suggested that coaches should not overexpose athletes' weaknesses and only provide athletes with feedback after positive performances, given athletes are likely to prefer this (Chiviacowsky *et al.* 2008).

Another key component of mental toughness, identified by Gucciardi *et al.* (2008), is sport intelligence. According to Gucciardi *et al.* (2008), sport intelligence in rugby would refer to a player's understanding of technical and tactical aspects of the game. Nicholls and Jones (2012) argued that coaches could enhance the sport intelligence of the players by providing detailed information on team tactics. For example, explaining tactics as opposed to just telling players where to stand and where to move.

Nicholls *et al.* (2008) found that the most mentally tough athletes were also the more optimistic, compared to athletes with lower mental toughness scores. Therefore, one way of enhancing mental toughness could be through providing an athlete with optimism training (Seligman 2006). Optimism refers to a person's outlook and whether he perceives good things will happen in his life. If a rugby player generally believes that he or she will play well and that good things will happen on the pitch, then he or she would be classified as optimistic, whereas players who think that negative things will happen to them, such as dropping high balls or getting injured, would be referred to as pessimistic. Seligman (2006) provided some excellent advice on teaching people to be more optimistic under the ABCDE acronym of Adversity, Belief, Consequences, Disputation, and Evidence.

All players experience adversity when they are in highly pressurised matches and make mistakes such as dropping a high ball or missing a kick, for example, which might influence their beliefs about being able to catch high balls. Every belief has a consequence, so players who believe they are not good at catching high balls may stand in positions at restarts which are less likely to receive the ball after a restart. It is essential that players dispute negative beliefs during times of adversity in order to remain optimistic. A player could use evidence to remember all of the times he or she has caught high balls and tell himself or herself that it was just a mistake that every player makes and that the next high ball will be caught.

Seligman (2006) suggested that players should also reduce pessimistic thoughts and can do so by using the three 'Ps' of pessimism: Personal, Permanent, and Pervasive. When pessimistic thoughts creep into a rugby player's mind during times of adversity (e.g. after dropping a high ball), he or she can eradicate these thoughts by attributing the mistake to an external source, such as the wind, rain, or a team-mate putting the player off rather than believing it was personal reason. Players who are pessimistic believe that they would always drop high balls, so they should be encouraged to think that dropping high balls was a temporary glitch and it will not be a permanent aspect of their performance. A pessimistic player would also believe that making mistakes would prevail in all parts of his or her game, so the coach could make pessimistic players aware that just because they have dropped a high ball, it does not mean that they will make mistakes when completing other skills such as passing and tackling. That is, mistakes are not pervasive to all parts of a player's game.

11.2.6 Team cohesion

Another important aspect of the psychological preparation for rugby players involves successfully bringing together a number of players to play within a team environment.

Team cohesion refers to a dynamic process which is reflected in the tendency for a group to stick together and remain united in the pursuit of its instrumental objectives and/or for the satisfaction of member affective needs (Carron *et al.* 1998, p. 213).

Team cohesion is important because it can lead to increased performance (Carron *et al.* 2002), reduced anxiety for team members (Prapavessis and Carron 1996), less jealousy (Kamphoff *et al.* 2005), and increased effort (Bray and Whaley 2001).

Providing information regarding building cohesion in a rugby team goes beyond the scope of this chapter; however, there are several strategies that coaches and sport psychologists can use such as team goal setting and team performance profiling. The same techniques mentioned in this chapter are used for individual goal setting and performance profiling, except that the whole team would be involved. Ryska *et al.* (1999) suggested that players should be integrated in a team through activities in which players spend time together away from rugby and get to know each other better. Ryska *et al.* (1999) also suggested that getting players to understand and accept their roles within the team is an important factor that can lead to a more cohesive team. It should be noted that building team cohesion takes time. A review by Martin *et al.* (2009) suggested that team building interventions lasting twenty weeks are much more effective than those lasting for much shorter periods. As such, it is important that coaches allow time for team cohesion to be developed where possible.

11.3 Summary

The research indicates that rugby players experience a variety of different stressors relating to performance (e.g. opponents) and their life outside of rugby (e.g. work). In order for players to experience psychological well-being and to perform at their best, it is important these players are mentally prepared to manage such demands. The techniques outlined in these chapters such as goal setting, performance profiling, mental toughness training, and coping effectiveness training have the potential to help rugby players.

Case study: a psychological case example and formulation framework

Andrew Rogers, Matt Thombs, James Bickley, and James Bell

Introduction

As applied practitioners, we would not advocate a 'one size fits all' approach. In our experience, support for the development of elite rugby players should be guided by a structured evaluation of individual risk and resilience factors (e.g. Gould *et al.* 2002), within the broader context of the developmental experience of the player.

One way of doing this is the use of a comprehensive psychological formulation 'framework' (e.g. Carr 2006; British Psychological Society (BPS) 2011), an approach adapted and piloted by the authors with international age-group rugby union players. It is important to recognize that this was implemented by a Health and Care Professions Council (HCPC) registered sport psychologist, who was embedded within the coaching and support team system and supported by a HCPC registered consultant clinical psychologist. We would not advocate the use of this framework without appropriate applied psychology support.

Having established the nature of the player's presenting concern(s) or question(s), the formulation 'framework' allows us to identify the immediate 'triggers' (precipitating factors) and historical predisposing factors that are associated with the onset of the difficulties. Precipitating factors might include a combination of sporting performance factors (e.g. being dropped), significant life events (e.g. peer rejection), and other acute factors (e.g. physical illness).

In understanding an athlete's predisposition to the presenting difficulties, it is deemed vital to consider his early life and developmental experiences, including family and peer relationships, as well as his early sporting career. Additional historical or predisposing factors can include the athlete's individual psychological and biological characteristics, such as cognitive ability, temperament, and any past illness or injury.

Once a shared understanding of the concern(s) or question(s) has been established, it is important to assess any on-going maintaining or protective factors. Maintaining factors are those that perpetuate or reinforce the presenting difficulties. Protective factors are likely to prevent further deterioration and have implications for prognosis and response to intervention (Carr 2006). Factors that are likely to maintain or protect against the presenting difficulties will again include individual psychological and biological characteristics (e.g. thinking style, temperament, physical development), as well as the athlete's family, peer, and environmental context (e.g. supportive family, peer group influence, coach-athlete relationship).

Formulation is acknowledged as a core competency of applied psychologists (BPS 2011). An effective formulation '…draws on psychological theory and research to provide a framework for describing a client's problem or needs, how it developed and is being maintained' (BPS 2010, p. 5-6). In this context, formulation involves the integration of a range of bio-psychosocial contributory factors, resulting in hypotheses that are open to scientific testing (BPS 2011). As such, the formulation should: (i) summarize the athlete's core concerns; (ii) suggest how the athlete's difficulties might relate to one another, by drawing on psychological theories and principles; (iii) aim to explain, on the basis of psychological theory, the development and maintenance of the athlete's difficulties, at this time and in these situations; (iv) indicate a plan of intervention which is based on the psychological processes and principles already identified; (v) be open to revision and re-formulation (Johnstone and Dallos 2006). An example of this process in action is described in the following case study.

Case presentation

The composite case study is fictional but draws on the experience of the authors' work with international age-group and adult rugby union players. It illustrates the potential application of the framework in practice.

Simon was a rugby player who was perceived to be highly talented, but was causing considerable management difficulties for the coaching and support team. Simon's presenting difficulties were described as: (i) expressing high levels of emotion and demanding of coach time, (ii) difficulties in accepting or accessing coaching support when offered, and (iii) frequently avoiding performance situations. Coaches described Simon often becoming agitated over minor changes to the coaching routine, refusing to follow instructions, and being 'overly dramatic'. He would approach coaches with the same question on many occasions and ask the same question of different members of the coaching and support team within a short period. This resulted in a large amount of time and resources from the coaching and support team being spent with Simon, generating a feeling that others were being neglected. Despite this, Simon's technical and tactical performance in training continued to be to a very high standard. It also appeared that the more time coaches spent with Simon trying to address his behaviour, the more challenging his behaviour became. Simon's behaviour was also beginning to be noticed by his peers, who were starting to make derogatory comments about him, highlighting his overall negative influence on the team.

The coaching and support team had numerous meetings to discuss Simon's presentation, which often went on beyond their allocated time. These meetings involved the coaching and support team discussing their frustrations, but at times concluded without any clear actions. This led to much frustration within the coaching and support team, with different people trying different approaches and an overall 'piece-meal' approach to managing Simon's presentation that was at times driven more by the emotional responses of staff rather than a rational appraisal of what may be helpful.

The coaching and support team was encouraged by the applied psychologist to use the framework as a way of thinking in a more structured way about Simon's presentation. Triggers for Simon's difficulties were thought to be a recent promotion to a more senior squad and perceived rejection from peers or the coaching team, his difficulties becoming more pronounced in the immediate period prior to selection decisions being made.

Individual predisposing factors included a history of high achievement and always having been one of the key squad members throughout his early career. From a contextual perspective, there was high expectation from others; a history of idealization from previous coaches, resulting in boundaries not being consistently employed (e.g. the rules do not apply to me); and a family environment that catered for his every need, despite being in late adolescence.

Individual maintaining factors included poor emotional regulation (especially in relation to anxiety) and overuse of avoidance strategies (e.g. withdrawal).

From a contextual standpoint, there were difficulties with peer interactions, the high level of reassurance provided by the coaching system, and high levels of emotion generated within the coaching and support team, with ongoing idealization from some and others strongly expressing negative views about him. This led to inconsistent management approaches being employed.

Protective factors included a high IQ, recognition from Simon that he was struggling, a capacity to respond well to praise, a good sense of humour, and a good relationship with a number of the coaching and support staff.

The applied psychologist, in collaboration with the coaching and support team, hypothesized that Simon's presentation was highly influenced by anxiety, triggered by the relatively 'new' experience of being out of his 'comfort zone'. His way of managing anxiety was based on seeking reassurance from others (that is likely to have developed from situations in the past when others have told him that 'everything is going to be okay'). Consequently, Simon became over-reliant on reassurance from others as a way of managing his own anxiety. Whilst helpful in the short term, this strategy was thought to reinforce Simon's anxiety in the longer term. In a similar way, Simon's history of high achievement meant that he had not developed effective strategies to manage 'not being the best' and had been protected in many ways from experiencing difficulty in a sporting context. Simon was desperately in need of others for reassurance, but his behaviour was generating inconsistent responses in others. His avoidance of high performance situations was a way of managing the high anxiety associated with not meeting expectations.

Based on this working hypothesis the following action plan was put in place:

1. Environmental interventions included coaching staff agreeing to consistent, firm, and fair responses to Simon's behaviour – that were in the context of boundaries and expectations of behaviour agreed with Simon.
2. Staff were encouraged to invest in regular and consistent time with Simon, rather than 'ad hoc' interactions. It was agreed that during every morning and evening meeting a key member of the coaching team, identified in collaboration with Simon, would offer a five minute outline on what had gone well and what had been difficult during the day. These meetings would focus on validating emotion (thus not triggering perceived rejection) and identifying patterns of thinking and behaviour that might be unhelpful. It was also agreed (with Simon's permission) to discuss this understanding of his difficulties with his wider support system.
3. Simon was offered individual intervention by the applied psychologist, who aimed to increase his awareness of anxiety and the reassurance cycle, along with simple strategies to manage thoughts and feelings associated with anxiety. Initially, the strategies focussed on relaxation techniques (centering and progressive muscle relaxation) and cognitive restructuring, which are in line with typical mental skills techniques used to enhance athletic performance.
4. A weekly review and evaluation of Simon's progress was to be undertaken over a six-week period.

It was noticeable that with this increased and 'agreed' understanding, the high emotion and strong feeling within the coaching and support team were reduced, and they were able to empathize more with Simon's presentation. As a result, they agreed a clear plan of action and the inconsistent management of Simon's presentation became more stable. Simon began to have more insight into the function of his behaviour and the role of anxiety within this. He responded quickly to the clear boundaries and consistent approach, and, although his anxiety was evident at times, he became more able to implement his own coping strategies and ask for support effectively, rather than resorting to excessive expressed emotion and constant attempts to seek clarification. Simon's relationship within his peer group also improved, and he began to share some of his anxieties with them. Consequently, they offered more support. Simon's avoidance of performance, by highlighting minor physical complaints, reduced significantly, and his overall performance improved and became more consistent.

Summary

As has been highlighted, promoting psychological characteristics and skills associated with excellence is fundamental for the development and performance of rugby players. However, in the experience of the authors, rugby union appears to present a unique set of pressures that might be associated with playing the sport itself, but can also be influenced by non-sport stressors. Talented rugby players can also at times present with behaviours that challenge the coaching and support team system and interfere with their sporting performance. Some of these behaviours might be linked to the emotional well-being of the player. One way of addressing this that seems promising is to take a holistic approach, focussing both on the environment as well as the individual. This approach incorporates a bio-psychosocial understanding or 'formulation' of the presenting challenges, in collaboration with the wider coaching and support team system, but overseen by appropriately qualified applied psychologist(s). There is clearly scope for future research to investigate the potential benefits of such an approach within rugby and the wider sporting community.

References

Amorose, A.J. (2007). Coaching effectiveness. In M.S. Hagger and N.L.D. Chatzisarantis (Eds.), *Intrinsic motivation and self-determination in exercise and sport* (pp. 209–28). Champaign, IL: Human Kinetics.

Beauchamp, P.H., Halliwell, W.R., Fournier, J.F, et al. (1996). Effects of cognitive-behavioural psychological skills training on motivation, preparation, and putting performance of novice golfers. *The Sport Psychologist*, 10, 157–70.

Bray, C.D. and Whaley, D.E. (2001). Team cohesion, effort, and objective individual performance of high school basketball players. *The Sport Psychologist*, 15, 260–75.

British Psychological Society (Division of Clinical Psychology). (2010). *The core purpose and philosophy of the profession*. Leicester: British Psychological Society.

British Psychological Society (Division of Clinical Psychology). (2011). *Good Practice Guidelines on the Use of Psychological Formulation*. Leicester: British Psychological Society.

Burton, D., Naylor, S., and Holliday, B. (2001). Goal setting in sport: Investigating the goal effectiveness paraadigm. In R. Singer, H. Hausenblaus and C. Janelle (Eds.), *Handbook of sport psychology* (pp. 497–28). NY: Wiley.

Butler, R.J. (1989). *The performance profile: Developing elite performance*. London: British Olympic Association Publication.

Callow, N. and Walters, A. (2005). The effect of kinaesthetic imagery on the sport confidence of flat-race horse jockeys. *Psychology of Sport and Exercise*, 6, 443–59.

Carr, A. (2006). *The handbook of child and adolescent clinical psychology: A contextual approach*. London: Routledge

Carron, A.V., Brawley, L.R., and Widmeyer, W.N. (1998). The measurement of cohesiveness in sport groups. In J. Duda (ed.), *Advances in sport and exercise psychology measurement* (pp. 213–26) Morgantown, WV: Fitness Information Technology.

Carron, A.V., Colman, M.M., Wheeler, J., *et al*. (2002). Cohesion and performance in sport: A meta-analysis. *Journal of Sport and Exercise Psychology*, 24, 168–88.

Chesney, M.A., Folkman, S., and Chambers, D.B. (1996). Coping effectiveness training for men living with HIV: preliminary findings. *International Journal of STD and AIDS*, 7, 75–82.

Chiviaacowsky, S., Wulf, G., Laroque de Medeiros, F., *et al*. (2008a). Learning benefits of self-controlled knowledge of results in 10-year-old children. *Research Quarterly for Exercise and Sport*, 79, 405–10.

Clough, P., Earle, K., and Sewell, D. (2002). Mental toughness: The concept and its measurement. In I. Cockerill (Ed.), *Solutions in Sport Psychology* (pp. 32–45) London: Thomson.

Clough, P.J. and Strycharczyk, D. (2011). *Applied mental toughness: A tool kit for the 21st Century*. London: Kogan Page.

Connaughton, D., Wadey, R., Hanton, S., *et al*. (2008). The development and maintenance of mental toughness: Perceptions of elite performers. *Journal of Sports Sciences*, 26, 83–95.

Dale, G.A. and Wrisberg, C.A. (1996). The use of a performance profiling technique in a team setting: Getting the athletes and the coach on the 'same page'. *The Sport Psychologist*, 10, 261–77.

D'Urso, V., Petrosso, A., and Robazza, C. (2002). Emotions, perceived qualities, and performance of rugby players. *The Sport Psychologist*, 16, 173–99.

Folkman, S. (1984). Personal control and stress and coping processes: A theoretical analysis. *Journal of Personality and Social Psychology*, 46, 839–52.

Gould, D., Eklund, R.C., and Jackson, S.A. (1993). Coping strategies used by US Olympic wrestlers. *Research Quarterly for Exercise and Sport*, 64, 83–93.

Gould, D., Dieffenbach, K., and Moffett, A. (2002). Psychological talent and its development in Olympic champions. *Journal of Applied Sport Psychology*, 14, 172–210.

Gould, D., Hodge, K., Peterson, K. and Petlichkoff, L. (1987). Psychological foundations of coaching: Similarities and differences among intercollegiate wrestling coaches. *The Sport Psychologist*, 1, 293–308.

Gucciardi, D.F., Gordon S. & Dimmock, J.A. (2008) Towards an understanding of mental toughness in Australian Football. *Journal of Applied Sports Psychology*, 20, 261–81.

Gucciardi, D.F., Gordon, S., Dimmock, J.A., *et al*. (2009a). Understanding the coach's role in the development of mental toughness: Perspective of elite Australian football coaches. *Journal of Sports Sciences*, 27, 1483–96.

Gucciardi, D.F., Gordon, S., and Dimmock, J.A. (2009b). Evaluation of a mental toughness training program for youth aged Australian footballers: I. A quantitative analysis. *Journal of Applied Sport Psychology*, 21, 307–23.

Holmes, P. and Collins, D. (2001). The PETTLEP approach to motor imagery: A functional equivalence model for sport psychologists. *Journal of Applied Sport Psychology*, 13, 60–83.

Holt, N.L. and Hogg, J.M. (2002). Perceptions of stress and coping during preparations for the 1999 women's soccer world cup finals. *The Sport Psychologist*, 16, 251–71.

Ievleva, L. and Orlick, T. (1991). Mental links to enhanced healing. *The Sport Psychologist*, 5, 25–40.

Jones, G. (1993). The role of performance profiling in cognitive behavioural interventions in sport. *The Sport Psychologist*, 7, 160–72.

Johnstone, L. and Dallos, R. (Eds.) (2006). *Formulation in psychology and psychotherapy: Making sense of people's problems*. London, New York: Routledge.

Kamphoff, C.S., Gill, D.L., and Huddleston, S. (2005). Jealousy in sport: Exploring jealousy's relationship to cohesion. *Journal of Applied Sport Psychology*, 17, 290–305.

Kelly, G.A. (1991). *The psychology of personal constructs: A theory of personality*. London: Routledge.

Kingston, K.M. and Hardy, L. (1997). Effects of different types of goals on processes that support performance. *The Sport Psychologist*, 11, 277–93.

Kowalski, K.C. and Crocker, P.R. (2001). Development and validation of the Coping Function Questionnaire for adolescents in sport. *Journal of Sport and Exercise Psychology*, 23, 136–55.

Lazarus, R.S. and Folkman, S. (1984). *Stress, appraisal and coping*. New York: Springer.

Locke, E.A. and Latham, G.P. (2002). Building a practically useful theory of goal setting and task motivation: A 35-year odyssey. *American Psychologist*, 57, 705–17.

Martin, L.J., Carron, A.V., and Burke, S.M. (2009). Team building interventions in sport: A meta-analysis. *Sport and Exercise Psychology Review*, 5, 3–18.

Munroe, K., Giacobbi, P., Hall, C., et al. (2000). The 4Ws of imagery use: Where, when, why, and what. *The Sport Psychologist*, 14, 119–37.

Murphy, S., Nordin, S., and Cumming, J. (2008). Imagery in sport, exercise, and dance. In T.S. Horn (Ed.), *Advances in sport psychology* (pp. 297–24). Champaign, IL: Human Kinetics.

Nicholls, A.R., Backhouse, S.H., Polman, R.C.J., et al. (2009). Stressors and affective states among professional rugby union players. *Scandinavian Journal of Medicine and Science in Sports*, 19, 121–8.

Nicholls, A.R. and Callard, J. (2012). *Focused for rugby*. Champaign, IL: Human Kinetics.

Nicholls, A.R., Holt, N.L., Polman, R.C.J., et al. (2006). Stressors, coping, and coping effectiveness among professional rugby union players. *The Sport Psychologist*, 20, 314–29.

Nicholls, A.R. and Jones, L. (2012). *Psychology in sports coaching: Theory and application*. London: Routledge.

Nicholls, A.R. and Polman, R.C.J., (2007). Stressors, coping, and coping effectiveness among players from the England under-18 rugby union team. *Journal of Sport Behavior*, 30, 199–218.

Nicholls, A.R., Polman, R.C.J., Levy, R.A., et al. (2008). Mental toughness, optimism, pessimism, and coping among athletes. *Personality and Individual Differences*, 44, 1182–92.

Poczwardowski, A. and Conroy, D.E. (2002). Coping responses to failure and success among elite athletes and performing artists. *Journal of Applied Sport Psychology*, 14, 313–29.

Polman, R., Nicholls, A.R., Cohen, J., et al. (2001). The influence of game location and outcome on behaviour and mood states among professional rugby league players. *Journal of Sport Sciences*, 25, 1491–500.

Prapavessis, H. and Carron, A.V. (1996). The effect of group cohesion on competitive state anxiety. *Journal of Sport and Exercise Psychology*, 18, 64–74.

Reeves, C.W., Nicholls, A.R., and Polman, J. (2009). Stressors and coping strategies among early and middle adolescent Premier League academy soccer players: Differences according to age. *Journal of Applied Sport Psychology*, 21, 31–48.

Reeves, C.W., Nicholls, A.R., and McKenna, J. (2011). The effects of a coping intervention on coping self-efficacy, coping effectiveness, and subjective performance among adolescent soccer players. *International Journal of Sport and Exercise Psychology*, 9, 126–42.

Richardson, A. (1969). *Mental imagery*. NY: Springer.

Ryska, T.A., Yin, Z., Cooley, D., *et al*. (1999). Developing team cohesion: A comparison of cognitive-behavioural strategies of U.S. and Australian sport coaches. *The Journal of Psychology*, 13, 523–39.

Seligman, M.E.P. (2006). *Learned optimism: How to change your mind and your life*. New York: Vintage Books.

Sheard, M. and Golby, J. (2006). Effect of a psychological skills training program on swimming performance and positive psychological development. *International Journal of Sport and Exercise Psychology*, 4, 149–69.

Smith, H.W. (1994). *The 10 natural laws of successful time and life management: Proven strategies for increased productivity and inner peace*. New York: Warner.

Weston, N.J.V., Greenlees, I.A., and Thelwell, R.C. (2011). The impact of a performance profiling intervention on athletes' intrinsic motivation. *Research Quarterly for Exercise and Sport*, 82, 151–5.

12

NOTATIONAL ANALYSIS FOR RUGBY FOOTBALL

Simon Eaves and Paul Worsfold

12.1 Introduction

Sports notational analysis is the systematic recoding and interpretation of a performance, with the intent of reducing the subjectivity and bias, inherent in human observation. It has been suggested that the earliest example of this form of sport analysis is Hugh Fullerton's 1910 paper, *The Inside Game: the Science of Baseball*. However, recent research has revealed notation systems developed by Fullerton, as early as 1894, and ideographic notations by Henry Chadwick, dating to the mid-1850s (Eaves 2013). An interesting and critical component in the development of these early analysis systems is that both Henry Chadwick and Hugh Fullerton were newspaper reporters. Similarly, the pioneers of rugby football notation were newspapermen, Maurice Martin of *La Petite Gironde* and Fernand Bidault writing for *La Vie Au Grand Air*. In what appears to be the first notation of a rugby game, Martin and Bidault situated themselves on the stadium roof to observe, and record, the 1907 French rugby championship final between Paris and Bordeaux (Figure 12.1).

The notation they produced (Figure 12.1) is extremely comprehensive, providing times of game actions, areas of movement on the pitch, and shorthand symbols to represent key game actions. The left and right sides of the diagram represent first and second halves, respectively, the different horizontal lines are the pitch areas (dead ball, goal, 22 m, and half way lines), and the symbols represent the specific game actions (try, penalty, scrum, lineout, etc.). The detail of this analysis is remarkable and yet there is scant evidence of any other rugby analyses, at this level, in the subsequent 75 years. However, the use of sports notation by both academic researchers and applied practitioners has grown markedly in the last few decades, coinciding with technological developments and the full professionalization of the games of rugby football.

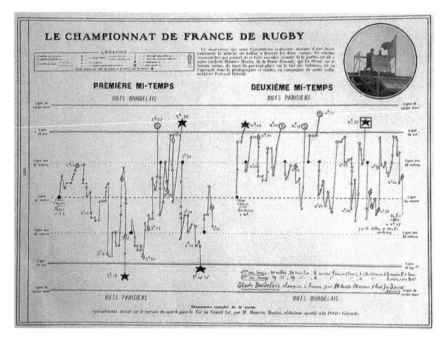

FIGURE 12.1 'Le Championnat de france de rugby, 1907' (Humbert 2010). Reproduced with kind permission from Frédéric Humbert

12.2 Rugby research

Many researchers have focussed on mapping the game over time (longitudinal analysis) in an attempt to understand how the games of rugby are continually evolving. In addition, researchers have sought to examine not only how the game has changed within a defined period, but also the impact of specific interventions, such as law changes and the introduction of professional playing status. In rugby union and, to a lesser extent, rugby league football, researchers have profiled both team and individual performances in an attempt to develop profiles that may act as predictors of successful performance. Often these are based on game outcomes; however, increasingly, researchers are now examining at a more micro-level and focussing on specific components of the game in relation to predefined success criteria, which is unrelated to a single game outcome.

12.2.1 Longitudinal analysis

In rugby union, most research which has sought to assess the game over a defined time period has done so, predominantly, in the context of changes between Rugby World Cups (Potter and Carter 2001a; Seuront 2013; Norton 2013), across Five and Six Nations Championships (Potter 1997; Eaves and Hughes 2003; Eaves et al.

2005; Williams *et al.* 2005a; Williams *et al.* 2005b), and Tri-Nations Championships (Williams *et al.* 2005a; Williams *et al.* 2005b). One of the first examinations of inter-tournament effects was undertaken by Potter and Carter (2001a), who assessed the relative frequencies of match and time indicators between the 1991 and 1995 Rugby World Cup tournaments. They reported an increase in scrum, ruck, and maul frequency in 1995 compared to 1991, which reflected the trend previously presented by Potter (1997). In addition, Potter and Carter indicated that the mean frequency of tries per game had increased from five to six, and goal kicking success from 52 to 61%, which they suggested was primarily due to conditions being drier underfoot in 1995, and law changes made in the inter-tournament period.

Some researchers (Seuront 2013; Norton 2013) have taken novel approaches to examining changes across Rugby World Cups (1987–2007). Norton examined ball speed, player density, tackles, and collisions, and presented a 'physicality metric' based on a calculation of collision intensity score and the number of players in a collision. He concluded that the game had changed from a 'kick to touch' game to a 'possession at all costs' game. This finding was consistent with previous research (Eaves *et al.* 2005), which suggested that in the 1988–92 Five Nations Championships, the average time between kicks to touch was only 45 seconds, but this had increased to 111 seconds by 1999. Norton (2013) also suggested that since 1987 there had been an increase in player density (more players playing within a five metre radius of the ball), but a decrease in the speed of the game, indicating a trend towards a more ruck dominated, less expansive game. This again was consistent with the findings presented by other researchers. Eaves and Hughes (2003), and Eaves *et al.* (2005) reported that, between 1988 and 2002, in Northern hemisphere international rugby, there was more than 100% increase in the frequency of rucks, which could not be explained, solely, by the increases in ball in play time over this period.

The importance of mapping ball in play time cannot be understated, since it is fundamental to normalising frequency data, and as such, enables researchers to fully understand and compare data sets. This important time variable has been presented by many researchers (McLean 1992; Potter 1997; Thomas 2001; Potter and Carter 2001a; Prim and van Rooyen 2013), and whilst there are inconsistencies in defining this variable, it is clear that in this code of rugby football, the ball in play time has increased, significantly, over the past 25 years. In the late 1980s, on average, the ball was in play for only 21 minutes, 14 seconds (Eaves *et al.* 2005) in Five Nations rugby, yet just over 20 years later the International Rugby Board (IRB) reported ball in play time of 39 minutes, 10 seconds in Six Nations rugby (Prim and van Rooyen 2013). This represents an increase of 84.5%, or very nearly 18 minutes, of playing time. William *et al.* (2005a) suggested that various law changes, implemented from January 2000 to April 2002, had a significant effect on ball in play time in Northern and Southern hemisphere games. They suggested that these changes were possibly due to law amendments implemented in January 2000, which were aimed at improving continuity and speeding up the game.

The changes to the laws of the game, instigated by the International Rugby Board (IRB), are often associated with a perceived need to speed up the game or improve spectator appeal. In the 1992–93 season the 'use it or lose it' law was introduced in an attempt to make the game 'more attractive'. Hughes and Clarke (1994) assessed the impact of this law change and suggested that this amendment resulted in more open play action, with the ball being released to the backs more frequently. More recently, van den Berg and Malan (2012) examined experimental law variations (ELVs) to determine whether these effected changes to the game that would increase spectator appeal in Super 14 matches. They reported that the law changes had resulted in scrum and lineout frequency decreasing, and metres gained, with tackle frequency and penalties conceded all increasing. The research suggested that these game changes had promoted continuity and, as such, increased spectator appeal.

It is clear that the IRB is cognisant of the importance of game continuity and spectator appeal, and many law amendments are directed at enhancing these aspects of the game. In 1999, the IRB introduced laws to nullify defending players preventing or slowing down the recycling of the ball at the tackle area. In an examination of this law change, Williams *et al.* (2005b) reported a reduction in the frequency and percentage of stoppages due to unplayable ball and scrums awarded in both Six Nations and Three Nations. In addition to laws changes at the breakdown, the IRB also introduced the 'use it or lose it' law at the scrum. According to Williams *et al.* (2005b), this was meant to improve the scrum by reducing the time spent on reformation, especially at the five metre scrum. They reported that the law change had an immediate effect in Six Nations rugby, increasing the percentage of clean scrums (those won directly by either team) from 13% in 1999 to 23% in the following year. However, in Tri-Nations rugby the law change had the opposite effect, reducing clean scrum percentages from 15% in 1999 to 7% in 2000. Whilst the implementation of law changes does have an impact in rugby union, the resultant changes might not be consistent across tournaments and playing hemispheres, and appear not to be permanent. Williams (2004) suggests that whilst law changes appear to have had an immediate effect, a period of acclimatization followed, and as such, they appear to have 'no real lasting effect'.

In rugby league, the examination of how the game has changed over time, and more specifically, the impact of law changes, has been less well researched than in the union code. Only the change from a 5 m to 10 m offside law (Meir *et al.* 1993; Meir *et al.* 2001; Eaves *et al.* 2008a; Eaves *et al.* 2008b) and the introduction of the 40–20 law (Eaves *et al.* 2008a) have been the subject of published research. Meir *et al.* (1993) hypothesized that 1992–93 law change regarding defensive players moving back 10 m after the tackle, compared to the previous law playing under a 5 m offside line, would result in significant changes in the game. This modification, they suggested, would effect a significant change in the distance covered by players during the game, and that such changes would be more evident in forwards than backs. In a later study, Meir *et al.* (2001) reported the distance covered by forwards increased by 3,282 m to just short of 10,000 m per game (49.4% increase), indicating that the introduction of this law had resulted in changes in player movement profiles.

Eaves *et al.* (2008a) also examined the impact of this law change, but from a more technical and tactical perspective. They reported that the change in the law resulted in a significant increase (11.6%) in the frequency of dummy half passes and a significant decrease (29.0%) in the frequency of ball kicks out of play. In addition, they suggested that the introduction of the 40–20 law also had an impact on kicking strategy, with a decrease in the percentage of ball kicks out of play. Eaves *et al.* (2008b) further reported that the law change (10 m offside) had resulted in a change at the ruck, reducing the time of the 'play the ball' by 18.6%. In addition, the law changes associated with the introduction of the summer playing season resulted in further decreases to the ruck time (13.7%). They concluded that these effects were probably a result of the change in the laws relating to increasing the number of interchanges from four to six, and a change in the rules preventing the marker at the 'play the ball' from striking for the ball.

Mapping the game, in both codes of rugby, continues to be an important research focus that acts to facilitate a deeper understanding of the games, and how they continue to evolve.

12.2.2 Identifying factors contributing to successful performance

Researches have focused on a number of indicators that might contribute to winning performance. In rugby union, most researchers have presented specific game action indicators (Hughes and Williams 1988; Hughes and White 1997; Potter and Carter 2001b; Jones *et al.* 2004; Ortega *et al.* 2009; Bishop and Barnes 2011; Vaz *et al.* 2010; Vaz *et al.* 2011, van Rooyen 2012), whilst some have examined technical variables (van Rooyen *et al.* 2014), and tactical strategies (Hunter and O'Donoghue 2001; James *et al.* 2005; Ortega *et al.* 2009; Sayers 2009; Wheeler 2010; van den Berg and Malan 2010; Bishop and Barnes, 2011; Diedrick and van Rooyen 2011; Bremner *et al.* 2013). In addition to studies that have focussed on assessing differences in performance related to score outcome (win or lose), researchers have also focussed on the success of performers in a specific game context, most notably in the contact area (McKenzie *et al.* 1989; Smythe *et al.* 1998; Jones *et al.* 2004; Sayers and Washington-King 2005; Wheeler *et al.* 2009; Sayers 2009).

Whilst the game of rugby union is continually changing, there are a number of factors that are consistent to successful performance. Evidence suggests that the lineout, kicking strategy, tackle area, and passing are all discriminating variables for a successful game outcome. Indeed, winning teams have fewer lineout throws (Potter and Carter 2001b), lose fewer of them (Ortega *et al.* 2009), win more lineouts when games are 'balanced' (Vaz *et al.* 2010), and win more on the opposition throws (Jones *et al.* 2004). From a more tactical standpoint, Hughes and White (1997) reported that successful teams varied their lineout pattern, winning more possession from the middle and the back of the lineout using a catch and drive/

peel, whereas, unsuccessful teams were more likely to use the tap down approach for securing possession. In terms of kicking, Bishop and Barnes (2011) reported winning teams kicked the ball out of hand more frequently than losing teams. This supported the view of Vaz *et al.* (2010), who suggested winning teams kicked away possession and kicked to touch more frequently than losing teams. This kicking strategy suggests a more conservative approach to the game, and supports the observation that winning teams are less likely to pass the ball than losing teams (Potter and Carter 2001b; Vaz *et al.* 2010). Vaz *et al.* (2010) and Ortega *et al.* (2009) also suggested that winning teams made more tackles than losing teams. Moreover, it appears that winning performance is determined, in part, by missing fewer tackles (Vaz *et al.* 2010), and that the percentage of tackles 'missed' by either the lock, winger, or fullback has an influential role in determining the game outcome (van Rooyen 2012).

Dominating the contact area and breaking the line of defence are viewed as highly important in determining team success (Ortega *et al.* 2009; Sayers 2009; van den Berg and Malan 2010; Wheeler *et al.* 2010; Diedrick and van Rooyen 2011; van Rooyen *et al.* 2014). Diedrick and van Rooyen (2011) and Ortega (2009) both reported that winning teams, on average, made significantly more line breaks than losing teams in the Rugby World Cup 2007. Furthermore, Diedrick and van Rooyen (2011) highlighted the importance of line breaks, reporting that 51% of all line breaks resulted in a try. Wheeler *et al.* (2010) also reported that the key determinants of try scoring were line breaks and offloading. This view was consistent with Sayers (2009), who suggested that 82% of line breaks were the result of an offload. In a more in-depth analysis of the contact situation, van Rooyen *et al.* (2014) reported that tackle 'effectiveness' was a characteristic of winning performance. They suggested that winning teams executed more tackles on or before the line of defence, or made tackles that drove the ball carrier backward. Moreover, from a technical standpoint, they suggested that the effective tackle was characterized by the tackler shifting his weight onto the front foot, adopting a forward lean into the torso and entering the tackle from either an oblique or front-on position.

In terms of assessing the effectiveness in the contact situation, researchers have focussed mainly on attacking the contact zone (McKenzie *et al.* 1989; Smythe *et al.* 1998; Wheeler *et al.* 2009; Sayers *et al.* 2009). Being able to maintain possession in contact is crucial in terms of offence continuity and pressurizing the defence. McKenzie *et al.* (1989) reported that whether teams advanced beyond the advantage line or not influenced the retention of the ball, with the ball being retained 67% of the time when the advantage line was crossed. McKenzie *et al.* (1989) and Smythe *et al.* (1998) suggested that ball retention improved when the body position was low, with the ball carrier turned towards supporting players. Similarly, Wheeler *et al.* (2009) suggested that in contact, tackle-breaks were achieved when players used a combination of low body position, strong leg drive, and good fending technique. They suggested that submissive contact, allied to poor body position, resulted in 69% of breakdown losses.

In addition to assessing success at the point of contact, the movement pattern into the contact area has been of interest (Sayers and Washington-King 2005; Sayers 2009). Sayers (2009) suggested that the attacker accelerating into the contact zone with the path at an oblique angle, and using stepping evasion techniques, determined positive outcomes. This evasion strategy was consistent with the views of Sayers and Washington-King (2005) who suggested that moving the ball beyond the defensive line and maintaining possession were achieved more often when the ball carrier attempted to avoid contact by stepping off the outside leg in a forward motion, and running oblique or angled (around the defender) lines. Moreover, this skill was strongly associated with the player breaking the tackle when executed at high speed, more than two body lengths from the defensive line, and followed by a straightening of the run.

In rugby league football, research focussing on identifying successful performance is scant by comparison. In terms of assessing winning and losing performance, the only published study (O'Connor 2004) assessed available statistics to identify which performance indicators contributed to success, in terms of whether or not a team qualified for the finals series of the National Rugby League (NRL). O'Connor (2004) reported that teams that reached the finals series used fewer players, achieved more line breaks and broke free of more tackles. Other researchers have focussed more on examining the contact area and subsequent 'play the ball'. The earliest published example of this is a 1995 article in *The New Scientist*, by Mick O'Hare. In this work, O'Hare, through the words of Andy Clarke (who was commissioned to undertake the research by the Rugby Football League), examined the differences between the playing performance of Australia and Great Britain. According to Clarke, the Australian team was successful by employing a strategy of running from greater depth, sprinting for (on average) 2.77 s prior to the collision, compared to the British players who sprinted for (on average) 1.69 s before collision. This meant the Australian players were more difficult to stop, moving nearly half a metre further in the collision and remaining on their feet for 0.63 s longer than the British players. A similar, but more comprehensive, time-based notational analysis, undertaken by Eaves and Evers (2007), examined how the speed of the 'play the ball' influenced the selection of the post-ruck playing pattern, and the development of scoring opportunities. They reported that whilst the speed of the 'play the ball' did not have a significant impact on the development of scoring opportunities, it did have a significant effect on the post-ruck event. In particular, hit ups were more likely to result from slow 'play the ball' and the dummy run more likely to result from quick 'play the ball'. In addition, it was identified that passing the ball beyond the first receiver resulted in a significant increase in scoring opportunities compared to when dummy runs, or hit ups were used. In a study that also examined scoring opportunities, Wheeler *et al.* (2011) reported that successful outcomes of the offload are more evident when the ball carrier moves beyond the advantage line before releasing the ball to his supporting player. In addition, the use of a 'pop' offload, rather than a 'wrap', 'flick', or 'conventional pass' offload was observed to be most associated with the successful outcome.

In terms of technical considerations, Wheeler *et al.* (2011) reported that the stability of the players' base is a significant factor in offload success, and suggested that players attempt to maintain a grounded base to dominate the collision. This idea of dominating of the contact area was also reported by Eaves and Broad (2007), who assessed the differences in playing patterns between Australian (NRL) and English (Super League; SL) domestic teams. They reported that teams in the NRL were more adept than teams in SL at confining their opponents to the defence zone, and were able to slow their opponents' play by utilizing the turtle tackle. Conversely, in attack, NRL teams played a more expansive game in the transition zone that enabled them to move more quickly into the attack zone, where they used a more direct style of play than teams in SL. The concept of dominance was also reported by Gabbett and Ryan (2009) who, as part of a wider study, coded tackle data and standardized technical tackling criteria. They reported that there were significant relationships between tackling technique and both the proportion of dominant tackles and proportion of missed tackles. In addition, they observed that players with better tackling techniques were involved in a greater number of tackle events.

The literature reviewed in this chapter is a small part of a much wider research area. For a more comprehensive review, the reader is referred to Prim and van Rooyen (2013). The depth and scope of research focussing on the performance analysis of rugby football, and the number of researchers who are active in this field, continues to grow. As a result, the evolving body of knowledge, and hence our understanding of the games of rugby football, continues to develop.

References

Bishop, L. and Barnes, A. (2011). Performance indicators that discriminate winning and losing in the knockout stages of the 2011 Rugby World Cup. *International Journal of Performance Analysis in Sport*, 13, 149–59.

Bremner, S., Robinson, G., and Williams, M.D. (2013). A retrospective evaluation of team performance indicators in rugby union. *International Journal of Performance Analysis in Sport*, 13, 461–73.

Diedrick, E. and van Rooyen, M.K. (2011). Line-break situations in international rugby. *International Journal of Performance Analysis in Sport*, 11, 522–34.

Eaves, S. and Hughes, M. (2003). Patterns of play in international rugby union teams before and after the introduction of professional status. *International Journal of Performance Analysis in Sport*, 3, 103–11.

Eaves, S.J., Hughes, M.D., and Lamb, K.L. (2005). The impact of the introduction of professional playing status on game action variables in international northern hemisphere rugby union football. *International Journal of Performance Analysis in Sport*, 5, 58–86.

Eaves, S.J. and Evers, A.L. (2007). The relationship between the 'play the ball' time, post-ruck action, and the occurrence of perturbations in professional rugby league football. *International Journal of Performance Analysis in Sport*, 7, 18–25.

Eaves, S. and Broad, G. (2007). A comparative analysis of professional rugby league football playing patterns between Australia and the United Kingdom. *International Journal of Performance Analysis in Sport*, 7, 54–66.

Eaves, S.J., Hughes, M.D., and Lamb, K.L. (2008a). Assessing the impact of the season change and rule changes on specific match and tactical variables in professional rugby league football in the United Kingdom. *International Journal of Performance Analysis in Sport*, 8, 104–18.

Eaves, S.J., Lamb, K.L., and Hughes, M.D., (2008b). The impact of rule and playing season changes on time variables in professional rugby league in the United Kingdom. *International Journal of Performance Analysis in Sport*, 8, 44–54.

Eaves, S.J. (2013). *Victorian and Edwardian journalists: Pioneers of sports notational analysis?* Unpublished paper presented at the British Society of Sports History conference, Weston, Cheshire.

Gabbett, T.J. and Ryan, P. (2009). Tackling technique, injury risk, and playing performance in high-performance collision sport athletes. *International Journal of Sports Science and Coaching*, 4, 521–33.

Hughes, M. and Clarke, A. (1994). Computerised notational analysis of the effects of the law changes upon patterns of play of international teams in rugby union. *Journal of Sports Science*, 12, 181.

Hughes, M. and White, P. (1997). An analysis of forward play in the men's Rugby Union World Cup, 1991. In M. D. Hughes (Ed.), *Notational Analysis of Sport I and II* (pp. 183–92). Cardiff: CPA, UWIC.

Hughes, M.D. and Williams, D. (1988). The development and application of computerized Rugby Union notation system. *Journal of Sports Sciences*, 6, 254–5.

Humbert, F. (2010, June 11). Broadcasted! Retrieved from http://rugby-pioneers.blogs.com/rugby/4_rugby_video/

Hunter, P. and O'Donoghue, P. (2001). A match analysis of the 1999 Rugby Union World Cup. In M. Hughes and I. Franks (Eds.), *Proceedings of the Computer Science and Sport III and Performance Analysis V Conference* (pp. 85–90). Cardiff: CPA, UWIC.

James, N., Mellalieu, S.D., and Jones, N.M.P. (2005). The development of position-specific performance indicators in professional rugby union. *Journal of Sports Sciences*, 23, 63–72.

Jones, N.M.P., Mellalieu, S.D., James, N., and Moise, J. (2004) Contact area playing styles of northern and southern hemisphere international rugby union teams. In P. O'Donoghue and M. Hughes (Eds.), *Performance Analysis of Sport VI* (pp. 114–9). Cardiff: UWIC.

McKenzie, A.D., Holmyard, D.J., and Docherty, D. (1989). Quantitative analysis of rugby: Factors associated with success in contact. *Journal of Human Movement Studies*, 17, 101–13.

McLean, D. (1992). Analysis of the physical demands of international rugby union. *Journal of Sports Science*, 10, 285–96.

Meir, R., Arthur, D., and Forrest, M. (1993). Time and motion analysis of professional rugby league: A case study. *Strength and Conditioning Coach*, 1, 24–9.

Meir, R., Colla, P., and Milligan, C. (2001). Impact of the 10-meter rule change on professional rugby league: Implications for training. *Strength and Conditioning Journal*, 23, 42–6.

Norton, K. (2013). Match analysis in AFL, Soccer and Rugby Union: patterns, trends and similarities. In H. Nunome, B. Drust and B. Dawson (Eds.), *Science and Football VII* (pp. 153–9). Abingdon: Routledge.

O'Connor, D. (2004). The relationship between performance of professional rugby league teams and game statistics. *Journal of Sports Science*, 22, 513.

O'Hare, M. (1995). In a league of their own. *New Scientist*, 30, 30–5.

Ortega, E., Villarejo, D., and Palao, J.M. (2009). Differences in game statistics between winning and losing rugby teams in the Six Nations Tournament. *Journal of Sports Science and Medicine*, 8, 523–7.

Potter, G. (1997). A case study of England's performance in the five nations championship over a three year period (1992–1994). In M. D. Hughes (Ed.), *Notational Analysis of Sport I and II.* 193–202. Cardiff: CPA, UWIC.

Potter, G. and Carter, A. (2001a). The four year cycle: A comparison of the 1991 and 1995 Rugby World Cup finals. In M. Hughes (Ed.), *Notational Analysis of Sport III* (pp. 216–9). Cardiff: CPA, UWIC.

Potter, G. and Carter, A. (2001b). The 1995 rugby world cup finals. From whistle to whistle: A comprehensive breakdown of the total game contents. In M. Hughes (Ed.), *Notational Analysis of Sport III* (pp. 209–15). Cardiff: CPA, UWIC.

Prim, S. and van Rooyen, M. (2013). Rugby. In T. McGarry, P. O'Donoghue and J. Sampaio (Eds.), *Routledge Handbook of Sports Performance Analysis* (pp. 338–56). Abingdon: Routledge.

Sayers, M. (2009). Development of an offensive evasion model for the training of high-performance rugby players. In T. Reilly and F. Korkusuz (Eds.), *Science and Football VI. The Proceedings of the Sixth World Congress on Science and Football* (pp. 278–84). Abingdon: Routledge.

Sayers, M.G.L. and Washington-King, J. (2005). Characteristics of effective ball carries in Super 12 rugby. *International Journal of Performance Analysis in Sport*, 5, 92–106.

Seuront, L. (2013) Complex dynamics in the distribution of players' scoring performance in Rugby Union word cups. *Physica A*, 392, 3731–40.

Smythe, G., O'Donoghue, P.G., and Wallace, E.S. (1998). Notational analysis of contact situations in rugby union. In M. Hughes and F. Tavares (Eds.), *Notational Analysis of Sport IV* (pp. 156–64). Cardiff: CPA, UWIC.

Thomas, C. (2001). The numbers game. *The RFU Technical Journal*, Spring, 28–33.

van den Berg, P.H. and Malan, D.D.J. (2010). Match analysis of the 2006 Super 14 Rugby Union tournament. *African Journal for Physical, Health Education, Recreation and Dance*, 16, 580–93.

van den Berg, P. and Malan, D.D.J. (2012). The effect of Experimental Law Variations on the Super 14 Rugby Union Tournaments. *African Journal for Physical, Health Education, Recreation and Dance*, 18, 476–86.

van Rooyen, M., Yasin, N., and Viljoen, W. (2014). Characteristics of an 'effective' tackle outcome in Six Nations rugby, *European Journal of Sports Science*, 14, 123–9.

van Rooyen, M. (2012). A statistical analysis of tackling performance during International rugby matches from 2011. *International Journal of Performance Analysis in Sport*, 12, 517–30.

Vaz, L., van Rooyen, M., and Sampaio, J. (2010). Rugby game-related statistics that discriminate between winning and losing reams in IRB and Super 12 close games. *Journal of Sports Science and Medicine*, 9, 51–5.

Vaz, L., Mouchet, A., Carreras, D., and Morente, H. (2011). The importance of rugby game-related statistics to discriminate winners and losers at the elite level competitions in close and balanced games. *International Journal of Performance Analysis in Sport*, 11, 130–141.

Wheeler, K. and Sayers, M. (2009). Contact skills predicting tackle-breaks in rugby union. *International Journal of Sports Science and Coaching*. 4, 535–44.

Wheeler, K.W., Askew, C.D., and Sayers, M.G. (2010). Effective attacking strategies in rugby union. *European Journal of Sports Science*, 10, 237–42.

Wheeler, K.W., Wiseman, R., and Lyons, K. (2011). Tactical and technical factors associated with effective ball offloading strategies during the tackle in rugby league. *International Journal of Performance Analysis in Sports*, 11, 392–409.

Williams, J. (2004). The effect of the wheeled scrum law in rugby union. *Journal of Sports Sciences*, 22, 520.

Williams, J., Hughes, M., and O'Donoghue, P. (2005a). The effect of rule changes on match and ball in play time in rugby union. *International Journal of Performance Analysis in Sport*, 5, 1–11.

Williams, J., Thomas, C., Brown, R., *et al.* (2005b). The effect of the wheeled scrum law in rugby union. In T. Reilly, J. Cabri, and D. Araujo (Eds.), *Science and Football V* (pp. 262–7). London: E. and F.N. Spon.

13

BIOMECHANICS OF RUGBY

Paul Worsfold and Doug McClymont

13.1 Introduction

Biomechanics applies the methods of mechanics to study the structure and function of biological systems to improve human movement performance and to reduce injury. To examine this, biomechanics is divided into the areas of kinematics (analysis of the movements of the body) and kinetics (analysis of forces acting on, or within the body). In every action, from passing, catching, running, jumping, and kicking and by applying force to the ground or onto other players, mechanics underpins every rugby skill.

13.2 Body collisions

With the primary purpose to prevent the advancement of the opposing team and to regain ball possession, collisions and tackling play a fundamental role in both rugby union and rugby league. The ability to win the tackle contest influences the outcome of both league and union matches (Gabbett and Ryan 2009; Wheeler *et al.* 2010); consequently, an understanding of the mechanics and effective, safe techniques are essential. Tackling techniques, frequencies, strategies, positional differences, and body contact locations have been investigated (Hendricks and Lambert 2010; Austin *et al.* 2011; King *et al.* 2010; Gabbett and Ryan 2009; Wheeler and Sayers 2009; Wheeler *et al.* 2010; Van Rooyen *et al.* 2014). However, the biomechanical assessment of complex multidimensional collisions between two or more bodies is problematic and consequently under-researched in rugby. Although limited research exists, the fundamental mechanical concepts of tackling and collisions will be discussed.

13.2.1 Momentum

When a force is applied from one player to another, there will be some change in motion of one or both players[1]. The success of the tackle is positively correlated with the amount of impact force a player can generate during the collision (Quarrie and Hopkins 2008), and consequently, the player's body kinematics and resultant force development is essential. One way players can increase their impact force is by increasing their momentum; this can only be influenced during a game by increasing their velocity (momentum = mass x velocity). When making comparisons between rugby codes, it is important to note the greater anthropometrical variance between positions within rugby union when compared to rugby league. The potential inequality in mass between union players entering into a collision will influence the momentum of the system, and therefore, the resultant impact between players. When body mass is comparable between the ball carrier and tackler, the ball carrier is often seen as having the advantage because he has the benefit of greater momentum – as he is often running faster than the tackler. As a result, the force applied by the ball carrier will be greater than the force applied by the tackler.

13.2.2 Rotation

A player tackled from the front at chest height will tend to rotate backward about the feet if the resistive force is greater than the force applied by the ball carrier. However, the tackler is disadvantaged because it is very difficult to maintain adequate forward momentum at chest height from a propulsive force at ground level. Simply, as a consequence of the shape of the human body, contact at chest height will always have a large vertical component, at the expense of the horizontal. If the ball carrier is moving forward, the advantage of momentum is with that player, and a chest high tackle usually results in a combination of rotation and backward translation of the tackler. The chest high tackle is therefore often mechanically inefficient. The ball carrier might also make further use of the principles of rotation by utilizing rotation about the long axis of the body. As the moment of impact approaches, the ball carrier needs only to move slightly off-line to change the point of impact of the tackle. At impact, the ball carrier may utilize the horizontal component of the eccentric force to 'spin' and evade the tackle to some extent.

13.2.3 Velocity and acceleration

The velocity and acceleration of the ball carrier and tackler entering into the tackle are also important determinants of the outcome of a tackle (Hendricks et al. 2012; McIntosh et al. 2010; Fuller et al. 2010; Wheeler et al. 2010; Gabbett 2008; Quarrie and Hopkins 2008). Within controlled testing conditions, the velocities of the ball carrier and tackler entering into a tackle have been reported to range between 1.5 to 5.9 m·s⁻¹ for the ball carrier, and 1.5 to 4.6 m·s⁻¹ for the tackler (Pain et al. 2008; Passos et al. 2008; Gabbett and Kelly 2007; Gabbett 2009; Gabbett and Ryan 2009; Wheeler and Sayers 2010). Such findings support the notion that, if body mass is comparable between players, the tackler is often disadvantaged at the point of impact (mass x velocity). Tackle velocities during competitive match, play have also been evaluated from video footage (Fuller et al. 2010; McIntosh et al.

2010; Quarrie and Hopkins 2008), and more recently, using video analysis combined with computer-generated algorithms (Hendricks *et al.* 2012).

Interestingly, Hendricks *et al.* (2012) identified that when tacklers enter the pre-tackle phase at a velocity considerably different to that of the ball carrier (whether higher or lower), tacklers adjusted their velocity accordingly to reach a suitable relative velocity before making contact with the ball carrier. In addition, Austin *et al.* (2011) identified the most frequent activity immediately before tackling was striding, implying that most tackles are not performed at a player's maximum running speed. A greater impact/momentum differential between the tackler and the person being tackled are reported to be a major risk factor for injury to the player with lower momentum (Garraway *et al.* 1999; Quarrie and Hopkins 2008; Posthumus and Viljoen 2008). Most players, who can see the oncoming player/tackler (50% of tackles are within the visual fields of the ball carrier; King *et al.* 2010), perceive the potential demands of the approaching collision and try to adapt their locomotive state prior to impact for performance gain or injury prevention. In part, this is achieved by modifying the kinematics of their body (height and location of center of mass, width of base of support, stride length, *etc.*). At slower speeds, players also increase their foot contact time (impulse) into the collision and therefore potentially increase the force/momentum production at the point of contact. The modification of acceleration and velocity of players prior to contact has been correlated with tackling proficiency (Gabbett 2009). Although tackle outcome was not measured in Gabbett's study, more proficient tacklers (assessed using a standardized technical criteria, see Gabbett 2008) were older, more experienced, shorter, lighter, and leaner, and therefore had greater acceleration and change of direction speed than poor tacklers.

13.2.4 Impact and impulse

The collision of two or more bodies during a tackle takes place under a force that exists only for a short time. The average collision force is connected to the mechanical impulse variation at impact ($Ft = mv_f - mv_i$), which depends on how long the contact lasts, the mass of the bodies, and the velocities immediately before and after collision. The impulse generated during the tackle will be determined through mechanical and technical adaptations during the contact phase. Maintaining foot contact with the ground and through the leg-drive are important factors that will enable the player some control over the velocity and the time in which they can apply the force (impulse) during the contact phase (Hendricks and Lambert 2010). The parameters of movement (impulse and kinetic energy) have very large variations (Budeseu and Iacob 2008) making it difficult to quantify during dynamic collisions. However, shoulder impact forces have been assessed during controlled tacking scenarios using customized force and pressure measuring sensors (Usman *et al.* 2011; Pain *et al.* 2008). Substantial collision forces were identified between the shoulder and opponent/target, with forces ranging between 1.00 and 2.31 body weight. Pain *et al.* (2008) reported the maximum impact force for rugby tackles from a crouch position (819 N) and from a run-up (1,283 N). Interestingly both Pain *et al.* (2008) and Usman *et al.* (2011) identified only small differences in shoulder impact forces when players wore shoulder pads and when they did not. Small differences were also identified between the shoulder forces produced on the dominant and non-dominant sides. Shoulder force did, however, reduce with tackle repetition, implying that fatigue diminishes tackling force and progressively influences technique (Gabbett 2008). It is important to note that past shoulder impact studies have quantified the impact forces against a tackle bag or a stationary player. The mass, zero velocity, and stiffness of the tackle bag/player will influence the force development in the resultant tackle. Therefore, shoulder forces in a match setting are likely to be much higher than those previously reported.

13.3 Ball Interactions

13.3.1 Kicking

Offensive and defensive kicking performance is an important skill in rugby and can determine the outcome of a game (Ortega *et al.* 2009; Vaz *et al.* 2010; Vaz *et al.* 2011). Although some kicking techniques and definitions differ between codes, principally there are two basic kicks. A kick released from the hand(s) and a stationary kick from the ground, and within those, several variations. When the ball is released from the hand(s), it falls towards the ground at a speed determined by gravity and whether or not the player pushed it down or simply dropped it. If we regard the ball and the foot as a system, then the momentum of the system is the product of the mass and speed of the two objects. The momentum will therefore influence the ball's release speed from the foot. As the size, shape, and resultant mass of rugby league and union balls are slightly different (see Table 13.1), the impact characteristics between the ball and foot will also be different.

When kicking from the hands, it has been suggested in other sports that the ball should be placed towards the foot with the hand ipsilateral to the kicking leg (Ball 2008; Carling 1994; McLeod and Jacques 2006; Robertson and Osborne 1984). Pavely *et al.* (2010) assessed the bilateral competency of players performing rugby clearance kicks. The study identified a tendency for players to use the contralateral hand or both hands together when guiding the ball to the non-preferred foot

TABLE 13.1 Official ball regulations

Ball characteristics	Union	League
Length (cm)	28 – 30	27
Circumference (cm)	58 – 62	60
Mass (kg)	0.41 – 0.46	0.38 – 0.44

(http://www.irblaws.com/index.php?law=2andlanguage=EN)
(http://media.rladmin.co.uk/docs/intl_rules_of_rugbyleague.pdf)

(i.e. right or both hands ball release for a left foot kick for a right handed/footed player). Interestingly, this hand dominance during the kick resulted in shorter kick distance and lower directional accuracy. When we consider place kicks from the ground, the mechanics change again. With a stationary ball, the kick becomes more of a closed skill. It will therefore be the kickers that dictate their approach routine (approach distance, velocity, angle, and subsequent body mechanics; Ball et al. 2013).

Whether the kick is from the ground or from the hands, many kicking situations will require the player to kick the ball as far as possible; therefore the speed of release from the foot is crucial. The speed of release of the ball is determined by two major factors. The first is the coefficient of restitution (e) of the ball and the foot/boot; this is determined by the characteristics of the two surfaces. Although the ball characteristics will not change significantly during a game, the rigidity of the foot at ball contact will have a large influence on the coefficient of restitution. The greater foot/ankle movement at contact, the lower the coefficient of restitution, and therefore, slower ball release speed. Therefore, the production and maintenance of isometric contractions to stabilize the ankle at ball contact are an important component of the kick. The second and by far the most important factor influencing the speed of ball release is the speed of contact of ball and boot; this is determined by a whole sequence of events that culminate in the force applied by the foot.

The ability to transfer kinetic energy from the body to the ball through the co-ordination of proximal to distal sequencing of body segments (sometimes referred to as the 'summation of speed principle') plays an important role in kicking. During the ball approach, the hips continue to move forward as a consequence of the running action, the pelvis rotates about the support hip, and the kicking leg accelerates about the hip. To maximize this acceleration, the kicking foot is left behind as the non-kicking foot is planted, with the lower leg flexed behind the thigh as in the recovery phase of running. This reduces the inertia of the whole leg and so increases the angular speed of the thigh until the appropriate moment when the knee slows in reaction to the shank being swung down in anticipation of ball contact. Like a cracking whip – kinetic link (Hay 1995) – the foot accelerates down and forward until at the moment of full extension, the rigid foot makes contact with the ball. Just prior to contact, the support-leg hip is extended to maintain stability and transfers momentum into the kicking-side hip, whilst the non-kicking side arm is extended to reduce contrary rotation (Bauer 1970; Bezodis et al. 2007). After contact the foot will follow-through in direction of the force, and the planted leg, which has fully extended during the final phase, will often leave the ground as a consequence of the principle of conservation of momentum.

Zhang et al. (2012) quantified the sequence and contributions of the motions of the individual segments to the final velocity of the foot using 3D motion capture. Proximal to distal sequences were identified with increasing segment velocity initiated at the hip – pelvis rotation ($2 \pm 1\%$), pelvis velocity ($9 \pm 1\%$), hip flexion ($13 \pm 2\%$), followed by knee extension ($75 \pm 8\%$). Further work by Ball et al. (2013) identified the knee to produce angular velocities at impact of $1044°/s$ and approach speeds (3 m·s⁻¹), which are comparable to soccer (Nunome *et al.* 2002; Kellis and Katis 2007), but the approach angle (31°) was much straighter than the 43° reported in soccer by Egan *et al.* (2007). A centre of mass (COM) velocity of 2.6 m·s⁻¹ towards the ball indicated that the body was continuing to move forward through ball contact. Importantly, the pelvis was also moving forward at the time of contact for all players, highlighting that the COM motion was not simply produced by the kicking leg moving rapidly, angularly upward. Although scientific understanding is limited, the mechanics and stability of the non-kicking hip and standing leg will also play an important role throughout the kicking sequence.

Upper body segments have also been found to contribute to kicking accuracy. Bezodis *et al.* (2007) assessed the determination of segmental contributions to whole–body angular momentum during kicking. The research identified rotations of the non-kicking-side arm; shoulder horizontal flexion and adduction during the downswing of the kicking leg were used to a greater extent by more accurate kickers. Angular momentum of the non-kicking-side arm about the Z axis opposed the motion of the kicking-leg, and momentum increased during maximal distance kicks for the participants who maintained their accuracy under these conditions.

The angle to the horizontal at which the ball leaves the kicking–foot is determined solely by the angle at which the boot makes contact. This angle is in turn determined by the stance of the kicker, the ball angle at impact, and the point at which the boot makes contact with the ball. Table 13.2 illustrates the different ball angles players use for different kick styles. Ball trajectories are reported between 1° – 53° depending on the type of kick (Table 13.2). Ball orientation and its resultant change through foot contact was evaluated by Ball *et al.* (2010), who identified the greatest change in place kicks (17°), with other kicks only moving through 5°. Interestingly, the variance between kicks from the most junior elite goal kicker was much higher (range of values 8 – 19°) when compared to the more senior kickers (range of values less than 2° for all three kickers). Furthermore, work by Ball and colleagues (2013) identified the most accurate kickers to have the most upright trunk angle (20° compared to 21–38°) during 40-metre goal kicks. It was hypothesized that a more upright trunk might allow for a leg-swing-plane more aligned with the intended path of the ball and a more balanced body and head position. To date, no optimal support foot positions, relative to the ball, have been identified.

13.3.2 Analysis of kick types

Comparisons of biomechanical variables between kick types are presented within Table 13.2. It can be seen that most variables are comparable across longer kick types within the elite groups. The highest ball velocity (28.06 m·s⁻¹) is seen for the spiral kick, a kick that is intended to travel maximum distance. Due to the grubber kick being intended to travel short distances along the ground, it is no surprise that the reported variables (ball velocity, trajectory, angle, and foot velocity) are

TABLE 13.2 A summary of kicking analysis research

Kick type, kick distance, and number of players	Homes et al. 2006		Bezodis et al. 2007		Ball et al. 2010		Zhang et al. 2012			Ball et al. 2013	
	Place (ME = ~ 54 m) (N=14)	Drop (ME = ~51 m) (N=14)	Spiral (ME = ~ 55 m) (N=14)	Place (ME = ~ 55.3 m) (N=5★)	Drop 45 m (N=7)	Bomb (N=4)	Field Goal 40 m (N=5)	Grubber 15 m (N=6)	Place (N=4)	Place (ME=7★) (N=7★)	40 m (N=4)
Foot velocity (m·s⁻¹) before BC					20.0±2.5	21.0±1.5	21.8±1.6	11±2.3	21.2±1.7	16.8±1.6	21±1
Ball velocity (m·s⁻¹) after BC	26.44±2.97	25.60±3.77	28.06±3.70	24.54±0.98	25.8±1.8	26.9±4.2	26.5±2.4	13.7±2.4	25.2±4.0	17.8±2.5	27±3
Ball foot ratio					1.30±0.13	1.28±0.12	1.22±0.11	1.27±0.25	1.20±0.20	1.06±1.6	1.26±0:16
Foot – ball velocity difference (%)					29.0	28.10	21.56	24.55	18.87	5.95	28.57
Ball contact time (ms)					7.2±0.6	6.8±0.2	7.1±0.5	8.8±0.7	7.4±0.3	0.27±0.04	
Ball displacement (m) during BC					0.20±0.02	0.20±0.01	0.23±0.04	0.12±0.03	0.22±0.02		
Work (J) during BC					290±49	342±50	316±48	68±17	306±71		

(Continued)

TABLE 13.2 (Continued)

Kick type, kick distance, and number of players	Homes et al. 2006 Place (ME = ~ 54 m) (N=14)	Drop (ME = ~51 m) (N=14)	Spiral (ME = ~ 55 m) (N=14)	Bezodis et al. 2007 Place (ME ~ 55.3 m) (N=5★)	Ball et al. 2010 Drop 45 m (N=7)	Bomb (N=4)	Zang et al. 2012 Field Goal 40 m (N=5)	Grubber 15 m (N=6)	Place (N=4)	Ball et al. 2013 Place (ME) 40 m (N=7★)	40 m (N=4)
Ball angle (°)											
Before BC				35	66±10	75±5	70±4	12±9	36±4		
After BC					70±8	77±9	65±17	20±25	53±8		
Change					4±8	2±10	5±17	8±19	17±4		
Foot trajectory (°) before BC					7±5	24±13	8±7	0±8	2±5		
Ball trajectory (°) after BC	30.2±4.4	35.8±4.3	43.9±4.6		32±11	53±12	39±9	1±2	36±3		
Support foot to ball distance (m)											
Horizontal					0.39±0.15	0.58±0.07	0.23±0.15	0.60±0.18	0.15±0.14		
Vertical					0.40±0.07	0.63±0.05	0.30±0.10	0.23±0.04	0.28±0.01		
Ball spin (rpm)	238.10±44.92	234.25±66.57	216.41±46.11								

★ sub-elite; BC = ball contact; ME = maximum effort

significantly different to other forms of kicking. It is noteworthy that the sub-elite groups reported in past studies produced lower ball (17.8–24.54 m·s⁻¹) and foot (16.8 m·s⁻¹) velocities and smaller ball to foot speed ratios (1.06) when compared to their elite counterparts (ball velocity 25.2–28.06 m·s⁻¹; foot velocity 20.0–21.8 m·s⁻¹; ball to foot ratio 1.20–1.30). Although only based on small data sets, it appears that elite players are able to repeatedly produce greater resultant ball velocity from the velocity of their kicking leg, as demonstrated with a higher percent change (18.87–29.0%) when compared to sub-elite players (5.95%).

13.3.3 Passing

Passing contributes more than any other skill, in terms of number of successful executions, to gains in attack (Sasaki *et al.* 2002). With the rules of the game requiring passes to be directed backwards, players need to be competent at passing bilaterally (Craven 1970). Using 3D motion capture, Sayers and Ballon (2011) assessed passes to the left and right at a target positioned five and eight metres away. Trials from the preferred side recorded significantly greater accuracy and pass velocities (12.01 ± 2.10 m·s⁻¹) than those from the non-preferred side (10.60 ± 1.71 m·s⁻¹). Asymmetries in upper body kinematics were evident with the rear shoulder and elbow actions, which correlated to pass velocity for passes to the non-preferred side. Results suggest that side dominance can have an influence on upper body passing technique, even for highly experienced rugby players.

There are various types of passes which players use, depending on their position, the amount of power required, the direction the ball is being passed, and the amount of time they have to complete the pass. The spin-pass is one of the most commonly used passes in rugby, because of its wide acceptance as the fastest, longest, and most accurate pass (Greenwood 1997; Crothers 1992). The spin-pass combines horizontal linear velocity with rotation around the longitudinal axis of the ball. The hand behind the ball generates spin and the front hand is used to guide the pass. The movement of the hands through the central plane of the ball provides the force needed to project the ball and the movement of the wrist and fingers imparts spin (Calverley 2009). Different variations in technique execution have been reported. Worsfold and Page (2014) assessed two distinct spin-pass styles when players made passes from their dominant and non-dominant hands over 4, 8 and 12 m. Players either lowered their centre of mass (body drop), then raised it again prior to ball release, utilizing the stretch–shortening cycle within the legs and trunk, or they maintained a more upright body position but incorporated greater arm movement. The research identified greater passing accuracy and ball velocity when a 'body drop' was used from both the dominant and non-dominant hands. However, the technique took significantly longer to execute when compared to an upright spin-pass technique. It is important to remember that the player's ability to select the most effective pass technique based upon the game situation, at that specific time, will often be the most important aspect that will determine the success of a pass.

13.3.4 Ball carrying

Running with the ball is an important skill used to maintain possession, to gain territory, and to score a try. Carrying the ball in two hands provides the player with more tactical options and is often recognized as the safest technique, as it makes it more difficult for defenders to remove the ball from an attacker's hands. Grant *et al.* (2003) compared sprint performance times of players carrying the ball in both hands, under the right and the left arms, and without the ball. The study identified that sprinting without the ball was the quickest, followed by single arm carry, whilst sprinting with the ball in two hands was the slowest. It was hypothesized that even though both arms can drive when holding the ball, their range of motion is restricted, resulting in a limited counter to body rotation around the pelvis. Further work by Walsh *et al.* (2007) assessed the influence of playing experience on ball carrying techniques. The research supported the previous work of Grant *et al.* (2003) with sprinting with the ball under one arm (whether left or right) pressed against the chest resulting in smaller decrements in speed than the two handed method. Playing experience decreased the extent to which running with the ball slowed the players down during the 10-m sprint. Sprinting with ball in two hands is difficult to do well, as it requires excellent pelvic control to maintain balance and efficient lower leg mechanics (Sayers 1999; 2000). Walsh and colleagues suggest that practicing the skill of running with the ball permits adaptation to the constraints of the task, limiting the negative effect ball carriage has on sprint speed.

The findings have important implications for training. Past research can only speculate the reasons why sprint times change when running with the ball, as to date no kinematic analysis has been conducted. Further investigation into the changes in kinematics (body positions, range of motion, stride length, etc.) whilst running with the ball is needed in this area to help develop appropriate coaching protocols.

13.4 Conclusions and future directions

It is evident that there has been some progress in the use of biomechanical measurement systems and analytical techniques, especially within the investigation of kicking and more recently the scrum in rugby union. However, with limited research in many areas of the game, it is important that the mechanics and risks of the game are explored further. Whilst the risk of injury is always going to be high in a collision sport, it is plausible that injury risk can be reduced through advancing our understanding of the mechanics of body collisions and subsequently educating and implementing safe and effective techniques.

Due to the required dynamic multi-directional actions of the body and its segments during rugby play, there is a need, where possible, to capture more advanced field-based biomechanical measurements (e.g. 3D motion capture; marker-less tracking; inertial sensors; segment location; acceleration/decelerations; force; pressure, etc.). Although complex, additional investigation into player interactions (with their environment and equipment) and collisions is also warranted. It is apparent from the reviewed research that significant technique variability exists between elite players in many rugby skills. Perhaps future research should reconsider the use of 'ideal' models of technique, and focus upon modelling individual movements and the variability of these to create normative profiles of performance outcome, which could then be utilized within coaching practice.

Case study: what does biomechanics feed into the rugby scrum?

Ezio Preatoni, Dario Cazzola, Keith Stokes, Michael E. England, and Grant Trewartha

Introduction

The Rugby Union scrum is viewed as an integral facet of the sport and has been the focus of attention from a player welfare and game management perspective. The scrum engagement is a critical phase of the scrum as it has traditionally involved an intense initial impact followed by a sustained push, both of which happen in a context characterized by multiple players' interactions, destabilising forces and movements in the three planes of motion, variable turf conditions, and the additional need of gaining possession of the ball (Milburn 1990; Preatoni *et al.* 2013). These factors generate very peculiar biomechanical demands on rugby forwards and make this event very interesting for both injury prevention and performance analysis. Being the shock absorption interface between the two forward packs whilst simultaneously receiving forward momentum from the second and back rows, it is front row players who are at higher risk for both acute injuries and overuse pathologies.

Case presentation

The 'Biomechanics of the Rugby Scrum' project was funded by the International Rugby Board (IRB) and was carried out by the Rugby Science group of the University of Bath (RS@Bath). The aims were to:

* Describe the kinematics and kinetics of the scrum
* Assess the effect of different scrum engagement techniques and playing standards on scrum mechanics
* Investigate possible routes to injury prevention

The research project was separated into two distinct phases. Phase 1 (June 2010– December 2011) studied the biomechanics of machine scrummaging, i.e. a forward pack against a sled-type scrum machine instrumented with strain gauges. Phase 2 (January 2012–May 2013) analysed the biomechanics of live scrummaging, i.e. two forward packs in live scrums simulating a contested match situation, with front-row players equipped with pressure sensors and accelerometers (Figure 13.1). Both studies

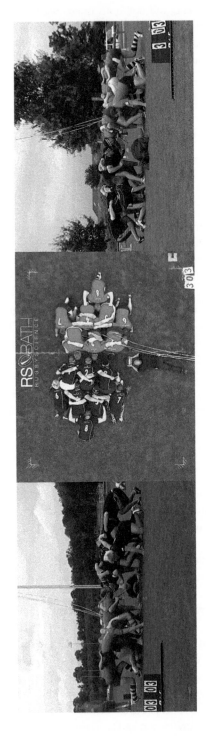

FIGURE 13.1 The camera views (left, right, top) for a typical experimental set-up from phase 2

attempted to maximize the ecological validity of the testing and to reduce the possible influence of the experimental setup. All sessions were carried out outdoors, on natural turf and without any substantial impact of measurement technologies on players' habits and freedom of movement. In both phases biomechanical outcome measures (a set of kinematic and kinetic variables) describing the mechanics of the scrum were analysed as a factor of playing standard and engagement techniques.

In Phase 1, 34 teams from six defined playing standards (International, Elite, Community, Academy, Women, and School) completed a testing protocol which involved performing scrums against the instrumented scrum machine using five different engagement techniques. These techniques included the scrummaging procedure in use until the 2011–12 season ('Crouch-Touch-Pause-Engage), which represented the baseline condition, and four modified techniques that differed from the baseline, either in the referee's calls (e.g. the three-stage sequence introduced by the IRB in the 2012–13 season as a law amendment trial) or in aspects aimed to modify the loading conditions on players (e.g. de-emphasizing the initial impact by introducing a fold-in procedure or sequential engagements where one or three back row players stood off the initial engagement).

The outcomes of Phase 1 drove the selection of three engagement techniques to be analysed in Phase 2, where 27 teams (54 forward packs) from five playing standards (the same as in Phase 1 except there was no 'School' group) performed simulated live scrums. The three techniques included the baseline condition ('Crouch-Touch-Pause-Engage'), the three-stage procedure ('Crouch-Touch-Set'), and a 'Pre Bind' condition (later adopted as a law amendment trial for the 2013–14 season). In this last condition, the front-row players maintained the bind with their opposition counterparts after the referee's 'Bind' call.

A bespoke control and acquisition system was devised to synchronize the multiple measurement devices and play pre-recorded audio files that simulated the referee's vocal commands with a consistent timing (Preatoni et al. 2013; Preatoni et al. 2012). Measures included: the players' movements from three different views (Figure 13.1), including displacements, angles, and their derivatives (Preatoni et al. 2012); forces in compression (for both machine and live scrummaging); lateral and vertical (for machine scrummaging only) directions, at the interface between the front-row players and the opposition; and accelerations on trunk and head segments of the six front-row players (for live scrummaging only).

Results from Phase 1 machine scrummaging tests showed that forces measured across all playing standards were considerably higher than the ones reported in past research (Milburn 1990). These differences might be associated with the changes in scrummaging techniques and players' physical characteristics over the last two decades (Quarrie and Hopkins 2007), and with the improvements in measurement technologies that have increased ecological validity (Preatoni et al. 2013; Preatoni et al. 2012). In the baseline condition, peak compression forces across the front row during the engagement phase ranged between 8,700 N for the Women teams and

16,500 N for the International male teams; sustained push was between 4,790 N (Women) and 8,300 N (International/Elite men); peak vertical forces during the early engagement were downward between -2,000 N (School) and -3,900 N (Elite). International and Elite men's groups generated significantly higher forces than all other groups, even after normalizing forces to the pack weight in order to take out the possible influence of inertia.

Changes in kinematic and kinetic measures due to scrum engagement condition were consistent across playing standards (Figure 13.2 and 13.3). De-emphasizing the initial impact, by means of either a fold–in procedure (machine scrummaging) or the pre-bind process (live scrummaging), significantly reduced engagement speed and peak compression forces without altering the magnitude of the sustained push. It also lowered other indicators of mechanical stress, instability, and potential hazard on players, such as: shear forces (e.g. peak downward, lateral excursion), peak decelera-tion at impact, and the combination of body misalignment with high force magni-tudes. It therefore appears that de-emphasizing the initial impact at engagement plus including a pre-bind prior to full engagement might go towards a more controlled scrummaging action without limiting the ability of forward packs to generate an effective sustained push.

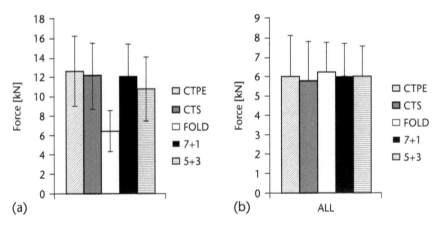

FIGURE 13.2 Some results from engagement technique comparison in Phase 1.
All teams from the different playing standards have been pooled together.
    CTPE = baseline condition, 'Crouch-Touch-Pause-Engage'
    CTS = 3-stage call condition, 'Crouch-Touch-Set'
    FOLD = 4-stage procedure with fold-in procedure and start of the push action, only after stable contact has been made
    7+1 = sequential engagement procedure with number 8 player not involved in initial engagement
    5+3 = sequential engagement procedure with the entire back row not involved in initial engagement
(a) peak of total compression force [kN]
(b) total sustained compression push [kN] from the scrum machine sensors embedded in the pusher arms

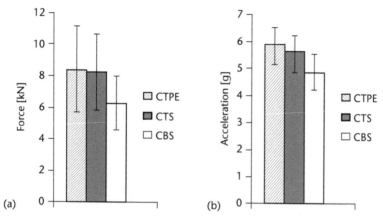

FIGURE 13.3 Some results from engagement technique comparison in Phase 2. All teams from the different playing standards have been pooled together.

    CTPE = baseline condition, 'Crouch-Touch-Pause-Engage'

    CTS = 3-stage call condition, 'Crouch-Touch-Set'

    CBS = Pre-bind process with the bind kept after 'Bind'

(a) Peak of total compression force [N] estimated from pressure sensors

(b) Average of the individual peaks of acceleration [g] from accelerometers on upper spine (C7) of front row players

Discussion

Combining the outcomes from the two phases of the research programme can draw a number of indications for both injury prevention and performance. Given the combined mass of the forward packs, the speed of the engagement, and the forces generated, it seems advisable to spend effort to reduce and/or add control over the dynamics of the early phases of the scrum. The fact that a consistent sustained push of similar magnitude was possible regardless of engagement technique further supports this view.

It is clear that there is a very important need to avoid uncontrolled scrum engagements which heighten the risk of catastrophic injuries. However, it is plausible that the magnitude and repetitiveness of the mechanical stresses acting on rugby forwards, associated with the possible misalignments and constraints of body-segment motion (head and trunk in particular) may also put forwards at risk of early degenerative changes to the spine. Further research is required to identify the precise mechanisms of how cervical spine injuries occur in scrum-specific contexts, and particularly the links between the external loads acting on the player and internal (i.e. at anatomical structures level) thresholds for such injuries.

This research programme has provided a thorough quantitative description of the biomechanics of rugby union scrummaging and has analysed the effects of playing standards and engagement conditions on the scrum outcomes. It has also provided an example of how a complex biomechanical investigation may inform practitioners and governing bodies about factors that may have an impact on performance and injury prevention. The outcomes of the study have indeed driven the identification and selection of new scrum engagement procedures, which have been progressively introduced into the laws of the game by the IRB, most recently the global trial of 'Crouch, Bind, Set', in use at all playing standards from September 2013.

Endnote

1   Newton's 1st and 2nd Laws

References

Austin, D., Gabbett, T., and Jenkins, D. (2011). Repeated high-intensity exercise in professional rugby union. *Journal of Sports Sciences*, 29, 1105–12.

Ball, K. (2010). Kick impact characteristics for different rugby league kicks. *28th International Society of Biomechanics in Sport*, 458–61.

Ball, K. (2008). Biomechanical considerations of distance kicking in Australian Rules football. *Sports Biomechanics*, 7, 10–23.

Ball, K., Talbert, D., and Taylor, S. (2013). Biomechanics of goal kicking in rugby league. In H. Nunome, B. Drust and B. Dawson (Eds.), *Science and Football VII: The Proceedings of the Seventh World Congress on Science and Football* (pp. 47–53). London: Routledge.

Bauer, T. (1970). *A biomechanical analysis of the rugby punt using the preferred and non-preferred foot*. Lakehead University.

Bezodis, N., Trewartha, G., Wilson, C., *et al.* (2007). Contributions of the non-kicking arm to rugby place kicking technique, *Sports Biomechanics*, 6, 171–86.

Budeseu, E.I. and Lacob, I. (2008). The human impact biomechanics in rugby game. ICCES, 8, 31–40.

Calverley, M. (2009). Biomechanics and skill analysis of scrum-half passing skills – *Part 2*. Retrieved from: www.attackingrugby.com/articles/SH%20Biomechanics%202.pdf.

Carling, W. (1994). *Rugby skills*. England: Queen Anne Press.

Craven, D. (1970). *Rugby handbook*. New Zealand: EP Publishing.

Crothers, D.S. (1992). Mathematics in sport I. *International Journal of Mathematical Education in Science and Technology*, 23, 117–26.

Cunniffe, B., Proctor, W., Baker, J.S., *et al.* (2009). An evaluation of the physical demands of elite rugby union using global positioning system tracking software. *Journal of Strength and Conditioning Research*, 23, 1195–1203.

Egan, C.D., Verheul, M.H., and Savelsbergh, G.J. (2007). Effects of experience on the coordination of internally and externally timed soccer kicks. *Journal of Motor Behavior*, 39, 423–32.

Fuller, C.W., Ashton, T., Brooks, J.H., *et al.* (2010). Injury risks associated with tackling in rugby union. *British Journal of Sports Medicine*, 44, 159–67.

Gabbett, T. (2008). Influence of fatigue on tackling technique in rugby league players. *Journal of Strength and Conditioning Research*, 22, 625–32.

Gabbett, T. and Kelly, J. (2007). Does fast defensive line speed influence tackling proficiency in collision sport athletes. *International Journal of Sport Science and Coaching*, 2, 467–72.

Gabbett, T. and Ryan, P. (2009). Tackling technique, injury risk, and playing performance in high-performance collision sport athletes. *International Journal of Sport Science and Coaching*, 4, 521–33.

Gabbett, T. (2009). Physiological and anthropometric correlates of tacking ability in rugby league players. *Journal of Strength and Conditioning Research*, 23, 540–8.

Garraway, W.M., Lee, A.J., Macleod, D.A., *et al*. (1999). Factors influencing tackle injuries in rugby union football. *British Journal of Sports Medicine*, 33, 37–41.

Grant, S.J., Oommen, G., McColl, J., *et al*. (2003). The effect of ball carrying method on sprint speed in rugby union football players. *Journal of Sport Sciences*, 21, 1009–15.

Greenwood, J. (1997). *Total rugby*. London: A and C Black.

Hay, J.G. (1995). *The biomechanics of sports techniques (5th ed)*. Englewood Cliffs, NJ: Prentice Hall.

Hendricks, S., and Lambert, M. (2010). Tackling in rugby: coaching strategies for effective technique and injury prevention. *International Journal of Sport Science and Coaching*, 5, 117–36.

Hendricks, S., Karpul, D., Nicolls, F., *et al*. (2012). Velocity and acceleration before contact in the tackle during rugby union matches. *Journal of Sports Sciences*, 30, 1215–24.

Holmes, C., Jones, R., Harland, A., *et al*. (2006). Ball launch characteristics for elite rugby union players. *The Engineering of Sport*, 1, 211–16.

Kellis, E., and Katis, A. (2007). Biomechanical characteristics and determinants of instep soccer kick. *Journal of Sports Science and Medicine*, 6, 154–65.

King, D., Hume, P.A., and Clark, T. (2010). Video analysis of tackles in professional rugby league matches by player position, tackle height, and tackle location. *International Journal of Performance Analysis in Sport*, 10, 241–54.

McLeod, A. and Jacques, T.D. (2006). *Australian Football: Steps to success (2nd ed)*. Champaign, Illinois: Human Kinetics.

McIntosh, A.S., Savage, T.N., McCrory, P., *et al*. (2010). Tackle characteristics and injury in a cross section of rugby union football. *Medicine and Science in Sports and Exercise*, 42, 977–84.

Milburn, P.D. (1990). The kinetics of rugby union scrummaging. *Journal of Sports Sciences*, 8, 47–60.

Nunome, H., Asai, T., Ikegami, Y., *et al*. (2002). Three-dimensional kinetic analysis of side-foot and instep soccer kicks. *Medicine and Science in Sports and Exercise*, 34, 2028–36.

Ortega, E., Villarejo, D., and Palao, J.M. (2009). Differences in game statistics between winning and losing rugby teams in the six nations tournament. *Journal of Sports Science and Medicine*, 88, 523–7.

Pain, M.T., Tsui, F., and Cove, S. (2008). In vivo determination of the effect of shoulder pads on tackling forces in rugby. *Journal of Sports Sciences*, 26, 855–62.

Passos, P., Araújo, D., Davids, K., *et al*. (2008). Manipulating constraints to train decision making in rugby union. *International Journal of Sports Science and Coaching*, 3, 125–40.

Pavely, S., Adams, R.D., Francesco, T.I., *et al*. (2009). Execution and outcome differences between passes to the left and right made by first-grade rugby union players. *Physical Therapy in Sport*, 10, 136–41.

Pavely, S., Adams, R.D., Francesco, T.I., *et al*. (2010). Bilateral clearance punt kicking in rugby union: effects of hand used for ball delivery. *International Journal of Performance Analysis of Sport*, 10, 187–96.

Preatoni, E., Stokes, K.A., England, M.E., *et al*. (2013). The influence of playing level on the biomechanical demands experienced by rugby union forwards during machine scrummaging. *Scandinavian Journal of Medicine and Science in Sports*, 23, e178–84.

Preatoni, E., Wallbaum, A., Gathercole, N., *et al*. (2012). An integrated measurement system for analysing impact biomechanics in the rugby scrum. Proceedings of the Institution of Mechanical Engineers, Part P: *Journal of Sports Engineering and Technology*, 226, 266–73.

Posthumus, M. and Viljoen, W. (2008). BokSmart: Safe and effective techniques in rugby union. *South African Journal of Sports Medicine*, 20, 64–70.

Quarrie, K.L. and Hopkins, W.G. (2007). Changes in player characteristics and match activities in Bledisloe Cup rugby union from 1972 to 2004. *Journal of Sports Sciences*, 25, 895–903.

Quarrie, K.L. and Hopkins, W.G. (2008). Tackle injuries in professional rugby union. *The American Journal of Sports Medicine*, 36, 1705–16.

Robertson, B. and Osborne, B. (1984). *Rugby coaching the New Zealand way.* New Zealand: Hutchinson Group.

Sasaki, K., Murakami, J., Shimozono, H., *et al.* (2002). Contributing factors to successful attacks in rugby football games. In W. Spinks, T. Reilly, and A. Murphy (Eds.). *Science and Football VI.* London: Routledge.

Sayers, M.G. and Ballon, R. (2011). Biomechanical analysis of a rugby pass from the ground. Paper presented at *7th World Congress of Science and Football*, Nagoya, Japan, 26–30 May.

Sayers, M.G. (1999). Running techniques for running rugby. *New Zealand Coach*, 7, 20–3.

Sayers, M.G. (2000). Running techniques for field sports players. *Sports Coach*, 23, 26–7.

Sayers, M.G. (2011). Kinematic analysis of lineout throwing in elite international rugby union. *Journal of Sport Science and Medicine*, 10, 553–8.

Usman, J., McIntosh, A.S., and Fréchède, B. (2011). An investigation of shoulder forces in active shoulder tackles in rugby union football. *Journal of Science and Medicine in Sport*, 14, 547–52.

van Rooyen, M., Yasin, N., and Viljoen, W. (2014). Characteristics of an 'effective' tackle outcome in Six Nations rugby. *European Journal of Sports Science*, 14, 123–9.

Vaz, L., van Rooyen, M., and Sampaio, J. (2010). Rugby game-related statistics that discriminate between winning and losing teams in IRB and Super 12 close games. *Journal of Sports Science and Medicine*, 9, 51–5.

Vaz, L., Mouchet, A., Carreras, D., *et al.* (2011). The importance of rugby game-related statistics to discriminate winners and losers at the elite level competitions in close and balanced games. *International Journal of Performance Analysis in Sport*, 11, 130–41.

Walsh, M., Young, B., Hill, B., *et al.* (2007). The effect of ball-carrying technique and experience on sprinting in rugby union. *Journal of Sports Sciences*, 25, 185–92.

Wheeler, K.W. and Sayers, M.G. (2009). Contact skills predicting tackle-breaks in rugby union. *International Journal of Sports Science and Coaching*, 4, 535–44.

Wheeler, K.W. and Sayers, M.G. (2010). Modification of agility running technique in reaction to a defender in rugby union. *Journal of Sports Science and Medicine*, 9, 445–51.

Wheeler, K.W., Askew, C., and Sayers, M.G. (2010). Effective attacking strategies in rugby union. *European Journal of Sport Science*, 10, 237–42.

Worsfold, P.R. and Page, M. (2014). The influences of rugby spin pass technique on movement time, ball velocity and passing accuracy. *International Journal of Performance Analysis in Sport*, 14, 296–306.

Zhang, Y., Liu, G., and Xie, S. (2012). Movement sequences during instep rugby kick: a 3D biomechanical analysis. *International Journal of Sports Science and Engineering*, **6**, 89–95.

14

INJURY EPIDEMIOLOGY IN RUGBY

Niki Gabb, Grant Trewartha, and Keith Stokes

14.1 Introduction

Rugby is a physically demanding game characterized by intermittent activity, with periods of low intensity movements, such as walking and jogging, punctuated by frequent bouts of high-intensity activities, such as running and sprinting, along with collision events such as tackling, scrummaging, rucking, and mauling (Roberts *et al.* 2008; Gabbett *et al.* 2008). These physical demands, in particular the regular exposure to collisions and physical contact, ensure that the inherent risk of injury in rugby is substantial (Williams *et al.* 2013; Gabbett 2004a). Indeed, rugby union and rugby league have some of the highest incidences of match injuries of professional team sports, albeit with rates similar to those of other full contact sports such as ice hockey (Lorentzon *et al.* 1988), American football (Meyers and Barnhill 2004), and Australian Rules football (Orchard and Seward 2002). Given the relatively high incidence of injuries in rugby and the potential long-term consequences [e.g. osteoarthritis (Drawer and Fuller 2001)], injury prevention/reduction is an important endeavour and is the joint responsibility of individual athletes, coaches, and sport regulatory bodies.

Injury surveillance seeks to describe the occurrence of, the circumstances around, and the factors associated with injury (Caine *et al.* 1996). The data collected from these epidemiological studies are considered essential for the continued development of injury prevention, treatment, and rehabilitation strategies (Brooks and Fuller 2006).

14.2 Match–related injuries in rugby league

There are a number of studies of match injuries in professional, semi-professional, and amateur men's rugby league, although very few pertaining to school level and the women's game (King *et al.* 2010). The results of many of these studies have been summarized by King and colleagues (2010) in a review of published studies, with match incidence rates for professional players ranging considerably from 58 (Walker 1985) to 211 (Estell *et al.* 1995) injuries per 1,000 player hours, compared with 115 (King and Gabbett 2009) to 825 (Gabbett 2003) injuries per 1,000 player hours for semi-professional players. Incidence rates for amateur players also vary greatly, with reports of match incidence rates from 114 injuries per 1,000 player hours (Stephenson *et al.* 1996) to 700 injuries per 1,000 player hours (King and Gissane 2009).

One of the reasons for the wide range of incidence values reported is that there has been little consensus in rugby league literature regarding a universal injury definition, with some preferring an all-encompassing definition (medical attention and time-loss injuries), and some preferring to only record time-loss injuries (Hodgson *et al.* 2007). Indeed, in a study by King and Gissane (2009) 372 injuries were sustained when both time-loss and medical attention injuries were reported, compared to 102 injuries when only time-loss injuries were reported (one missed match/training week). The resulting incidence rates were 405 compared with 111 injuries per 1,000 player hours, respectively. However, reporting only missed matches (or missed weeks of training) is believed to under-report medical treatments by as much as 70% (Stephenson *et al.* 1996), whereas reporting all injuries (including transient injuries) results in very high rates, as transient injuries might account for as many as 93% of all injuries reported (Gabbett 2004b).

A second issue lacking consensus is a common definition for injury severity. King *et al.* (2009) proposed that injury severity should be based on the 'actual number of matches missed per injury' rather than using time (days absent). However, unless matches are played at regular intervals (e.g. every seven days), this not only makes cross-study comparisons impossible, but the same injury (e.g. an ankle sprain requiring three weeks to recover) could result in varying reported severity (i.e. number of missed matches) (Orchard and Hoskins 1997). There are also the challenges of categorizing the severity of injuries that are not resolved during the regular season (i.e. when there are no matches).

Based on the variation in reporting of injury incidence and severity, it is very difficult to make any clear comparison between the findings of different studies in rugby league. However, some general conclusions can be drawn, including that the injury incidence rate is higher for match-play compared to training, the incidence of injury increases as playing standard increases, and being tackled is responsible for the greatest number of injuries regardless of the standard of participation (King *et al.* 2010).

14.3 Match-related injuries in rugby union

14.3.1 Men's elite rugby

There is a relative wealth of data pertaining to injuries in elite men's rugby union with papers published as far back as the 1950s (O'Connell 1954). However, the game has changed greatly since these initial studies, in particular since the adoption of professionalism in 1995. From an injury surveillance perspective, a consensus statement regarding appropriate definitions and methodologies for the recording and reporting of injuries in rugby union was published in 2007 (Fuller *et al.* 2007b). This was a major step in facilitating cross-study comparisons.

Although pre-dating the consensus statement, Brooks and Fuller (2005a) used methodologies consistent with the statement when observing injuries in English Premiership players, and reported a match injury incidence of 91 injuries per 1,000 player hours (95% CI: 87 to 96). Comparable data (i.e. injury resulting in more than 24 hours time-loss/one day lost) from Southern hemisphere competitions, provide similar incidence rates from the 2008 Super 14 Competition (96 injuries per 1,000 player hours) and the Vodacom Cup (71 injuries per 1,000 player hours) (Fuller *et al.* 2009). Furthermore, incidence figures from the Rugby World Cup (RWC) tournaments indicate a similar injury profile with 84 injuries per 1,000 player hours noted at the 2007 RWC (Fuller *et al.* 2008) and 89 injuries per 1,000 player hours at the 2011 RWC (Fuller *et al.* 2012). Indeed, a meta-analysis of injuries in men's elite professional rugby union reports a match injury incidence of 81 per 1,000 player hours (95% CI: 63–105) (Williams *et al.* 2013).

Mean injury severity figures for English Premiership data between 2002–2003 and 2011–2012 ranged from 16 to 27 days lost per injury (Kemp *et al.* 2013). Similarly, mean severity of injuries sustained by players competing in the Vodacom Cup was 21 days; however, players competing in the 2008 Super 14 competition experienced, on average, 13 days absence from training/playing with each injury (Fuller *et al.* 2009). The meta-analysis described above reported a mean severity for match injuries of 20 days (95% CI: 14–27) (Williams *et al.* 2013). Mean values for severity tend to be inflated by a (small) number of very severe injuries, whilst median values tend to be considerably lower in terms of days absence per injury.

The product of injury incidence and mean injury severity, referred to variously as 'injury burden', 'injury risk', or 'absolute risk' (Fuller *et al.* 2007a), gives an estimate of the overall cost of injuries to a team in terms of days absence resulting from a given period of exposure. Brooks and Kemp (2011) reported injury burden in professional rugby in England of 1,569 days absence per 1,000 player–hours for forwards and 1,507 days absence per 1,000 player–hours for backs. These figures equate to 33 days absence per match for forwards and 28 days absence per match for backs.

The contact nature of rugby is highlighted by the finding that 456 contact events occur per game in elite level rugby (Fuller *et al.* 2007a). These events include tackling, being tackled, mauls, rucks, collisions, lineouts, and scrums (Fuller *et al.* 2007a), and when grouped together these events are responsible for approximately 80% of all match injuries (Williams *et al.* 2013). Being tackled is associated with more injuries than any other event, with an incidence of 29 per 1,000 player hours, followed by tackling and the ruck/maul (17 and 19 per 1,000 player hours, respectively), and then collisions, scrums, other contact events, and lineouts (11, 7, 6, and 1 per 1,000 player hours, respectively) (Williams *et al.* 2013).

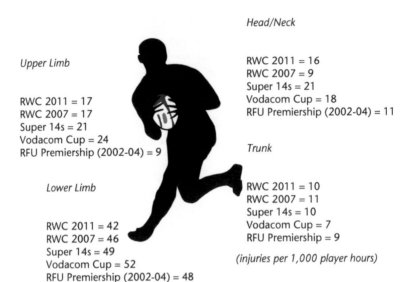

Head/Neck

RWC 2011 = 16
RWC 2007 = 9
Super 14s = 21
Vodacom Cup = 18
RFU Premiership (2002-04) = 11

Upper Limb

RWC 2011 = 17
RWC 2007 = 17
Super 14s = 21
Vodacom Cup = 24
RFU Premiership (2002-04) = 9

Trunk

RWC 2011 = 10
RWC 2007 = 11
Super 14s = 10
Vodacom Cup = 7
RFU Premiership = 9

Lower Limb

RWC 2011 = 42
RWC 2007 = 46
Super 14s = 49
Vodacom Cup = 52
RFU Premiership (2002-04) = 48

(injuries per 1,000 player hours)

FIGURE 14.1 Injury incidence by body region for men's elite rugby (Fuller *et al.* 2009; Brooks *et al.* 2005b; Fuller *et al.* 2008; Fuller *et al.* 2012)

The tackle event is consistently reported to be responsible for the highest number of injuries in rugby union. There are, however, reported to be 221 tackle events per game, thus it could be argued that the high number of injuries simply reflects the number of events (Fuller *et al.* 2007a). Fuller *et al.* (2007a) reported the tackle to be associated with a propensity of six injuries per 1,000 events; however, the scrum (not collapsed) had a higher propensity to cause injury with a reported rate of nine injuries per 1,000 events. Reporting injury propensity is useful when developing targeted injury prevention strategies, since it identifies the risk per individual event.

The body region sustaining the greatest number of injuries is consistently found to be the lower limbs (Figure 14.1). Williams *et al.* (2013), collating epidemiological data across the senior men's professional game, found that the lower limb (47 injuries per 1,000 player hours; 95% CI: 26–84) was significantly more likely to sustain an injury than the upper limb (14 injuries per 1,000 playing hours; 95% CI: 8–25), head (13 injuries per 1,000 playing hours; 95% CI: 7–23), and trunk (9 injuries per 1,000 playing hours; 95% CI: 5–16).

14.3.2 Men's community rugby

'Community' rugby refers to the non-elite level of the game, usually at least one level below a country's top tier of club rugby, and played in the most part on an amateur basis. Surprisingly, despite the vast majority of the world's playing population competing at community level, there is currently limited injury epidemiology information on this group. Community rugby is more difficult to study than the

TABLE 14.1 Incidence and severity in community rugby literature

Author	Injury incidence (using published data)	Time-loss injury incidence (>24 hours) Injuries per 1,000 player hours (*recalculated where required)	Injury severity outcome	Injury severity
Hughes and Fricker (1994)	Medical Attention Only and Time-Loss Injuries	1 injury per 16.7 player-games (*time loss only*)	*Unable to recalculate for > 24 h time-loss only*	No. of days lost: Minor ≤ 1 week Intermediate = 1 to 3 weeks Serious > 3 weeks	% of Injuries classified as: Minor = 59% Intermediate = 29% Serious = 13%
Garraway and Macleod (1995)	Included injuries <24 hours in duration	14 injuries per 1,000 player hours	*Unable to recalculate for > 24 h time-loss only*	Transient – <7days Mild – <28 days Moderate – 29–84 days Severe – >84 days	Transient = 22% Mild = 38% Moderate = 24% Severe = 16%
Bird et al. (1998)	Medical Attention Only and Time-Loss Injuries	9.9 injuries per 100 player games	*Unable to recalculate for > 24 h time-loss only*	Not reported	Not reported
Schneiders et al. (2009)	Medical Attention Only and Time-Loss Injuries	52 injuries per 1,000 player hours	34*	No. of days lost: Slight – 0–1 days Minimal – 2–3 days Mild – 4–7 days Moderate – 8–28 days Severe – >28 days	% of Injuries classified as: Slight = 35% Mild = 17% Moderate = 30% Severe = 7% Season Ending = 8% Career Ending = 4%
Roberts et al (2013)	Time-Loss Injuries >7 days	16.9 per 1,000 player hours#	*Unable to recalculate for > 24 hr time-loss only*	Mean no. of matches missed	6.6 per injury

Incidence rates for RFU levels 9–3 ranged from 14.2 to 21.7 injuries per 1,000 player hours based on ≥ 8 days time-loss

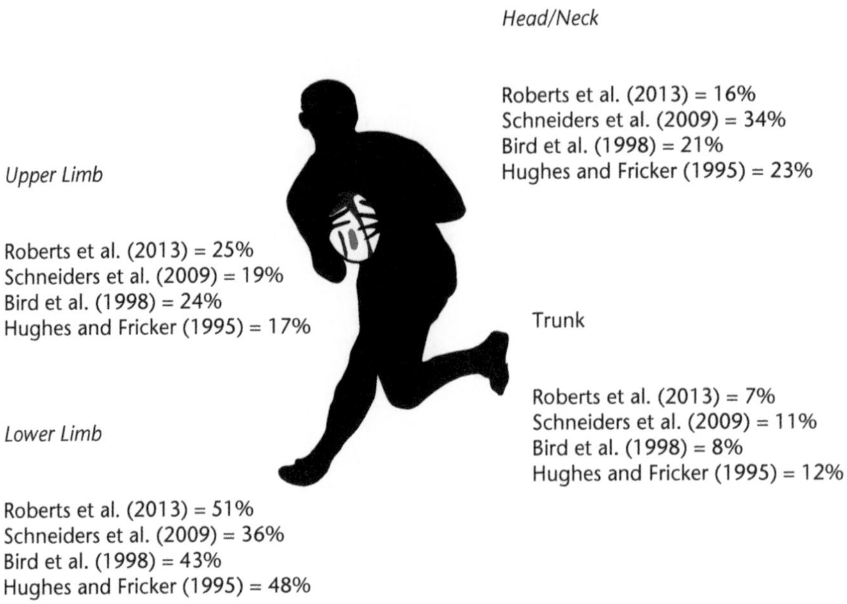

Head/Neck

Roberts et al. (2013) = 16%
Schneiders et al. (2009) = 34%
Bird et al. (1998) = 21%
Hughes and Fricker (1995) = 23%

Upper Limb

Roberts et al. (2013) = 25%
Schneiders et al. (2009) = 19%
Bird et al. (1998) = 24%
Hughes and Fricker (1995) = 17%

Trunk

Roberts et al. (2013) = 7%
Schneiders et al. (2009) = 11%
Bird et al. (1998) = 8%
Hughes and Fricker (1995) = 12%

Lower Limb

Roberts et al. (2013) = 51%
Schneiders et al. (2009) = 36%
Bird et al. (1998) = 43%
Hughes and Fricker (1995) = 48%

FIGURE 14.2 Injury proportion by body region for community-level men's rugby

elite game, due mainly to the amateur nature of the players and typically less inter-action between players and coaching/medical staff. Nevertheless, it is important to establish whether differences exist in injury patterns between the elite and com-munity game in order to determine whether it is appropriate to transfer injury surveillance findings and injury prevention messages from the elite to the commu-nity game.

The range of published incidence rates for time-loss injuries in the community rugby population is 14 to 45 per 1,000 player hours, but this range is due to variations in injury definition (Table 14.1). Irrespective of this, the incidence values reported using equivalent definitions are lower than those reported for the professional game, which is not unexpected as the intensity of play is likely to be very different between the elite and community populations. Moreover, there is some evidence that higher levels generally result in a greater incidence of time-loss injuries than lower levels of community rugby (Bird *et al.* 1998; Roberts *et al.* 2013).

There is inconsistent reporting of injury severity within the community rugby literature that prevents easy comparison between studies. The most recent literature by Roberts and colleagues (2013) reported that community players miss on average eight weeks of rugby match-play as a result of each ≥8 days time-loss injury sus-tained. In a small proportion of these injuries, the absence might also correspond with absence from employment, which potentially has a cost for the individual, the employer, and health providers.

In terms of the body region injured (Figure 14.2), the lower limb accounts for between 35 and 48% of all injuries at this playing level (Chalmers *et al.* 2012; Hughes and Fricker 1994; Bird *et al.* 1998; Schneiders *et al.* 2009). The head is often reported to sustain a relatively high number of injuries (Hughes and Fricker 1994; Bird *et al.* 1998; Schneiders *et al.* 2009), but Schneiders and co-workers (2009) noted that injuries to this site mainly comprised medical attention injuries (e.g. cuts and lacerations) for which the player was minimally absent.

Consistent with the elite game, contact between players results in the greatest number of injuries in community rugby with the tackle cited as the most common injury-causing event, accounting for between 40 and 59% of all injuries, followed by injuries associated with rucks and mauls (29–30%) (Bird *et al.* 1998; Hughes and Fricker 1994; Schneiders *et al.* 2009). Interestingly, Schneiders *et al* (2009) reported that tackling (29%) resulted in a greater number of injuries than being tackled (19%), whereas Roberts *et al.* (2013) reported results more consistent with the elite game, with the ball carrier sustaining significantly more injuries than the tackler (28% versus 22%, respectively). Again, caution must be taken when using these figures for direct comparison due to differences in injury definitions.

14.3.3 Youth rugby

Participation in rugby at youth level is increasing both within Tier 1 rugby nations such as England (RFU 2012) and developing rugby nations such as the United States of America (Chadwick *et al.* 2010). The risk of injury is reported to be higher for those young people exposed to high level sports participation compared with their peers (Caine *et al.* 2003), and injuries may have a significant effect on the health of these young athletes (Caine *et al.* 2006). There is currently a broad array of injury surveillance literature concentrating on youth rugby, yet, unfortunately, there is very little consistency in terms of the injury definitions and data collection methods, and consequently it is difficult to make meaningful comparisons (Bleakley *et al.* 2011). Concentrating on those studies that have reported injury incidence rates for time-loss injuries sustained throughout the season (i.e. not during an international tournament), incidence ranges from 16 to 49 injuries per 1,000 player hours (Table 14.2) (Palmer-Green *et al.* 2013; Kerr *et al.* 2008; Haseler *et al.* 2010).

Despite using similar injury definitions, there are a number of contextual differences between the published youth rugby studies, which might explain in part the variation in injury incidence figures. These factors include different standards of play, with significant differences found between Tier 1 and Tier 2 nations at the respective Junior Rugby World Championship/Trophy tournaments (Fuller and Taylor 2012b), and between school and English Premiership academy rugby cohorts (Palmer–Green *et al.* 2013). Age must also be considered, as it has been found that the risk of injury increases with age through youth rugby (Haseler *et al.* 2010).

TABLE 14.2 Injury incidence in youth rugby

Author	Injury definition	Age range	Collection method	Injury incidence time-loss (per 1,000 player hours)
Kerr et al. (2008)	Requiring medical attention. Resulting in any restriction of the player's participation for ≥ 1 day beyond the injury event.	USA collegiate ~17–21 y	Medics/team coaches/ identified player	16★
Haseler et al. (2010)	IRB Consensus statement definition – Time-loss injuries (≥ 24h absence)	English Clubs U16–U17	Team coach/first aider	40
Haseler et al. (2010)	IRB Consensus statement definition – Time-loss injuries (≥ 24h absence)	English Clubs U17	Team coach/first aider	49
Brown et al. (2012)	Time-loss Injuries – absence from more than one match in tournament or one day of normal/planned activity after the tournament.	U16 (South Africa-Tournament)	Team reported to tournament medic	20
Brown et al. (2012)	Time-loss Injuries – absence from more than one match in tournament or one day of normal/planned activity after the tournament.	U18 – Academy (South Africa-Tournament)	Team reported to tournament medic	25
Brown et al. (2012)	IRB Consensus statement definition – Time-loss injuries (≥ 24h absence)	U18 (Craven) (South Africa – Tournament)	Team reported to tournament medic	29
Palmer-Green et al. (2013)	IRB Consensus statement definition – Time-loss injuries (≥ 24h absence)	English Schools (16–18)	School medic	35
Palmer-Green et al. (2013)	IRB Consensus statement definition – Time-loss injuries (≥ 24h absence)	England Premiership Academies (16–18)	Academy team physio	47
Fuller and Taylor (2012a)	IRB Consensus statement definition – Time-loss injuries (≥ 24h absence)	U20 Tier 1 nations (International Tournament)	Team medic	47 to 87†
Fuller and Taylor (2012b)	IRB Consensus statement definition – Time-loss injuries (≥ 24h absence)	U20 Tier 2 nations (International Tournament)	Team medic	20 to 50†

★Re-calculated to report time-loss incidence rate only; † Range of injury incidence rates observed from 2008–2012

As with both elite and community senior rugby, the tackle is the most common match event associated with injury in the youth game (Garraway *et al.* 1999; Kerr *et al.* 2008; Collins *et al.* 2008; Palmer-Green *et al.* 2013), with between 50 and 58% of all injuries occurring in the tackle (Fuller and Taylor 2012b; Palmer-Green *et al.* 2013; Haseler *et al.* 2010). There does not, however, appear to be consensus when reviewing which region of the body has the highest incidence of injury. This is an area that needs further investigation to inform comprehensive injury reduction strategies for this rugby population.

14.3.4 Women's rugby

Despite the growth in the women's game, relatively little evidence is available from this population as to the incidence, causes, or severity of injuries sustained during match-play or practice. Indeed, a search of current literature yields only seven injury surveillance papers examining the incidence of injuries in the women's game (Carson *et al.* 1999; Taylor *et al.* 2011; Doyle and George 2004; Kerr *et al.* 2008; Bird *et al.* 1998; Schick *et al.* 2008). Unfortunately, similar to other populations, the ability to generalize and make cross–study comparisons is restricted due to the variability in the methodologies adopted within these papers (Table 14.3).

The incidence rate for injuries sustained in women's rugby in studies complying with the IRB consensus document ranges from 16 to 38 injuries per 1,000 hours, which is lower than elite men's rugby but is very similar to the range for both community men's and youth rugby (Kerr *et al.* 2008; Taylor *et al.* 2011). The only reported mean severity of injuries within the women's game is 55 days per injury sustained, based on injuries sustained at the 2010 Women's RWC (Taylor *et al.* 2011). Unfortunately, other studies have not reported mean injury severity, with many not reporting severity at all (Table 14.3). Women's rugby remains, for the most part, amateur and consequently the level of medical cover and rehabilitation opportunities might hamper the time it takes a player to return to play. Thus it is perhaps not a surprise that the mean severity reported for the 2010 women's RWC was significantly higher than that reported for the 2007 men's RWC (Taylor *et al.* 2011; Fuller *et al.* 2008).

Similar to the men's game, the tackle is responsible for the greatest proportion of injuries, with figures ranging from 38 to 66% per cent (Kerr *et al.* 2008; Taylor *et al.* 2011; Schick *et al.* 2008). Closer study of the tackle event shows that being tackled (33–36% of all injuries) accounts for proportionally more injuries compared with tackling (5–21%) (Schick *et al.* 2008; Kerr *et al.* 2008; Taylor *et al.* 2011). Further description of injury causation is limited in women's rugby.

The lower limbs are again the region of the body sustaining the greatest proportion of injuries, with a range from 41 to 67% (Kerr *et al.* 2008; Carson *et al.* 1999; Bird *et al.* 1998; Schick *et al.* 2008; Taylor *et al.* 2011; Doyle and George 2004). Again, these studies utilize various injury definitions and cover a range of playing standards (collegiate, school, international).

TABLE 14.3 Injury incidence and injury severity in women's rugby

Author	Competitive level	Injury definition	Incidence	Time-loss injury incidence (>24 hours) injuries per 1,000 player h	Severity
Bird et al. (1998)	Community/ School	Medical attention or causing the player to miss at least one scheduled match or practice.	6.1 per 100 player-games	*Unable to recalculate for >24 h time-loss only*	% of Injuries per severity AIS* category: AIS-1 – minor = 76.7% AIS-2 – moderate = 22.8% AIS-3 – serious = 0.5%
Carson et al. (1999)	National and Regional (Canadian)	Rugby-related event that kept a player out of practice or competition for > 24h or required attention of a physician.	21 per 1,000 player-game hours	*Unable to recalculate for >24 h time-loss only*	% of Injuries per severity category: NTO = 4% 1 day = 7.2% 2–3 days = 17.1% 4–7 days = 20.7% >7days = 51%
Doyle and George (2004)	National (England)	Rugby-related event that kept a player out of practice or competition for > 24h or required attention of a physician.	3.6 per 1,000 playing hours (Match and training injuries combined)	*Unable to recalculate for >24 h time-loss only*	% of Injuries per severity category: <1 week – 43% 1–3 weeks – 20% >3 weeks – 37%
Kerr et al. (2008)	Collegiate	Requiring medical attention. Resulting in any restriction of the player's participation for ≥ 1 day beyond the injury event.	17.1 per 1,000 player-game hours	16.4	% of Injuries per severity category: No time loss – 11% 1 week absence – 37% 2 week absence – 7% >2 week absence – 44%
Schick et al. (2008)	World Cup	IRB Consensus statement definition – Time-loss injuries (≥ 24h absence)	37.5 per 1,000 player-game hours	37.5	Severity not reported due to incomplete data.
Taylor et al (2011)	World Cup	IRB Consensus statement definition – Time-loss injuries (≥ 24 h absence)	35.5 per 1,000 player-game hours	35.5	No. of days lost from play: Mean = 55 days per injury Median = 9 days per injury
Peck et al. (2013)	Military Collegiate	Any new event occurring during rugby practice or match that required medical attention.	29.1 per 10,000 Athletic-Exposures	*Unable to recalculate for >24 h time-loss only*	Severity not reported

*AIS – Abbreviated Injury Scale

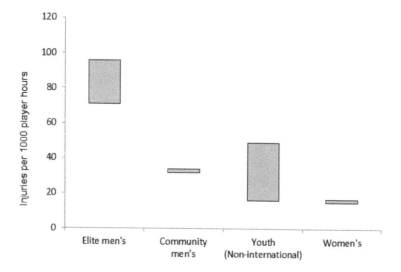

FIGURE 14.3   Comparison of the range of incidence rates recorded across the rugby playing population.

These data are for injuries sustained across at least one season (i.e. not during a tournament) and the injury definition used is that of time-loss with >24 hours lost from training or match-play.

14.4 Summary and conclusion

Rugby Union is a sport played worldwide by a diverse population of men, women, and youth players. Injury definitions, reporting measures, and general methodologies vary greatly across the existing rugby injury surveillance literature making cross-study comparisons difficult to perform. The publication of a consensus statement for reporting injuries in Rugby Union alleviates some of these challenges, although comparisons with past studies might remain difficult. Importantly, the injury surveillance process is not static, and as the game/population evolves, so should the definitions/methodologies used for injury surveillance, and thus regular reviews of the consensus statement would be prudent.

Rugby Union is played at varying levels from amateur through to fully professional. Injury incidence varies greatly between playing levels, with the highest reported in the elite men's game and the lowest reported in the women's game (Figure 14.3). In the youth population, the risk of injury increases with age (Haseler *et al.* 2010) and with the level of rugby being played (Palmer–Green *et al.* 2013). Although the incidence of injuries is important, the severity of injuries, as well as the time a player is unable to play or fully train, also has a large impact on the individual and the team. Whilst the incidence of injuries increases at higher playing standards, it appears that severity increases as the playing level decreases, which might be indicative of a number of factors including the amount of medical support, time given to rehabilitation, and player and club priorities.

Case study: boksmart – turning science into practice; work in progress

Wayne Viljoen, Clint Readhead, James Brown, and Mike Lambert

Introduction

The BokSmart National Rugby Safety Programme (Viljoen and Patricios 2012) in South Africa is a prime example of a national sporting body adopting an evidence-based and evidence-driven approach to dealing with rugby injuries, especially catastrophic head, neck, and spine injuries. Albeit a relatively young programme, significant progress has already been made towards active injury prevention through compulsory coach and referee education, scientific research programmes, medical protocol development and implementation, local rugby safety regulations and Law changes made over the last four years in South African rugby structures. The following case study will provide some insight as to how the programme has used science to guide its decision making process to make a safer game for all, and ultimately attempt to lower the number of catastrophic injuries associated with the game of rugby union.

Case presentation

The BokSmart programme was borne from concerns around an increasing number of serious and catastrophic spinal cord injuries, especially in 2006 (n = 16) and 2007 (n = 20), which showed a need for a more pragmatic and scientific approach to address these concerns. Following stakeholder workshops that were held during this period, it was decided that an educational approach similar to that of RugbySmart New Zealand (Quarrie *et al.* 2007; Gianotti *et al.* 2009) would be the most prudent method to reduce injury within the South African rugby environment (South African Rugby Union 2013a; Viljoen and Patricios 2012). In 2008, a programme manager was appointed and the development process began, with the joint support of the Chris Burger/Petro Jackson Player's Fund (Chris Burger Petro Jackson Player's Fund 2013) and the South African Rugby Union (SARU) (South African Rugby Union 2013b).

An 18 month process of content research and programme development was performed, before officially launching on July 9, 2009. The programme is based on the four main pillars of injury prevention, injury management, player safety, and performance. The vehicle for implementation is through various platforms such as mandatory coach and referee education (Quarrie et al. 2007; Gianotti et al. 2009), scientific research processes, development of medical protocols and policies, legislation, and marketing and communication. More on the structure of the programme and its subcomponents can be found described in the published literature (Viljoen and Patricios 2012).

In 2008, BokSmart introduced a systematic and standardized way of capturing catastrophic injury data and implemented this with immediate effect. The thought process was to capture data prospectively on a national register and analyse and review the data annually, whilst simultaneously exploring potential associated factors related to these injuries. The logic was to make evidence-driven decisions and develop and implement interventions based on these identified factors.

The first major step of the programme was to make the biennial rugby safety education and training component a compulsory requirement for all coaches and referees, across all South African Rugby structures (South African Rugby Union 2011a). This major step towards rugby safety was in line with the evidence demonstrated by New Zealand in their local rugby safety initiative, RugbySmart (Quarrie et al. 2007; Gianotti et al. 2009).

Whilst prospectively collecting serious and catastrophic rugby injury data during the early stages of programme development, the practice of senior clubs using players younger than 18 years old to make up numbers in adult rugby teams was identified as an immediate concern which needed to be addressed. In response to this, under-age rugby regulations were developed, accepted, and implemented in 2010 by the South African Rugby Union, to restrict this practice (South African Rugby Union 2011b). This is in line with similar initiatives internationally (Scottish Rugby Union 2013; Australian Rugby Union 2013) and also with other evidence provided for in the scientific literature (Bohu et al. 2009). Since these regulations have been implemented, there have been no further incidents of this nature reported to date.

Over the first four years of BokSmart's development and implementation (2008–2011) catastrophic injuries were regularly monitored and analysed. It became evident that there were concerns emerging associated with (1) the hooker playing position, (2) the senior or adult rugby playing population, and (3) the scrum phase of play (Brown et al. 2013). Match-related spinal cord injuries in the scrum were steadily increasing over this period with the majority of these ending up in permanent injury outcomes; seven permanent scrum injuries were recorded in 2011. Most (95%) of the scrum injuries were related to impact upon engagement (58%) and the subsequent scrum collapse (37%). After a few expert panel discussions on the matter, it was felt that if one could remove or reduce the impact on engagement (the 'hit') from the scrum, this would potentially remove all of the impact on engagement injuries and even some of the scrum collapse injuries that South African rugby were experiencing in the amateur game. In addition, it was felt that the same change could improve the spectator value of the game by possibly reducing the number of scrum collapses, resets, and increasing the ball in play time.

BokSmart then assembled an expert Scrum Smart working group at SARU to explore different options to improve the safety of the scrums, especially in the amateur game. This panel consisted of national coaches with scrum expertise, and also had representation from BokSmart, and medical and referee departments. Before recommending specific changes to the scrum in amateur rugby, the existing scientific literature was first reviewed to see if there was any research evidence to support the Scrum Smart working group's proposed direction. In direct consultation with the Bath University Research Group, the IRB's Phase 1 Biomechanics of the Scrum Research Report (Preatoni et al. 2012) was reviewed and discussed.

A novel French paper had shown positive results in reducing catastrophic injuries using amateur scrum law modifications, together with a front row licensing procedure in amateur rugby (Bohu et al. 2009). New Zealand data (Quarrie et al. 2007) showed similar results to the French, using the educational approach that SARU adopted with BokSmart.

However, it was felt that the current educational approach used in South Africa, albeit supported by research evidence from New Zealand (Quarrie et al. 2007; Gianotti et al. 2009), would initially take too long to embed itself in the rugby culture and would result in too many unwarranted scrum injuries in the interim. Whilst Bohu et al. (2009) recommended removing the 'hit' on engagement completely from all levels of the French amateur game, the expert Scrum Smart working group considered that such a move would create potential for serious injuries when players were later exposed to the 'full hit' at the elite standard. Hence a modified version, which required front rows to come closer to each other, i.e. ear-to-ear distance apart across the mouth of the scrum, with a pre-bind, and a reduced or 'mini-hit' on scrum engagement, was recommended by the panel. It was expected that this change would provide better stability to the scrum and remove the danger of the large number of impact on engagement related catastrophic injuries that formed part of the amateur game in South Africa and even some of the scrum collapse injuries.

As a result, a long-term player development pathway was proposed which progressed from (1) uncontested scrums with no hit, to (2) contested scrums with no hit, to (3) contested scrum with a closer distance pre-engagement, pre-bind, and mini-hit, to (4) the full hit IRB version of the scrum for elite players. These were accepted and implemented as of January 2013 in SA (South African Rugby Union 2012). Only one permanent scrum collapse and no impact on engagement injuries has been recorded to date since implementation of these new amateur scrum laws.

Summary

The BokSmart programme has used an evidence-based and evidence–driven approach to help make game changing decisions that have improved the player safety in South African rugby. The programme has used both a global and local consultative approach to develop pragmatic prevention solutions to address catastrophic head, neck, and spine injuries in South African rugby. This has been achieved by exploring the available scientific evidence, and prospectively collecting and analysing serious injury data, which BokSmart continues to re-evaluate and assess. Furthermore, BokSmart incorporates expert panels, end–user feedback, random safety audits, and any other issues that arise via consultation with rugby stakeholders to explore and implement pragmatic solutions to identified problems.

A consistent finding across the entire rugby playing spectrum is that contact mechanisms account for the greatest number of injuries; in particular, much of the literature cites 'being tackled' as the most common cause of injuries. In contrast, when injury risk per event is considered, the scrum has a higher propensity to cause injury than the tackle (Fuller *et al.* 2007a). Whilst strategies can be put in place in an attempt to minimize the number and severity of injuries in rugby union, the game remains a high intensity full contact sport, and as such, injuries are unlikely to be eradicated. Consequently, it is crucial to develop an accurate picture of those areas where injury prevention, rule changes/reinforcement, and/or coaching can have an impact to maximise approaches to injury reduction and enhance the welfare of players.

References

Australian Rugby Union (2013). Junior age limits. Available at: http://www.rugby.com.au/ tryrugby/Administration/JuniorAgeLimits.aspx.

Bird, Y.N., Waller, A.E., Marshall, S.W., et al. (1998). The New Zealand rugby injury and performance project: V. Epidemiology of a season of rugby injury. *British Journal of Sports Medicine*, 32, 319–25.

Bleakley, C., Tully, M., and O'Connor, S. (2011). Epidemiology of adolescent rugby injuries: A systematic review. *Journal of Athletic Training*, 46, 555–65.

Bohu, Y., Julia, M., Bagate, C., et al. (2009). Declining incidence of catastrophic cervical spine injuries in French Rugby: 1996–2006. *The American Journal of Sports Medicine*, 37, 319–23.

Brooks, J. and Fuller, C. (2006). The influence of methodological issues on the results and conclusions from epidemiological studies of sports injuries: illustrative examples. *Sports Medicine*, 36, 459–72.

Brooks, J.H., Fuller, C.W., Kemp, S.P., et al. (2005a). Epidemiology of injuries in English professional rugby union: Part 1 match injuries. *British Journal of Sports Medicine*, 39, 757–66.

Brooks, J.H. and Kemp, S.P. (2011). Injury-prevention priorities according to playing position in professional rugby union players. *British Journal of Sports Medicine*, 45, 765–75.

Brown, J.C., Lambert, M.I., Verhagen, E., et al. (2013). The incidence of rugby-related catastrophic injuries (including cardiac events) in South Africa from 2008 to 2011: a cohort study. *BMJ Open*, 3: e002475.

Brown, J.C., Verhagen, E., Viljoen, W., et al. (2012). The incidence and severity of injuries at the 2011 South African Rugby Union (SARU) Youth Week tournaments. *South African Journal of Sports Medicine*, 24, 50–4.

Caine, D., DiFiori, J., and Maffulli, N. (2006). Physical injuries in children's and youth sports: reasons for concern? *British Journal of Sports Medicine*, 40, 749–60.

Caine, D., Knutzen, K., Howe, W., et al. (2003). A three-year epidemiological study of injuries affecting young female gymnasts. *Physical Therapy in Sport*, 4, 10–23.

Caine, D.J., Caine, C.G., and Lindner, K.J. (1996). Epidemiology of sports injuries. *The Nurse Practitioner*, 21, 142.

Carson, J., Roberts, M., and White, A. (1999). The epidemiology of women's rugby injuries. *Clinical Journal of Sports Medicine*, 9, 75–8.

Chadwick, S., Semens, A., Schwarz, E.C., et al. (2010). Economic impact report on global rugby. Part III: Strategic and emerging markets. http://www.irb.com/mm/document/ newsmedia/mediazone/02/04/22/88/2042288_pdf.pdf (Accessed 31 Aug 2012).

Chalmers, D.J., Samaranayaka, A., Gulliver, P., et al. (2012). Risk factors for injury in rugby union football in New Zealand: a cohort study. *British Journal of Sports Medicine*, 46, 95–102.

Chris Burger/Petro Jackson Player's Fund. Chris Burger Petro Jackson Player's Fund Available at: http://www.playersfund.org.za/ (accessed 14/11/13).

Collins, C.L., Micheli, L.J., Yard, E.E., et al. (2008). Injuries sustained by high school rugby players in the United States, 2005–2006. *Archives of Pediatrics and Adolescent Medicine*, 162, 49–54.

Doyle, C. and George, K. (2004). Injuries associated with elite participation in women's rugby over a competitive season: an initial investigation. *Physical Therapy in Sport*, 5, 44–50.

Drawer, S. and Fuller, C. (2001). Propensity for osteoarthritis and lower limb joint pain in retired professional soccer players. *British Journal of Sports Medicine*, 35, 402–8.

Estell, J., Shenstone, B., and Barnsley, L. (1995). Frequency of injuries in different age groups in an elite rugby league club. *Australian Journal of Science and Medicine in Sport*, 27, 95–97.

Fuller, C., Laborde, F., Leather, R., *et al.* (2008). International Rugby Board Rugby World Cup 2007 injury surveillance study. *British Journal of Sports Medicine*, 42, 452–9.

Fuller, C. and Taylor, A. (2012a). Junior World Championship, Injury Epidemiology Results: 2008 to 2012. International Rugby Board, Injury Surveillance Studies.

Fuller, C. and Taylor, A. (2012b). Junior World Rugby Trophy. Injury Epidemiology Results: 2008 to 2012. International Rugby Board, Injury Surveillance Studies.

Fuller, C.W., Brooks, J.H., Cancea, R.J., *et al.* (2007a). Contact events in rugby union and their propensity to cause injury. *British Journal of Sports Medicine*, 41, 862–7.

Fuller, C.W., Molloy, M.G., Bagate, C., *et al.* (2007b). Consensus statement on injury definitions and data collection procedures for studies of injuries in rugby union. *British Journal of Sports Medicine*, 41, 328–31.

Fuller, C.W., Raftery, M., Readhead, C. (2009). Impact of the International Rugby Board's experimental law variations on the incidence and nature of match injuries in southern hemisphere professional rugby union. *South African Medicine Journal*, 99, 232–7.

Fuller, C.W., Sheerin, K., and Targett, S. (2012). Rugby World Cup 2011: International Rugby Board Injury Surveillance.

Gabbett, T. (2003). Incidence of injury in semi-professional rugby league players. *British Journal of Sports Medicine*, 37, 36–44.

Gabbett, T., King, T., and Jenkins, D. (2008). Applied physiology of rugby league. *Sports Medicine*, 38, 119–38.

Gabbett, T.J. (2004a). Incidence of injury in junior and senior rugby league players. *Sports Medicine*, 34, 849–59.

Gabbett, T.J. (2004b). Influence of training and match intensity on injuries in rugby league. *Journal of Sports Sciences*, 22, 409–17.

Garraway, M. and Macleod, D. (1995). Epidemiology of rugby football injuries. *Lancet*, 345, 1485–7.

Garraway, W.M., Lee, A.J., Macleod, D.A., *et al.* (1999). Factors influencing tackle injuries in rugby union football. *British Journal of Sports Medicine*, 33, 37–41.

Gianotti, S.M., Quarrie, K.L., and Hume, P.A. (2009). Evaluation of RugbySmart: A rugby union community injury prevention programme. *Journal of Science and Medicine in Sport*, 12, 371–5.

Haseler, C.M., Carmont, M.R., and England, M. (2010). The epidemiology of injuries in English youth community rugby union. *British Journal of Sports Medicine*, 44, 1093–9.

Hodgson, L., Gissane, C., Gabbett, T., *et al.* (2007). For debate: consensus injury definitions in team sports should focus on encompassing all injuries. *Clinical Journal of Sports Medicine*, 17, 188–91.

Hughes, D. and Fricker, P. (1994). A prospective survey of injuries to first-grade Rugby Union players. *Clinical Journal of Sports Medicine*, 4, 249–56.

Kemp, S.P., Brooks, J.H., Fuller, C.W., *et al.* (2013). England Professional Rugby Injury Surveillance Project 2011–2012 Season Report. RFU.

Kerr, H., Curtis, C., Micheli, L., *et al.* (2008). Collegiate rugby union injury patterns in New England: a prospective cohort study. *British Journal of Sports Medicine*, 42, 595–603.

King, D. and Gabbett, T., (2009). Injuries in the New Zealand semi-professional rugby league competition. *New Zealand Journal of Sports Medicine*, 36, 6–15.

King, D., Gabbett, T., Gissane, C., *et al.* (2009). Epidemiological studies of injuries in rugby league: Suggestions for definitions, data collection, and reporting methods. *Journal of Science and Medicine in Sport*, 12, 12–19.

King, D. and Gissane, C. (2009). Injuries in amateur rugby league matches in New Zealand: a comparison between a Division 1 and a Division 2 Premier Grade team. *Clinical Journal of Sport Medicine*, 19, 277–81.

King, D.A., Hume, P.A., Milburn, P.D., *et al.* (2010). Match and training injuries in rugby league a review of published studies. *Sports Medicine*, 40, 163–78.

Lorentzon, R., Wedren, H., Pietilä, T., *et al.* (1988). Injuries in international ice hockey: A prospective, comparative study of injury incidence and injury types in international and Swedish elite ice hockey. *The American Journal of Sports Medicine*, 16, 389–91.

Meyers, M.C. and Barnhill, B.S. (2004). Incidence, causes, and severity of high school football injuries on fieldturf versus natural grass: a 5-year prospective study. *The American Journal of Sports Medicine*, 32, 1626–38.

Milburn, P.D. (1990). The kinetics of rugby union scrummaging. *Journal of Sports Sciences*, 8, 47–60.

O'Connell, T. (1954). Rugby football injuries and their prevention: a review of 600 cases. *Journal of the Irish Medical Association*, 34, 20.

Orchard, J. and Hoskins, W. (1997). Rugby league injuries at State of Origin level [Online]. Available from URL: http://www.injuryupdate.com.au/images/research/Origininjuries 20002006.pdf [Accessed 7 Oct 2013].

Orchard, J. and Seward, H. (2002). Epidemiology of injuries in the Australian Football League, seasons 1997–2000. *British Journal of Sports Medicine*, 36, 39–44.

Palmer-Green, D.S., Stokes, K.A., Fuller, C.W., *et al.* (2013). Match injuries in English youth academy and schools rugby union an epidemiological study. *The American Journal of Sports Medicine*, 41, 749–55.

Preatoni, E., Stokes, K., England, M., *et al.* (2012). Biomechanics of the rugby scrum, Phase 1 report: Biomechanics of the machine scrummaging.

Peck, K.Y., Johnston, D.A., Owens, B.D., *et al.* (2013). The incidence of injury among male and female intercollegiate rugby players. *Sports Health: A Multidisciplinary Approach*, 5, 327–33.

Quarrie, K.L., Gianotti, S.M., Hopkins, W.G., *et al.* (2007). Effect of nationwide injury prevention programme on serious spinal injuries in New Zealand rugby union: ecological study. *British Medicine Journal*, 334, 1150.

RFU, 2012. Rugby participation up by 26,000 in England. http://www.rfu.com/news/2012/ june/newsarticles/220612_participation_grainger, [Accessed 4 Oct 2013].

Roberts, S.P., Stokes, K.A., and Trewartha, G. (2013). Epidemiology of time-loss injuries in English Community level Rugby Union. Unpublished.

Roberts, S.P., Trewartha, G., Higgitt, R.J., *et al.* (2008). The physical demands of elite English rugby union. *Journal of Sports Sciences*, 26, 825–33.

Schick, D.M., Molloy, M.G., and Wiley, J.P. (2008). Injuries during the 2006 Women's Rugby World Cup. *British Journal of Sports Medicine*, 42, 447–51.

Schneiders, A.G., Takemura, M., and Wassinger, C.A. (2009). A prospective epidemiological study of injuries to New Zealand premier club rugby union players. *Physical Therapy in Sport*, 10, 85–90.

Scottish Rugby Union (SRU) (2013). Age banding policies. Available at: http://www.scottishrugby.org/sites/default/files/editor/docs/male_u18_in_adult_rugby_policy_-_policy_overview_-_june_2013_0.pdf.

South African Rugby Union (2011a). South African Rugby Union (SARU) Regulations. Available at: http://images.supersport.com/SARU%20Regulations%20on%20BokSmart %20Rugby%20Safety%20Workshops%20Amended%20June%202011.pdf.

South African Rugby Union (2011b). South African Rugby Union (SARU) regulations for under-aged rugby. Available at: http://images.supersport.com/BokSmart%202011-SARU%20Regulations%20for%20Under-aged%20rugby%20April%202011.pdf.

South African Rugby Union (2012). South African Modified Amateur Scrums Laws. Available at: http://images.supersport.com/SARU%20Modified%20Amateur%20Rugby%20Scrum%20Laws%20accepted%206%20December%202012.pdf.

South African Rugby Union (2013a). BokSmart website. Available at: http://www.boksmart.com (accessed 09/10/12).

South African Rugby Union (2013b). South African Rugby Union. Available at: http://www.sarugby.co.za/default.aspx (accessed 15/11/13).

Stephenson, S., Gissane, C., and Jennings, D. (1996). Injury in rugby league: a four year prospective survey. *British Journal of Sports Medicine*, 30, 331–4.

Taylor, A.E., Fuller, C.W., and Molloy, M.G. (2011). Injury surveillance during the 2010 IRB Women's Rugby World Cup. *British Journal of Sports Medicine*, 45, 1243–5.

Viljoen, W. and Patricios, J. (2012). BokSmart – implementing a National Rugby Safety Programme. *British Journal of Sports Medicine*, 46, 692–3.

Walker, R. (1985). Sports injuries: rugby league may be less dangerous than union. *The Practitioner*, 229, 205.

Williams, S., Trewartha, G., Kemp, S., *et al.* (2013). A meta-analysis of injuries in senior men's professional rugby union. *Sports Medicine*, 43, 1043–55.

15

TALENT IDENTIFICATION, DEVELOPMENT, AND THE YOUNG RUGBY PLAYER

Steve Cobley and Kevin Till

15.1 Introduction

Attaining excellence in rugby, like in other sports and domains, is valued by particular nations, sub-regions, cultures, and communities. An aspiration for many is to follow in the footsteps of local and national iconic players like Dan Carter and Brian O'Driscoll in rugby union; Sam Tomkins and Darren Lockyer in rugby league, or players who successfully traversed both codes of the game like Jason Robinson and Jonathan Davis. But also within the last twenty years, rugby has changed markedly in a way that is intricately related to professionalization, growing local and international media interest, and associated commercialism. A consequence of such trends has been the emergence of 'top–down' economic and competitive demands, as well as growth in 'bottom-up' social demands. For instance, there is inherent interest in wanting to watch and participate in the game(s) at grass-roots levels, whilst at the same time, local and national teams are attempting to systematically identify, train, and develop future players (i.e. top-down demand). This latter process has become more popularly known as: Talent Identification and Development (TID).

15.2 Talent defined?

In an effort to acknowledge the potential range of cognitive, psychological, motor skill, anthropometric, and physical characteristics that could contribute in accelerating learning and development in sport, talent has recently been defined by Cobley *et al.* (2012) as 'the presence or absence of particular skills or qualities identified at early time points that correlate or predict exceptionality in the future'. However, there are other definitions, as well as differing descriptions and applications of the word 'talent' that depend on the perspective (e.g. researchers, practitioners, popular press) and domain of interest (e.g. music vs. rugby). Understanding is not helped by popular media and press predominantly associating talent (wrongly in our view) with 'innate predispositions', 'giftedness', and an 'apparent capability to perform without prior practice'. Coaches and practitioners often apply the term interchangeably (e.g. 'he has raw talent'), sometimes referring to a general ability (i.e. across skills) or using the term as a description of overall performance, such as a player's performance relative to others in a given age group or standard of competition. Yet in other circumstances, talent is used to refer to a specific capability of executing a learned skill exceptionally well (e.g. decision-making in a game scenario; scrummaging). Either way, multiple meanings do not promote clarity.

In research terms, 'talent' – whether it exists is still contested, as well as how we define and measure it. In fact, researchers are possibly guilty of not addressing these challenges, something not aided by the perennial 'nature–nuture' debate (e.g. Howe *et al.* 1998; and responses). Although this debate has somewhat been superseded by emerging evidence and acceptance that nurture is able to shape nature and *vice versa* (e.g. Davids and Baker 2007; Ridley 2003). This implies that exceptionality in athlete characteristics or skills might potentially be able to emerge without necessarily TID system training. These characteristics might also be highly responsive and adaptable to TID system training, or potentially be constrained (i.e. limited degree of response and adaptability) by TID training.

If talent is task-specific, but still often multi-faceted, then multiple factors can potentially exert their influence at different developmental time points. These might also include socio-cultural and environmental settings (Baker and Horton 2004; Champagne 2010; Slavich and Cole 2013). Although by no means exhaustive, factors affecting talent might include the genetic constraints within the human species (e.g. biological growth and ageing processes), phenotype potential adaptability (i.e. anthropometric and physical composition; e.g. height, muscle mass). Talent might also be affected by the volume and intensity of training (e.g. deliberate practice framework; Ericsson *et al.* 1993), psychological characteristics and skills of the player, family social support and facilitation, coaching expertise (i.e. social/cultural factors), and school and club provision (e.g. environmental factors to support rugby participation).

15.3 TID systems

TID systems represent the contact point and transition between youthful interest and participation and adult, professional competition. Representing what has become a common and accepted sports practice, national rugby governing bodies and professional clubs are deploying TID systems of various durations, intensities, and sophistication.

TID systems can be lengthy, commencing in junior ages (i.e. pre 11 years old) and continue into early adulthood (i.e. 18 years of age), and they commonly consist of two basic, related processes. First, identification attempts to recognize young players (presently participating or not) who illustrate 'potential' in becoming adult elite players (Williams and Reilly 2000). Then development attempts to accelerate learning and performance of those identified through provision of optimal training conditions and environments (Abbott and Collins 2004).

The popularity of TID systems is currently high, based on the social perception and assumption that TID involvement provides a 'good opportunity', and increases the likelihood of attaining the elite echelons of the sport. Access to TID systems is regulated by coaches, scouts, and administrator selections, informed by subjective (e.g. game observations) and objective (e.g. fitness tests, game analysis) assessments conducted within age (e.g. Under 16s) and/or stage (e.g. representative county/ state standard) matched competition. Rugby TID programme resources are usually concentrated, provided by professional club 'academies' or national governing bodies at centralized sites.

To illustrate an example of a modern TID system, Table 15.1 gives an overview of the Rugby Football League's (RFL's) Player Development Pathway (2010–2016). The pathway has evolved based on prior research evidence and best practice (see Till *et al.* 2012 for an overview). At its base, the pathway emphasizes the inclusion and participation of a wider pool of players at earlier ages (e.g. 6–12 years) prior to eventual 'pyramidialization' (Güllich and Emrich 2012), eventually evident in all TID systems. The participation base is achieved by integrating local schools and club organizations, structuring the game around skill development as opposed to competition, and with consideration to the psychological, social, and developmental needs of the player (see Table 15.1; purpose, competition, volume/intensity). Together, these strategies attempt to delay the onset of adult–like performance, competition, and the accompanying (de)selection, though these features still occur from Phase 3 onward (ages 13 to 16). The pathway stands against the current tide of team sport contexts implementing TID systems earlier with features of competition and (de)selection, and is aligned with research recommendations associated with holistic athlete development (e.g. Baker *et al.* 2009; Côte *et al.* 2009; Moesch *et al.* 2011).

The question of whether or not athletes need to partake in 'early specialized training' as part of a TID system has attracted research attention. On the matter of need, there is a suggestion on the one hand that 'early specialized training' invokes specific skill development, such as technical proficiency and accuracy in movement, as well as cognitive expertise like anticipation, 'positional knowledge', 'ability to read the game play' and decision-making, all of which are beneficial to long-term development (e.g. Chase and Simon 1973; Ford *et al.* 2009; Ford and Williams 2012). On the other hand, early high volume, intensity, and repetition in physical training are not deemed beneficial, but rather are often associated with negative psycho-social health, injury outcomes, and overtraining/burnout concerns (e.g. Malina 2010; Rongen *et al.* 2014; Wiersma 2000). In team sports (e.g. rugby) where peak professional performance most often occurs between 20–30+ years of age, the need for physical training specific to rugby at an early age has been challenged, when there appears to be long-term benefit from a diverse sporting engagement in the earlier years (e.g. Baker *et al.* 2003; Capranica and Millard-Stafford 2011).

TABLE 15.1 An overview of the RFL player development pathway (2010–2016).

Phase	Where	Stage	Environment	Purpose	Competition	Volume/Intensity
1	School and Club	6–8 years	School	Developing fundamental movement skills	No formal competition	Mini Rugby Festivals
2	School and Club	8–12 years	Club (*PESSYP*[1] *and Sustain*)	Developing fundamental sport skills and core Rugby League skills	Youth and Junior Leagues Champion Schools	U11 Modified games U12 Full
3	Service Area and Regions	13–16 years	Talent Development Groups	Developing the athlete and position specific skills and Talent Identification	Youth and Junior Leagues Champion Schools FE Colleges	League and cup
4	Professional Club	15–16 years	Scholarship	Preparation for elite competition and Talent Confirmation (*6–8 years from elite*)	National Youth League FE Colleges Scholarship Games	Six games
5	Professional Club	17–20 years	Academy	Individual specialisation and enhancement for maximal performance at elite level (*3–6 years from elite*)	National Youth League Super 6 University U18 Academy Games U20 Valvoline Cup	U18 16 Games 20 Rounds + Grand Final
6	Professional Club	18–30 years	1st Grade	Delivering and sustaining elite performance	Championship Super league	27 Rounds + Grand Final Northern Rail Cup 27 Rounds + Grand Final Challenge Cup
7	International	15–30 years	Elite Training Squads	Individualised preparation for elite performance at a world class level	U16 England Youth U18 England Academy U20 England Knights Full International	International Fixtures European Nations Cup 4 Nations World Cup

Physical Education School Sport and Young People, Youth Sport Trust

TID system processes have also been critiqued due to their low ability to forecast (Durand-Bush and Salmela 2001) and their ineffectiveness (i.e. low percentage) in retaining/developing athletes into the adult elite stage (see Vaeyens *et al.* 2008). Likewise, the capability to identify and differentiate 'talented' young athletes from normative population variation has been questioned. For instance, TID systems in 'later specialising sports' like rugby often deploy identification and selection processes with an emphasis on a player's 'current performance' relative to others. This offers an alternative method with a more narrowed focus for defining 'talent' than that offered earlier. Furthermore, these identification and selection processes often occur during times of substantial growth and developmental variability (i.e. maturation) that bring about ongoing change (e.g. anthropometric and physical). There is ample evidence to suggest that markers of athleticism – such as speed, power, and body size – are substantially confused by growth and maturation (see Meylan *et al.* 2010; Pearson *et al.* 2006), thus making the differentiation of 'athletic talent' in youth populations difficult.

15.4 Biological age: growth and maturational variability

As children develop from birth to adulthood, growth and maturation occur, and although these processes are inter-related, they have fundamental differences (Baxter-Jones and Sherar 2007). Growth is predominantly genetically determined, and refers to changes in the size of the body or its parts including height, body mass, fat tissue, and organ size (Malina *et al.* 2004). Height and body mass are the most commonly used measurements of growth and, to indicate health status, individuals can be compared against large databases of chronologically aged matched healthy children using growth charts or reference data (see Freeman *et al.* 1995; RCPCH 2013). Growth charts allow individuals to be compared against reference percentiles, such as the 50th = average, 75th = top 25%, and 25th = lowest 25% at specific chronological age points (e.g. 4–18 years of age).

At around 12 to 15 years of age for males (11–14 for females), a rapid growth spurt occurs, typified by a period of dynamic anthropometric and physical change known as maturation (Baxter-Jones *et al.* 2005). Maturation is regarded as growth towards the mature adult state (Malina 1994), and has two components: timing and tempo. Timing indicates the age when specific maturational events occur, such as age of pubic hair appearance or age of maximum growth in height. Tempo refers to the rate at which maturation progresses. Both the timing and tempo of maturation can vary significantly, with individuals of similar chronological age potentially differing dramatically in terms of their biological maturity. The maturational growth spurt, where height gain per year increases substantially, is the age of peak height velocity (PHV), and is the most commonly used measure to assess maturation in childhood longitudinal growth studies (Baxter-Jones *et al.* 2005).

Mirwald *et al.* (2002) also developed a regression equation permitting a practical method of calculating age at PHV using the anthropometric characteristics of height, sitting height, weight, and chronological age. Age at PHV can be used to ascertain an individual's maturational age (i.e. Years from PHV; aka – YPHV). Years from PHV is calculated by subtracting age at PHV from chronological age to determine how far players are from their PHV. For example, a player who reaches PHV at 13.8 years has a maturational age of -2.0 years at 11.8 years, 0.0 at 13.8 years and 2.0 at 15.8 years. Research data suggests that age at PHV usually occurs around 14 years of age in adolescent boys (e.g. Bell 1993; Beunen and Malina 1988; philippaerts *et al.* 2006), but can occur anywhere between 12.0–15.8 years of age (based on UK data; Malina *et al.* 2004) because of variability in maturation onset.

Maturational variation of young players of similar chronological age is illustrated in Figure 15.1. On the left half are hypothetical examples from Tanner (1962) showing how three males of similar chronological age (i.e. 14.75 years) differ substantially in terms of maturational stage. On the right, a practical comparison of three male rugby league players of differing maturational stages (i.e. pre, mid, post maturation), but residing within the same chronological age category (i.e. Under 15s). Within a physically demanding sport like rugby, it is these inter-player variations that can significantly influence performance and TID opportunities at this stage.

15.4.1 The chronological age – biological age mismatch

For purposes of attempting to ensure equal competition and opportunities, sport governing bodies and TID systems routinely allocate players into chronological (bi) annual age categories. For example, United Kingdom education and sport systems use a September 1st cut-off date to demarcate players into chronological age groups (e.g. Under 13s, 14s, *etc.*). Inadvertently, this form of categorization permits 364 days for normative growth discrepancy (when comparing a 1st September – 31st August), which can then be further heightened during the maturation phase. The potential of increased time for growth and entering of maturation earlier compared to age-group peers (Musch and Grondin 2001) bring clear anthropometric and physical advantages such as size, strength, speed, and endurance (Baxter-Jones *et al.* 1995). For instance, 'early maturers' usually outperform 'later maturers' when comparing results across chronological age-matched norms (Armstrong *et al.* 1998; Beunen *et al.* 1997). This results in consistently more 'relatively older and early maturing boys' having increased participation and selection opportunities in TID systems within youth sport, as they are perceived as being more talented (Sherar *et al.* 2007; Simmons and Paull 2001).

In terms of a TID system sample of young rugby league players (aged 13–16 years; n=683), Till *et al.* (2010a) recently compared their growth status against UK reference percentiles (Freeman *et al.* 1995). For height, 92.4% of players were taller than the age-match 50th percentile (or average), and 33.3% were above the 97th percentile (top 3% of the UK). In terms of weight, similar findings were evident, with 96% and 30.3% of players above the 50th and 97th percentiles, respectively. These figures show an orientation towards the selection of taller and heavier players when set against the age-matched UK normal population. A similar pattern is identified for maturational status, whereby players had an age at PHV of 13.61 ± 0.58 years. This indicates

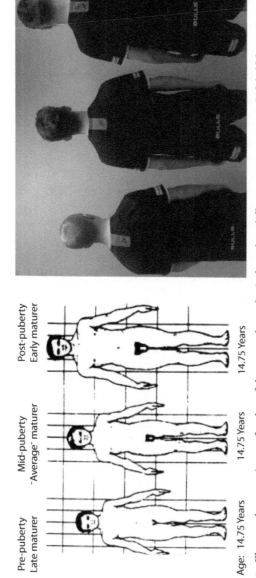

FIGURE 15.1 Illustrated comparisons of males of the same chronological age but differing maturity status (left half from Tanner, J. [1962]. *Growth at adolescence*. Oxford: Blackwell Scientific Publications).

earlier rates of maturation when referenced against the average age of PHV in European boys, which occurs between 13.8–14.2 years (Malina *et al.* 2004). Studies in other junior team sports contexts have consistently replicated these trends (e.g. soccer – Malina *et al.* 2004; ice-hockey – Sherar *et al.* 2007).

15.4.2 Relative age effects

Confirmation of the described 'chronological–biological age mismatch' is provided by Relative Age Effects (RAEs; Wattie *et al.* 2008). RAEs represent the interaction between a player's 'birth date' and the dates used for chronological age grouping. Therefore, a 'relatively older' (i.e. born in the 1st quartile of the year) player, compared to a 'relatively younger' player born in the last quartile (e.g. August 28th in the UK), is more likely to participate in local junior community, representative, and national standard rugby due to the benefits of advanced growth and maturation. To illustrate, Figure 15.2 shows RAE trends within UK junior rugby league (Till *et al.* 2010b). From the local community (n=4,829; aged 13–15) to the national standard (n=88; aged 13–15), participation and selection inequalities are evident, with RAE trends increasing significantly across the TID system. Other studies by Abernethy and Farrow (2005) and Till *et al.* (2010b) confirm that RAE biases are evident in junior, adult professional, and international standards of rugby. Further, a review by Cobley *et al.* (2009) suggested that RAEs are most prevalent in male representative team sports, with the highest discrepancies between Quartile 1–4 occurring at approximately 14–18 years of age.

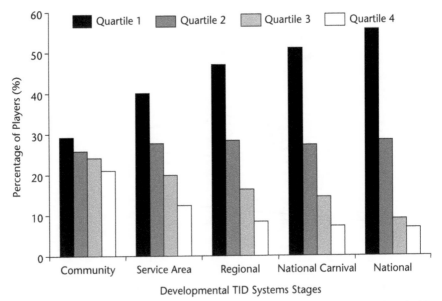

FIGURE 15.2 Relative age distribution of junior rugby league players (i.e., Under 13–15s combined) according to generic TID system stages (Till *et al.* 2010b).

Taken together, findings from studies assessing growth, maturation, and RAEs suggest TID systems presently need to be more open-minded and responsive to the developmental changes and the variability of these changes that occur in the lives of young rugby players. TID systems are placing great emphasis on 'current performance', and, in doing so, are not recognising the confounding influences of growth and maturation on performance. These points are substantiated when considering the possibility that anthropometric and physiological 'gaps' between junior players are changeable, potentially decreasing to the point of becoming non-existent in later stages of maturation and adulthood (Till *et al.* 2013; Till *et al.* 2014). Our broader notion in terms of TID is that the systems are under–valuing and unnecessarily excluding many athletically and skilful, talented players early due to their latent growth and maturation. The following cases illuminate the concern.

Case study: biological variability and changing development

Introduction

To illustrate variability and changing developmental trajectories in young rugby players, Till *et al.* (2013) examined cases of two rugby league players who were part of a broader TID selected group (n=1,172; aged 13–15). Over a two-year period, case player anthropometrics, (i,e., height, sitting height, weight, sum of skinfold thickness), maturational (i.e. age at PHV and YPHV) and fitness measures (i.e. vertical jump, medicine ball throw, running speed [10–60 m sprints], agility and estimated VO_{2max}) were compared against the broader group using z-scores and radar graph plots (see Figure 15.3). Z-scores identify whether, for example, a case player's score on vertical jump is similar, below, or above the mean average of all players, and helps identify how far away a score is from the group mean. Z-scores were generated using the calculation $x - \mu/\alpha$, where x is the raw score, μ is the average and α is the standard deviation of all player scores. Z-scores of -3, -2, -1, 0, 1 and 2 were used to represent the mean and standard deviations of all players. So for instance, z-score values for height were -3 (151.7 cm), -2 (159.0 cm), -1 (166.7 cm), 0 (174.4 cm), 1 (182.1 cm), and 2 (189.8 cm). As three measurements were taken repeatedly over a two-year period, z–scores could assess whether a case players improved or regressed over time compared to all other players.

Case presentation

The following describes two cases from Till *et al.* (2013): Case Player 1 – at the time of writing – is a professionally contracted UK Super League player, and Case Player 2 is now an age-matched adult amateur.

At Under 13s, Case Player 1 was an 'average–late maturer', shorter and lighter compared to the rest of the TID group of players with z-scores of around -1 (see Case Player 1 in Figure 15.3). Fitness characteristics at Under 13s were approximately 0 (i.e. average). Perhaps on initial reading, indicator measures do not suggest a 'shining

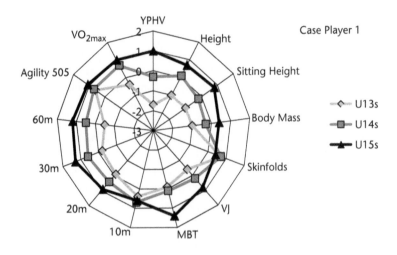

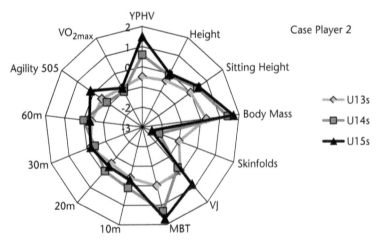

FIGURE 15.3 Anthropometric and fitness profile for two young rugby league players within a rugby league TID system.

Key: YPHV = Years from Peak Height Velocity

Skinfolds = Sum of 4 Skinfolds

VJ = Vertical Jump

MBT = Medicine Ball Throw; 10m = 10 m sprint, 20m = 20 m sprint etc.

VO_{2max} = Estimated VO_{2max}

star in the making' at this point in time. However, from Under 13s–15s, z-scores for height (-1.0 to 0.7), sitting height (-1.0 to 0.8), and body mass (-1.0 to 0.4) improved noticeably, whilst sum of four skinfolds remained constant. At Under 15s, fitness characteristics were also indicating an improving trajectory compared to all other players with z-scores approximating 1. By contrast, Case Player 2 at Under 13s was relatively 'earlier maturing' (i.e. close to average in Under 13s), and scored approximately 0 on anthropometric measures (see Case Player 2 in Figure 15.3). Fitness characteristics z–scores were also between 0 and -1 at the Under 13s age category. Between Under 13s-15s, z–scores for height (-0.4 to 0) and sitting height (0 to 0.5) improved slightly, but weight (0.3 to 1.7) and sum of four skinfolds (-1 to -2.5) increased (i.e. more body fat), with the latter higher than the average for all players. Over the same period, improvements in some fitness characteristics occurred (e.g. vertical jump -0.1 to 0.8). However, speed, agility, and estimated VO_{2max} did not change across the two year period (see Figure 15.3). This case represents an example of what appears to be a 'good-average performer' at Under 13s, perhaps beyond their chronological age, but who showed minimal anthropometric and fitness improvement over the subsequent two years. Overall, Case Player 2's future trajectory appears less positive relative to Player 1. It is likely that many of the measures which regressed between 13 to 15 years of age would detrimentally affect onward performance, as the nature of the game (e.g. speed and intensity) changes with age and representative stage.

Findings from Till *et al.* (2013) highlight that even within a group of relatively homogenous rugby players developmentally distinct from the normal age-matched population, the potential for changing trajectories based on differing initial maturation status can still occur. It appears that there is merit and value in individually monitoring longitudinal change in growth, maturation, fitness, and performance compared to other young rugby players. If players are not assessed, or only assessed in a one-off manner, such change might not be captured and/or understood, and the same problems may continue. Namely, that 'early maturing' players will be immediately selected and overvalued, even though 'later maturing' players might exhibit more accelerated development in later adolescence.

Here we also need to provide forewarning. In these case analyses, case players were deliberately identified to show developmental change as a function of varying initial maturational status. This does not equate to saying that every 'late maturing' player will become a better athlete in a two year period or in the longer term. Nor are we stating that all 'early maturers' will not go on to succeed. We do not suggest that growth or maturational indices single handedly predict long-term performance *per se*. If alternative player cases were examined, we would likely see 'more average' performance scores as well as differing trajectory profiles. Graphically 'more average' translates to z–scores within +1 to -1 on a radar plot. That said, it is feasible that a common trajectory change may occur between early and late maturers even though at a slower tempo. For now, we can consider the cases presented as identifying changing developmental trajectories, which begins to acknowledge that the matter of long-term athlete development is complicated.

Summary

This chapter has been written from the dual perspectives of researcher and coach practitioner. From this 'insider – outsider' stance, we have discussed topics of knowing concern and awareness to those in the field, whilst as researchers we have independently used research methodologies to examine such concerns. In our roles, one of our aims is to help 'best implement' and utilize the most up to date evidence (i.e. evidence based practice) and applied knowledge (i.e. practice based evidence) to hopefully benefit TID systems. We acknowledge that sport TID systems, like others (e.g. medical and educational training) trying to optimize human development, necessarily have to work within day to day, 'real world' constraints and might have difficulty in changing practice or culture. Like maturing players, systems possess strengths and weaknesses that need to evolve over time. To this end, we attempt to provide some specific recommendations for governing bodies, clubs, coaches, and athlete development staff, although there could be many other recommendations offered.

For anyone working with young players in rugby, our first recommendation has to be the acknowledgement and recognition of the relationships between growth, maturation, development, and performance. The unstable variability of the maturational years affects anthropometric and fitness characteristics, and subsequent physical performance in junior/development rugby. This challenges the ability to accurately assess athletic potential relative to peers, and predict future performance. One-off assessments (e.g. coaching/scouting judgements) predominantly reliant upon physical capability could very likely be inaccurate in identifying future 'talented' potential. What might be deemed as 'exceptional' at one age and stage might not remain the same for the same individual at a later age and stage. For example, later maturing players could close the 'fitness and performance gap'.

The second recommendation emphasizes the need to monitor young players over time, and should be prioritized above cross-sectional one-off trials and selections. To aid tracking and monitoring of developmental change, z-scores and radar graphs could not only aid individual profiling, but permit comparisons against the development of other players, such as those of similar chronological age, maturational, and performance stages. The differing developmental trajectories (e.g., emerging, regressing) can then be used to better inform training, development, and (de)selection within TID systems. For instance through longitudinal tracking, a 'later maturing player' (e.g. Case Player 1) is more likely to be retained, and his trajectory and progress could be reviewed at a later time point (i.e. post-maturation). Still, with emphasis towards onward development as opposed to de-selection, the trajectory of an 'earlier maturing – non-developing' player (e.g. Case Player 2) might be used to inform player specific decisions and interventions. This could include manipulation of training factors (e.g. volume and intensity of endurance) alongside other supporting factors (e.g. nutrition advice) to help the player maintain a 'progressive trajectory'.

If organizations feel they cannot effectively consider and implement these two recommendations due to resources or time constraint factors, then it remains difficult to justify early player differentiation, and (de)selection within grass-roots and TID system rugby during the pre-maturation and maturational years. Based on research data presented, our third recommendation is for rugby coaches, clubs, administrators, and governing bodies to develop and implement initiatives that provide as many participation and developmental opportunities to as many junior players as possible.

Possibly up to under 16 to 18 years of age, rugby could more greatly emphasize participation, inclusion, and personal and team development and improvement, as opposed to winning and competition alone. Practitioners should develop a 'mind-set' of longer-term, inclusive player development instead of an emphasis on immediate performance success. Like the TID system that the RFL Player Development Pathway (2010–2016) has initiated, broad base participation can be extended to above the maturational years, allowing more opportunities for more players to develop in the long term. On current understanding, we propose that such a recommendation would not detrimentally affect the likelihood of developing elite adult rugby players. Further, TID systems would be less likely to miss out on '[later] emerging shining stars' via early assessment, differentiation, and de-selection.

TID systems are charged with the task of achieving the 'top down demands' of developing future athletes. However, through attention to only junior athlete biological growth and maturation, we have shown that athlete development is more complicated than current TID practices appear to consider and recognize. Also consider that rugby development is multi-faceted, and that other developmental paths (e.g. movement and technical skills) contribute their own challenges, which need to be navigated by both young players and TID systems. Further, multiple contributory factors likely underpin later accelerated learning and onward player development (e.g. psychological, cognitive, social, etc.). Taken together, these ideas highlight the challenges ahead, and demonstrate the necessity of a multi-disciplinary understanding to inform beneficial, valid, and effective player development.

References

Abbott, A. and Collins, D. (2004). Eliminating the dichotomy between theory and practice in talent identification and development: considering the role of psychology. *Journal of Sports Sciences*, 22, 395–408.

Abernethy, A, and Farrow, D. (2005). *Contextual factors influencing the development of expertise in Australian athletes.* Paper presented at the *ISSP 11th World Congress of Sport Psychology: Promoting Health and Performance for Life,* Sydney, Australia, 14–19 August.

Armstrong, N., Welsman, J.R., and Kirby, B.J. (1998). Peak oxygen uptake and maturation in 12 year olds. *Medicine and Science in Sports and Exercise*, 30, 165–9.

Baker, J., Cobley, S., and Fraser-Thomas, J. (2009). What do we know about early sport specialization? Not much! *High Ability Studies*, 20, 77–89.

Baker, J., Côté, J., and Abernethy, B. (2003). Sport-specific practice and the development of expert decision-making in team ball sports. *Journal of Applied Sport Psychology*, 15, 12–25.

Baker, J. and Horton, S. (2004). A review of primary and secondary influences on sport expertise. *High Ability Studies*, 15, 211–228.

Baxter-Jones, A., Eisenmann, J., and Sherar, L. (2005). Controlling for maturation in pediatric exercise science. *Pediatric Exercise Science*, 17, 18–30.

Baxter-Jones, A., Helms, P., Maffulli, N., *et al.* (1995). Growth and development of male gymnasts, swimmers, soccer and tennis players: a longitudinal study. *Annals of Human Biology*, 22, 381–94.

Baxter-Jones, A., and Sherar, L. (2007). *Growth and maturation.* Philadelphia, PA: Elsevier Limited.

Bell, W. (1993). Body size and shape: A longitudinal investigation of active and sedentary boys during adolescence. *Journal of Sports Sciences*, 11, 127–38.

Beunen, G. and Malina, R. (1988). Growth and physical performance relative to the timing of the adolescent spurt. *Exercise and Sport Sciences Reviews*, 16, 503–40.

Beunen, G., Malina, R., Lefevre, J., *et al.* (1997). Prediction of adult stature and non-invasive assessment of biological maturation. *Medicine and Science in Sports and Exercise*, 29, 225–30.

Capranica, L. and Millard-Stafford, M.L. (2011). Youth sport specialization: How to manage competition and training? *International Journal of Sports Physiology and Performance*, 6, 572–9.

Champagne, F.A. (2010). Early adversity and developmental outcomes interaction between genetics, epigenetics, and social experiences across the life span. *Perspectives on Psychological Science*, 5, 564–74.

Chase, W.G. and Simon, H.A. (1973). Perception in chess. *Cognitive Psychology*, 4, 55–81.

Cobley, S., Baker, J., and Schorer, J. (2012). Identification and development of sport talent: A brief introduction to a growing field of research and practice. In J. Baker, S. Cobley, and J. Schorer (Eds.), *Talent identification and development in sport: International perspectives* (pp. 1–10). London: Routledge.

Cobley, S., Baker, J., Wattie, N., *et al.* (2009). Annual age-grouping and athlete development: A meta-analytical review of relative age effects in sport. *Sports Medicine*, 39, 235–56.

Côté, J., Baker, J., and Abernethy, B. (2003). From play to practice: A developmental framework for the acquisition of expertise in team sports. In J. Starkes and K.A. Ericsson (Eds.), *Expert performance in sports: Advances in research on sport expertise* (pp. 89–114). Champaign, Illinois: Human Kinetics.

Davids, K. and Baker, J. (2007). Genes, environment and sport performance: Why the Nature–Nurture dualism is no longer relevant. *Sports Medicine*, 37, 961–80.

Durand-Bush, N., and Salmela, J. (2001). The development of talent in sport. In R. Singer, H. Hausenblas and C. Janelle (Eds.), *Handbook of Sport Psychology*, 2, (pp. 269–89). New York: Wiley.

Ericsson, K.A., Krampe, R.T., and Tesch-Römer, C. (1993). The role of deliberate practice in the acquisition of expert performance. *Psychological Review*, 100, 363–406.

Ford, P.R., Ward, P., Hodges, N.J., *et al.* (2009). The role of deliberate practice and play in career progression in sport: the early engagement hypothesis. *High Ability Studies*, 20, 65–75.

Ford, P.R. and Williams, A.M. (2012). The developmental activities engaged in by elite youth soccer players who progressed to professional status compared to those who did not. *Psychology of Sport and Exercise*, 13, 349–52.

Freeman, J., Cole, T., Chinn, S., *et al.* (1995). Cross sectional stature and weight reference curves for the UK, 1990. *Archives of Disease in Childhood*, 73, 17–24.

Güllich, A. and Emrich, E. (2012). Individualistic and collectivistic approach in athlete support programmes in the German high-performance sport system. *European Journal of Sport and Society*, 9, 243–68.

Howe, M.J., Davidson, J.W., and Sloboda, J.A. (1998). Innate talents: Reality or myth? *Behavioural and Brain Sciences*, 21, 399–407.

Malina, R.M. (1994). Physical growth and biological maturation of young athletes. *Exercise and Sport Sciences Reviews*, 22, 280–4.

Malina, R.M. (2010). Early sport specialization: Roots, effectiveness, risks. *Current Sports Medicine Reports*, 9, 364–71.

Malina, R.M., Bouchard, C., and Bar-Or, O. (2004). *Growth, maturation, and physical activity*. Champaign, IL: Human Kinetics.

Meylan, C., Cronin, J., Oliver, J., et al. (2010). Talent identification in soccer: The role of maturity status on physical, physiological and technical characteristics. *International Journal of Sports Science and Coaching*, 5, 571–92.

Mirwald, R.L., Baxter-Jones, G.A.D., Bailey, D.A., et al. (2002). An assessment of maturity from anthropometric measurements. *Medicine and Science in Sports and Exercise*, 34, 689.

Moesch, K., Elbe, A., Hauge, M., et al. (2011). Late specialization: the key to success in centimetres, grams, or seconds (cgs) sports. *Scandinavian Journal of Medicine and Science in Sports*, 21, 282–90.

Musch, J. and Grondin, S. (2001). Unequal competition as an impediment to personal development: A review of the relative age effect in sport. *Developmental Review*, 21, 147–67.

Pearson, D., Naughton, G., and Torode, M. (2006). Predictability of physiological testing and the role of maturation in talent identification for adolescent team sports. *Journal of Science and Medicine in Sport*, 9, 277–87.

Philippaerts, R.M., Vaeyens, R., Janssens, M., et al. (2006). The relationship between peak height velocity and physical performance in youth soccer players. *Journal of Sports Sciences*, 24, 221–30.

RCPCH. (2013). UK 2–18 years growth chart resources. Available at: http://www.rcpch. ac.uk/growthcharts. [Accessed 15th July 2013].

Ridley, M. (2003). *Nature via nurture: Genes, experience, and what makes us human*: Harper-Collins.

Rongen, F., Cobley, S., McKenna, J., et al. (2014). Talent identification and development: The impact on athlete health? In J. Baker, P. Safai and J. Fraser-Thomas (Eds.), *Health and elite sport: Is high performance sport a healthy pursuit?* London: Routledge.

Sherar, L.B., Baxter-Jones, A.D.G., Faulkner, R.A., et al. (2007). Do physical maturity and birth date predict talent in male youth ice hockey players? *Journal of Sports Sciences*, 25, 879–86.

Simmons, C. and Paull, G.C. (2001). Season-of-birth bias in association football. *Journal of Sports Sciences*, 19, 677–86.

Slavich, G.M. and Cole, S.W. (2013). The emerging field of human social genomics. *Clinical Psychological Science*, 1, 331–48.

Tanner, J. (1962). *Growth at adolescence*. Oxford: Blackwell Scientific Publications.

Till, K., Chapman, C., Cobley, S., et al. (2012). Talent identification, selection and development in UK junior Rugby league: An evolving process. In J. Baker, S. Cobley and J. Sehorer (Eds.), *Talent identification and development in sport: International perspectives* (pp. 106–18). London: Routledge.

Till, K., Cobley, S., O'Hara, J., et al. (2013). An individualized longitudinal approach to monitoring the dynamics of growth and fitness development in adolescent athletes. *The Journal of Strength and Conditioning Research*, 27, 1313–21.

Till, K., Cobley, S., O'Hara, J., et al. (2014). Considering maturation status and relative age in the longitudinal evaluation of junior rugby league players. *Scandinavian Journal of Medicine and Science in Sports*, 24, 569–76.

Till, K., Cobley, S., O'Hara, J., et al. (2010a). Anthropometric, physiological, and selection characteristics in high performance UK Junior Rugby League players. *Talent Development and Excellence*, 2, 193–207.

Till, K., Cobley, S., Wattie, N., et al. (2010b). The prevalence, influential factors, and mechanisms of relative age effects in UK Rugby League. *Scandinavian Journal of Medicine and Science in Sports*, 20, 320–9.

Vaeyens, R., Lenoir, R., Williams, A.M., et al. (2008). Talent identification and development programmes in sport: Current models and future directions. *Sports Medicine*, 38, 703–14.

Wattie, N., Cobley, S., and Baker, J. (2008). Towards a unified understanding of relative age effects. *Journal of Sports Sciences*, 26, 1403–9.

Wiersma, L. (2000). Risks and benefits of youth sport specialization: Perspectives and recommendations. *Pediatric Exercise Science*, 12, 13–22.

Williams, A., and Reilly, T. (2000). Talent identification and development in soccer. *Journal of Sports Sciences*, 18, 657–67.

INDEX